W9-CSB-170

PSYCHIATRIC DISORDERS

Executive Editor: *Richard A. Weimer*
Production Editor: *Elizabeth S. Burns*
Art Director: *Don Sellers, AMI*
Typesetting: *Bookmakers, Inc., Washington, DC*
Typeface: *Bodoni Book*
Printing: *R. R. Donnelley, Harrisonburg, Virginia*

PSYCHIATRIC DISORDERS
Diagnosis and Treatment

Patrick T. Donlon, M.D.
Don A. Rockwell, M.D.

ROBERT J. BRADY CO.
A Prentice-Hall Publishing and Communications Company
Bowie, Maryland 20715

Psychiatric Disorders: Diagnosis and Treatment

Library of Congress Cataloging in Publication Data

Donlon, Patrick T.
　　Psychiatric disorders.

　　Includes index.
　　1. Psychiatry.　　I. Rockwell, Don.
II. Title.　[DNLM:　1. Mental disorders—
Diagnosis.　2. Mental disorders—Therapy.
WM　100　D684p]
RC454.D66　　　　616.89　　　　81-10191
ISBN 0-89303-034-1　　　　AACR2

Prentice-Hall International, Inc., London
Prentice-Hall of Australia, Pty., Ltd., Sydney
Prentice-Hall of India Private Limited, New Delhi
Prentice-Hall of Japan, Inc., Tokyo
Prentice-Hall of Southeast Asia Pte. Ltd., Singapore
Whitehall Books, Limited, Petone, New Zealand

Printed in the United States of America

82　83　84　85　86　87　88　89　90　　　10　9　8　7　6　5　4　3　2　1

TO

Patti and Fran—supportive spouses

AND TO

Se´ann and Grant and Chad—super sons

Contents

III. TREATMENT CONCERNS

Foreword

There is general concern today that the primary care physician has an essential role as a principal provider of mental health services, especially in the prevention, diagnosis, and management of common mental disorders. Over one-half of all patients with mental health disorders are cared for solely by the primary care sector.

The utility of a psychobiomedical model of disease and health care as advocated by Engel is gaining increasing acceptance in medical education and among primary care physicians in view of the important influence of psychosocial factors upon the occurrence and natural history of disease. It is now well documented that patients with mental health disorders have a higher incidence of organic illness than others without such problems. There is therefore a definite need for readily accessible literature which bridges the historical gap between mental health problems and organic illness.

Psychiatric Disorders: Diagnosis and Treatment addresses an important subject area in everyday medical practice and should be of wide interest and value to medical students, residents in training, and practicing physicians, especially in the primary care specialties. The range of psychiatric disorders which are covered in this volume represents a sizable portion of primary medical care.

Despite a plethora of previous books on various aspects of psychiatry, including some attempting to focus on psychiatry in primary care, there have been serious deficits in most of these books from the standpoint of the primary care physician. Most are unduly oriented to the psychodynamics (often controversial) of psychiatric disorders, are laden with jargon, and fail to adequately represent those problems commonly encountered in primary care. Most available books are of limited value for immediate reference purposes.

This book is a refreshing change. The editors have approached the subject on an eclectic basis. The content of the book represents a broad range of problems commonly encountered in daily medical practice, with an emphasis on ambulatory care. In addition to coverage of the traditional psychiatric disorders, thorough attention is directed to a number of subjects not usually well covered, including suicide, grief, life crises, sexual dysfunction, rape, and alcoholism. Psychiatric jargon has been carefully avoided, and a genuine effort has been made to make the book useful for ready reference, including specific coverage of drug therapy. Biomedical and psychosocial factors have been well integrated to provide a practical approach to problems as they present to the physician in the office. A chapter dealing with the tired patient represents an excellent example of the psychobiomedical approach to such problems.

It is a privilege to welcome this new volume as the first edition of what is likely to become a series of editions addressing a central need in medical practice.

John P. Geyman, M.D.
Professor and Chairman,
Department of Family Medicine, School of Medicine,
University of Washington, Seattle, Washington

Preface

It is the bane of every medical educator's life to have to select a text for his or her students or colleagues. It is the curse of that life to discover there is no text that meets specific needs and then to have to sit down and write that "great American" text. This text grew out of the need to meet the demands of our various "student" bodies. It was designed with several factors in mind.

First and foremost the need addressed most directly is the one for a practical text designed for the clinician or clinician-to-be. It is not a text for the sophisticated psychiatric practitioner. It is a text for clinicians on the spot in primary medical care. Of prime importance to us clinically and editorially is the issue of "does it work?" The book is designed to let you know what we do in the most concrete terms possible. In this text our posture is then one of aggressive pragmatics.

A second factor of importance to us is the patient's perspective and how this presents to the real world clinician. This view dictates a systems approach with intervention aimed at the system most likely to change in a way beneficial to the patient.

A third factor is the significance of preventive ideas. We do not delude ourselves into thinking we know "the cause" of mental and emotional illness, but we do believe in pursuing prevention aggressively. Many "problems in living" found in the clinician's office can in fact be softened or avoided through primary preventive approaches outlined herein.

A fourth factor is our concern for comprehensive yet not encyclopedic coverage of a wide range of topics. The typical clinician may buy the encyclopedia but uses a practical manual. The student clinician may be "required" to read the lengthy tome but uses the practical text.

We started with the premise that every clinician seeing patients needed to know more about each area we covered. We see the information we provide as an irreducible core. Each chapter is designed to provide the reader with a succinct organized overview of an aspect of psychiatric disorders. Diagnosis is focused upon as a necessary prelude to effective treatment. We eschew "diagnostic acumen" which does not lead to clear cut practical therapy. The focus then is upon the care of the patient.

We have freely used DSM-III and just as freely have left out some aspects of DSM-III we consider clinically less germane.

Finally, and importantly, this is a continuing effort. Feedback about the text from the practicing physician will assist us in further refining our educational efforts and subsequent editions.

Patrick T. Donlon, M.D.
Don A. Rockwell, M.D.

Contributors

Robert M. Bittle, M.D.
  Associate Clinical Professor
  Department of Psychiatry
  University of California at Davis
Kay H. Blacker, M.D.
  Professor and Vice-Chairperson
  Department of Psychiatry
  University of California at Davis
William Burr, M.D.
  Associate Professor
  Department of Family Practice
  Unviversity of California at Davis
Patrick T. Donlon, M.D.
  Associate Clinical Professor
  Department of Psychiatry
  University of California at Davis
Lena K. Ericksen, Ph.D.
  Sacramento, California
John P. Geyman, M.D.
  Professor and Chairman
  Department of Family Medicine
  School of Medicine
  University of Washington

Gabe J. Maletta, Ph.D., M.D.
  Program Director
  Geriatric Research, Education and Clinical
    Center
  V.A. Medical Center
  Minneapolis, Minnesota
Donna Stringer-Moore, Ph.D.
  Director of Office of Women's Rights
  Seattle, Washington
Fran Pepitone-Arreola-Rockwell, Ph.D.
  Assistant Professor-In-Residence
  Department of Psychiatry
  University of California at Davis
Don A. Rockwell, M.D.
  Professor, Department of Psychiatry, Asso-
    ciate Dean for Student Affairs
  University of California at Davis
Hobart Sewell, M.D.
  Assistant Clinical Professor
  Department of Psychiatry
  University of California at Davis
Mark Willenbring, M.D.
  Post Doctoral Trainee
  Department of Psychiatry
  University of Wisconsin—Madison

I

ASSESSMENT AND DIAGNOSIS

1

Psychiatric Assessment

PATRICK T. DONLON, M.D.

Diagnosis in psychiatry must be as precise as it is in other specialties in medicine. To this end each patient must be carefully assessed, and a comprehensive historical review, mental status examination, and indicated diagnostic tests must be completed. Although pathognomonic biologic signs have not yet been identified for the majority of psychiatric disorders and the diagnosis remains clinical, most patients still require a physical examination, review of medical symptoms and agents administered, and routine laboratory tests at the initial assessment to best aid in the differential diagnosis.

PSYCHIATRIC INTERVIEW

The initial assessment normally requires about 60 minutes to complete. Privacy and a quiet and pleasant setting are essential. It is helpful also to begin by explaining to the patient the importance of the comprehensive psychiatric assessment and the need for reliable information so that the preferred treatment approach can be most readily identified and implemented.

Following this the patient should be asked to discuss his current psychiatric concerns and then be allowed to describe the course and nature of the symptoms in his own words and with relatively few interruptions. This is the most important part of the evaluation. The remainder of the assessment should be used to gather additional information on the present illness, to obtain comprehensive background data, and to complete the mental status examination.

During the interview, steps should be taken to place the patient at ease. The techniques used will vary and depend on the patient's complaints and presentation. A nod or a yes will help most patients continue their description of their concerns and history. Many patients have trouble with direct questions, and it is best to use open-ended questions like . . . "tell me more about . . . " or "what effects did this have on you?" The interview should be a positive emotional experience for the patient. The doctor's concern and willingness to help can indeed provide beneficial effects and offset the anxiety associated with the assessment.

When terminating the interview, it is helpful to summarize and review the salient historical facts and symptoms with the patient for further comment. The patient should then be asked if there is other important information to be discussed. Before concluding, the physician should make some comments on diagnostic impression, need for additional diagnostic tests, and the tentative treatment plans and be prepared to answer questions. At this time it is also helpful to meet with family members or friends who escorted the patient to supplement the history and, if appropriate, discuss treatment.

Either during or immediately following the interview, the history and observation should be recorded. It is also helpful to record many of the comments and responses to questions in the mental status examination verbatim in the record.

Psychiatric History

What follows is a sample outline for obtaining the psychiatric history:

identification data: Name, age, sex, marital and employment status. Important addresses and phone numbers. Referral source.

chief complaint: Reason for referral—includes verbatim statement of patient; if unreliable, from relatives.

present illness: Indicate source of history and reliability.

  symptoms—description, onset, circumstances under which they occur, precipitating factors, degree of incapacity, previous episodes, course, treatment and response.

family history: mother—Age, health; if dead, age of patient and response to death; mental illness, type of person, interaction with patient.

  father: Same as above—occupation, parents interaction. Dominance/discipline—how? who?

  siblings:—Number, place of patient in family, interaction of patients and siblings.

  other: Mental illness, interaction with those significant in home and life of patient, e.g., grandparents. Family response to psychiatric treatments including drugs.

past history: birth and early development—Age of walking, speaking, toilet training, enuresis, nightmares; sleep-walking, temper tantrums. *School*—age beginning, ending, failures, missed school, class standing, truancy, behavior problems, extracurricular activities; teachers and peer interaction.

work: Type, progress, relationship with co-workers, with authority figures.

military: Dates, rank, type discharge.

psychosexual development: Knowledge of sex; how obtained; attitudes toward sex in family; early sex experience; masturbation; homosexual and heterosexual activity and fantasies.

marital relationship: Wife, personality, age, background, interaction, number of children, health, adjustment, role of patient in family, sexual activity.

religion: Affiliation, activity, change.

medical history: Previous and present illnesses.

drug history: Note proprietary and illicit; extent, effects, residual, allergies, interactional effects.

mental status exam: As described separately.

physical: Emphasize neurological.

differential diagnosis: Prioritize. List facts supporting each diagnosis. For new patients, provide only a provisional diagnosis.

formulation: Outline possible etiologic factors including genetic, biologic, and dynamic.

recommendations: Diagnostic work-up, treatment strategies, dispositional plans.

The evaluation begins with a thorough discussion of the present illness and the outlining of possible etiologic factors, degree of incapacity, course, phenomena, treatment and response, and reason for current assessment. Every psychiatric history should include family, social-occupational, medical and drug histories. It is often essential to obtain additional information from friends and family members and to review past psychiatric and medical records if available.

Appetite and sleep disturbances are common in psychiatric patients, and detailed information is essential in the differential diagnosis (See Tables 1-1 and 1-2).

Also there are several medical disorders and adverse effects from psychotropic drugs such as the following that can masquerade as primary psychiatric disorders,* and which make early recognition imperative:

Infections
Most common viral illnesses
Mononucleosis

Infectious hepatitis
Tuberculosis
Chronic pyelonephritis

---

*Adapted from an unpublished list prepared by Charles B. Schaffer, M.D., University of California at Davis. Printed with permission.

Table 1-1. Appetite and Weight Disturbances.

Clinical Picture	Appetite	Weight and Course
I. Associated With Mental Illness and Affective States		
Anxiety	Often increased.	Often weight gain.
Reactive or situational depression	Often increased.	Often weight gain.
Clinical depressions	Moderate to severe anorexia.	Significant recent weight loss.
Manic states	Often increased appetite.	Stable weight due to increased activity.
Schizophrenia	Erratic appetite.	Stable to reduced weight.
Anorexia nervosa	Anorexia. Often hoard food and eat privately. Self-induced vomiting.	Significant weight loss to emaciated state and even death by starvation.
Organic brain disease	Often appetite reduction. Problems obtaining and preparing food.	Progressive weight loss.
II. Psychotropic Agents		
Neuroleptics, lithium, tricyclic antidepressants	Increased.	Weight gain common.
Marijuana	Temporary increase.	Weight stable unless chronic abuse.
CNS stimulants (amphetamines, cocaine)	Reduced.	Significant reduction with continued abuse.
III. Medical Disorders		
Many acute medical and surgical illnesses.	Sudden decrease.	Limited to course of illness.
Chronic medical disorders	Reduced.	Progressive weight loss.

Infections (continued)
  Subacute bacterial endocarditis
  Encephalitides
  Brucellosis
  Parasitic infestations
Endocrine Disorders
  Hypothyroidism
  Hyperparathyroidism
  Diabetes mellitus

Hypo and hyperadrenalism
Hypopituitarism
Cushing's disease
Metabolic Disorders
  Uremia (any etiology)
  Metabolic acidosis (any etiology)
  Hepatic encephalopathy
  Acute intermittent porphyria

(text continues on page 11)

Table 1-2. Sleep Disorders.

PRIMARY

(Disordered sleep is the only sign and symptom of abnormality.)

Disorder	Clinical Findings	EEG Findings	Treatment
Cataplexy	Sudden decrease or loss of muscle tone, often generalized. May be precipitated by laughter, anger, or surprise. Eye muscles are not paralyzed. If person supine, sleep may follow.	Ensuing sleep lapses directly into REM state.	Imipramine.
Hypersomnia (chronic)	Excessive sleep at night or during day. None of the findings associated with *narcolepsy*. Post sleep confusion. Increased cardiac and respiratory rates. *Depression* may be present. Can occur with *central nervous system damage*.	Normal sleep EEG.	Treatment for any other disorder present.
Insomnia	Inability to fall asleep and difficulty staying asleep including early morning awakening. As a primary sleep disorder, it occurs in the absence of physical or psychological illness.	Longer time before sleep onset. Short sleeping time. Greater physiologic arousal during sleep. Increased REM sleep.	Hypnotic drugs and supportive treatment.
Kleine-Levin Syndrome	Periodic episodes (about every 6 months) of hypersomnia. First appears in *adolescence*, usually in boys, and is accompanied by *bulimia*.	Various findings. Some show absence of sleep spindles.	Eventual spontaneous disappearance of syndrome.
Narcolepsy	Uncontrollable, recurrent, brief episodes of sleep associated with *cataplexy*; sleep paralysis (inability to move occurring at waking) and *hypnagogic hallucinations* (occurs as the person falls asleep). Disturbed nocturnal sleep is also present.	REM episode begins with sleep onset.	Amphetamines or methylphenidate.

Table 1-2. Sleep Disorders **(continued).**

PRIMARY

(Disordered sleep is the only sign and symptom of abnormality.)

Disorder	Clinical Findings	EEG Findings	Treatment
Nightmares (dream anxiety attacks)	Mild anxiety and *autonomic* reactions. Good recall of dream. Contrast with *night terrors.*	Occurs during REM sleep.	Reassurance. Psychotherapy if severe.
Night Terrors (pavor nocturnus)	Extreme panic, verbalizations, *autonomic activity,* confusion, poor recall for event. *Psychopathology* rare in children, common in adults with the disorder. Contrast with *nightmares.*	Occurs during stage 4 sleep.	Children—reassure parents. Adults—possible use of medication to suppress stage 4 sleep.
Pickwickian Syndrome	Obesity, respiratory irregularities and *hypersomnia.* Sleep associated with periods of apnea (no breathing). Sleep is discontinuous.	EEG signs of arousal at end of each apneic period. Little or no slow wave of REM sleep.	

SECONDARY

(Clinical problems accompanied by specific or nonspecific sleep disturbances.)

Disorder	Clinical Findings	EEG Findings	Treatment
Alcoholic Psychoses	Variable.	Slow wave and REM sleep suppressed during acute alcoholic state, following an initial increase. Withdrawal results in rebound	

Disorder	Clinical Findings	EEG Findings	Treatment
Anorexia Nervosa	Decreased total sleep time.	of slow wave and REM sleep.	
Depression	Less sleep time, more awakenings.	Decreased stages 3, 4 and REM sleep. Increased time before onset of stage 1, 3 and REM sleep. Less slow wave sleep. REM state findings vary. Decreased time before REM sleep and decreased intervals between REM periods.	
Hyperthyroidism	Insomnia.	Stages 3 and 4 increased.	
Hypothyroidism	Increased somnolence.	Stages 3 and 4 decreased.	
Schizophrenia	Variable.	Much less slow wave sleep. REM debt related to symptoms.	

PARASOMNIAS

(Waking type behavior occurring during sleep.)

Disorder	Clinical Findings	EEG Findings	Treatment
Bruxism (teeth grinding)	Loud noises and eventual damage to teeth and supporting structures.	Occurs during stage 2 sleep. Sleep stages not disturbed.	Removal of dental problems. Use of dental prosthesis to discourage biting.
Enuresis	In boys and men predominantly. May be familial. Excessive bladder contractions during sleep and higher heart rates.	Can occur during all sleep stages but often associated with stage 4. Not related to daydreaming.	Parental guidance, training, imipramine.

***Table 1-2. Sleep Disorders* (continued).**

PARASOMNIAS

(Waking type behavior occurring during sleep.)

Disorder	Clinical Findings	EEG Findings	Treatment
Sleep Talking	Very common by itself or as part of other sleep disorders, psychological or organic disorders.	Mainly during NREM sleep. Occasionally during REM sleep.	
Sleep Walking (somnabulism)	Mainly in boys and men. Often accompanied by night terrors and enuresis. Forced awakening accompanied by confusion.	Occurs during stage 4 sleep.	Children often outgrow. Adults often have psychiatric disturbances.

SLEEP EXACERBATED DISORDERS

Disorder	Clinical and EEG Findings	Treatment
Bronchial Asthma	In adults, attacks unrelated to sleep stage. In children, attacks generally do not occur during first part of night when stage 4 sleep predominates. Adults and children have decreased amounts of stage 4 sleep and less total sleep time.	
Coronary Artery Disease	REM sleep associated with changes in heart rate, respiration and blood pressure. Nocturnal angina associated with REM sleep.	Avoid drugs which result in REM rebound.
Duodenal Ulcer	Greatly increased gastric acid secretion at night compared to normal people. Peak acid secretion during REM sleep.	Avoid drugs which result in REM rebound.

From Frazier, SH, et al. (eds): *A Psychiatric Glossary*, 4th ed.. Washington, D.C., American Psychiatric Association, 1975. Printed with permission.

Nutritional
  Pellagra
  Iron deficiency anemia
  Hypervitaminosis D
  Nutritional deficiencies secondary
    to fad diets
  General malnutrition
Neoplasm
  Pancreas
  Frontal lobe
  Lung
  Temporal lobe
Collagen Vascular
  Rheumatoid arthritis
  Lupus erythematosus
  Polyarteritis nodosa
  Scleroderma
Neurological
  Parkinson's disease
  Most dementing processes
  Huntington's chorea
  Amyotrophic lateral sclerosis
  Multiple sclerosis

Epilepsy (temporal lobe)
Delirium
Drugs
  Hypertension medication (reserpine,
    methyldopa, clonidine, proprano-
    lol, beta-adrenergic blocking
    agents)
  Steroids
  Oral contraceptives
  CNS depressants (sedative/hypnot-
    ic/minor tranquilizers/alcohol)
  CNS stimulants (amphetamines, co-
    caine)
  Hallucinogenic agents and sub-
    stances of abuse)
  Caffeinism
  Chronic bromism
  Levodopa
  Digitalis
  Anticonvulsants
  Antituberculous drugs
  Phenylbutazone and indomethacin

Mental Status Examination

An outline for the mental status examination is given below:

general appearance, attitude and behavior:

Clothes—tidy, slovenly, neat, careless, dirty, decorative, mourning.
Facies—smiling, crying, blank, tense, sad, mask-like, inappropriate for content.
Attitude—cooperative, resistive, sociable, reserved, seclusive, belligerent, negativistic, suspicious, apathetic, fearful, confident, over-confident, sarcastic, superior.
Motor Activity—hyperactive, hypoactive, bizarre gesture, mannerisms, posture, gait, paralysis, tremor.

stream of thought and speech:

Intensity—loud or soft. Pitch—monotonous, high. Speed—slow, rapid. Ease of speech—pressure (hypomanic). Blocking (psychotic). Relevance—logical, distractable, flight of ideas (hypomania), tangential (psychotic). Manner—formal, relaxed. Deviation—neologism, clang associations, word salad (all psychotic) and perseveration, confabulation, echolalia (all organic). Vocabulary and diction (intelligence and education). Attention defect.

content of thought
>   Preoccupation, areas of concern, delusions (fixed false belief), hallucination (false perceptions), anxiety, phobias, compulsions, obsessions, ideas of refer- ence, feelings of unreality and depersonalization, passive feelings, ideas of influence, somatic trends, self-condemnatory trends, expansive trends, thought and feeling insertion or withdrawal.

mood (sustained affect) **and affect** (subjective-feeling part of emotion):
>   Elated, euphoric, calm, placid, depressed, isolated, anxious, flattened, labile, inappropriate.

sensorium and intellectual resources:
>   *Orientation*—place, date, person, situation.
>   *Memory*
>   a. Remote—dates, military service, marriage, jobs, birthdates
>   b. Recent—account of past 24 hours
>   c. Immediate—numbers, name objects, digits forward and backward, serial 7's subtraction
>   *Grasp of General Information*—5 presidents, governor, wars, news headlines.
>   *Calculation*—arithmetic test.
>   *Abstraction Ability*—Similarities: bird-butterfly, mouse-elephant, car-train, literature-painting, ball-sun. Differences: lie-mistake, dwarf-child, idleness- laziness, poverty-misery, character-reputation.
>   *Judgment*—(ability to make reasonable plans and appraise past performance)— find sealed addressed envelope; what do you do in a theatre if someone yells "fire?"
>   *Proverbs*—cat's away, mice will play; never rains but it pours; rolling stone gathers no moss; don't count chickens before they are hatched; proof of the pudding is in the eating.
>   *Intelligence and Comprehension*—reading and explaining, education, occupa- tion, testing.

insight into illness:
>   Realization, recognition, degree and nature of illness.

Commonly used psychiatric terms in the examination and the psychological defense mechanisms will be found on page 17 for easy reference.

Special Diagnostic Tests

Many patients require additional diagnostic tests and periods of extended obser- vation before the diagnosis is established. An outline of commonly administered psychological tests is given in Table 1-3. Additional medical and neurologic examinations are often necessary.

Psychiatric Diagnosis

The third edition of the Diagnostic and Statistical Manual of Mental Disorders (DSM-III) of the American Psychiatric Association became the official psychiatric

Table 1-3. Psychologic Tests.

Test	Type	Assesses	Age of Patient	Output	Administration
Bayley Scales of Infant Development	Infant development.	Cognitive functioning and motor development.	1–30 months.	Performance on subtests measuring cognitive and motor development.	Individual.
Bender Visual-Motor Gestalt Test	Projective visual-motor development.	Personality conflicts. Ego function and structure. Organic brain damage.	5–Adult.	Patient's reproduction of geometric figures.	Individual.
Benton Visual Retention Test	Objective performance.	Organic brain damage.	Adult.	Patient's reproduction of geometric figures from memory.	Individual.
Cattell Infant Intelligence Scale	Infant development.	General motor and cognitive development.	1–18 months.	Performance on developmental tasks.	Individual.
Children's Appercep-tion Test (CAT)	Projective.	Personality conflicts.	Child.	Patient makes up stories after viewing pictures.	Individual.
Draw-A-Person Draw-A-Family House-Tree	Projective.	Personality conflicts. Self-Image (DAP). Family perception (DAF). Ego functions. Intellectual functioning (DAP). Visual-motor coordination.	2–Adult.	Patient's drawings on a blank sheet of paper.	Individual.
Frostig Developmental Test of Visual Perception	Visual perception.	Eye-motor coordination. Figure ground perception. Constancy of shape. Position in space. Spatial relationships.	4–8 years.	Performance on paper and pencil test measuring five aspects of visual perception.	Individual or group.

Table 1-3. Psychologic Tests (continued).

Test	Type	Assesses	Age of Patient	Output	Administration
Gesell Developmental Schedules	Preschool development.	Cognitive, motor, language and social development.	1–60 months.	Performance on developmental tasks.	Individual.
Halstead-Reitan Neuropsychological Battery and Other Measures	Brain functioning.	Cerebral functioning and organic brain damage.	6–Adult.	Various subtests measure aspects of cerebral functioning.	Individual.
Illinois Test of Psycholinguistic Ability (ITPA)	Language ability.	Auditory-vocal, visual-motor channels of language; receptive, organizational, and expressive components.	2–10 years.	Performance on 12 subtests measuring various dimensions of language functioning.	Individual.
Michigan Picture Stories	Defensive structure.	Personality conflicts.	Adolescent.	Patient makes up stories after viewing stimulus pictures.	Individual.
Minnesota Multiphasic Personality Inventory (MMPI)	Paper and pencil; personality inventory.	Personality structure. Diagnostic classification.	Adolescent–Adult.	Personality profile reflecting nine dimensions of personality. Diagnosis based upon actuarial prediction.	Group.
Nebraska Luria	Brain functioning.	Cerebral functioning and organic brain damage.	6–Adult.	Various subtests measure aspects of cerebral functioning.	Individual.
Otis Quick Scoring Mental Abilities Tests	Intelligence.	Intellectual functioning.	5–Adult.	Performance on verbal and nonverbal dimensions of intellectual functioning.	Group.

Test	Type	Assesses	Age	Description	Administration
Rorschach	Projective.	Personality conflicts. Ego function and structure. Defensive structure. Thought processes. Affective integration.	3–Adult.	Patient's associations to inkblots.	Individual.
Senior Apperception Test (SAT)	Projective.	Personality conflicts.	Over 65.	Patient makes up stories after viewing stimulus pictures.	Individual.
Stanford-Binet	Intelligence.	Intellectual functioning.	2–Adult.	Performance on problem solving and developmental tasks.	Individual.
Tasks of Emotional Development (TED)	Projective.	Personality conflicts.	Child and Adolescent.	Patient makes up stories after viewing stimulus pictures.	Individual.
Thematic Apperception Test (TAT)	Projective.	Personality conflicts.	Adult.	Patient makes up stories after viewing stimulus pictures.	Individual.
Vineland Social Maturity Scale	Social maturity.	Capacity for independent functioning.	0–25+ years.	Performance on developmental tasks measuring various dimensions of social functioning.	Interview patient or guardian of patient, occasional self-report.
Wechsler Adult Intelligence Scale (WAIS)	Intelligence.	Intellectual functioning.	16–Adult.	Performance on 10 subtests measuring various dimensions of intellectual functioning.	Individual.

Table 1-3. Psychologic Tests (continued).

Test	Type	Assesses	Age of Patient	Output	Administration
Wechsler Intelligence Scale for Children (WISC)	Intelligence.	Intellectual functioning. Thought processes. Ego functioning.	5–15.	See above.	Individual.
Wechsler Preschool Primary Scale of Intelligence (WPPSI)	Intelligence.	Intellectual functioning. Thought processes. Ego functioning.	4–6½ years.	See above.	Individual.

From: *A Psychiatric Glossary*, 5th ed., Washington, D.C., American Psychiatric Association, 1980, pp. 71-75. Printed with permission.

diagnostic classification for mental disorders in 1980 (Table 1-4). The International Classification of Diseases (ICD-9) was modified (ICD-9-CM) to include the DSM-III and since January 1979 has been the official classification system for recording diseases in the United States. DSM-III is a multiaxial classification and each case must be assessed on each of 5 "axes" (Table 1-5). The first three axes constitute the official diagnostic assessment and the last two provide supplemental information. Axis IV notes the severity of psychosocial stressors on a scale of (1) "none" to (7) "catastrophic." Axis V rates the highest level of adaptive functioning over the past year on a scale of (1) "superior" to (7) "grossly impaired."

Diagnosis in psychiatry must follow very careful assessment with emphasis being placed on accuracy. The diagnosis should be based on positive supportive data and not simply on the exclusion of organic findings.

*Terms Used in the Mental Status Examination**

affect—The outward manifestation of a person's feelings, tone, or mood. Affect and emotion are commonly used interchangeably.

anxiety—Apprehension, tension, or uneasiness from anticipation of danger, the source of which is largely unknown or unrecognized. Primarily of intrapsychic origin, in distinction to fear, which is the emotional response to a consciously recognized and usually external threat or danger. May be regarded as pathologic when it interferes with effectiveness in living, achievement of desired goals or satisfactions, or reasonable emotional comfort.

apathetic—Showing lack of interest, or indifference, lacking feeling.

association—Relationship between ideas or emotions by contiguity, continuity, or similarity.

autism—A developmental disability caused by a physical disorder of the brain appearing during the first three years of life. Symptoms include disturbances in physical, social, and language skills; abnormal responses to sensations; and abnormal ways of relating to people, objects, and events.

blocking—A sudden obstruction or interruption in spontaneous flow of thinking or speaking, perceived as an absence or deprivation of thought.

catatonic—A marked psychomotor disturbance which may involve particular forms of stupor, rigidity, excitement, or posturing. Sometimes where there is a rapid alternation between the extremes of excitement and stupor, associated features include negativism, stereotypy, and waxy flexibility. Mutism is common.

character disorder (character neurosis)—A personality disorder manifested by a chronic, habitual, maladaptive pattern of reaction that is relatively inflexible, limits the optimal use of potentialities, and often provokes the responses from the environment that the subject wants to avoid. In contrast to symptoms of neurosis, character traits are typically ego-syntonic.

(text continues on page 23)

---

*A Psychiatric Glossary, 5th ed. Washington, D.C., American Psychiatric Association, 1980. Printed with permission.

Table 1-4. DSM-III Classifications: Axes I and II Categories and Codes.

All official DSM-III codes and terms are included in ICD-9-CM. However, in order to differentiate those DSM-III categories that use the same ICD-9-CM codes, unofficial non-ICD-9-CM codes are provided in parentheses for use when greater specificity is necessary.

DISORDERS USUALLY FIRST EVIDENT IN INFANCY, CHILDHOOD OR ADOLESCENCE

Mental retardation
(Code in fifth digit: 1 = with other behavioral symptoms (requiring attention or treatment and that are not part of another disorder), 0 = without other behavioral symptoms.)
317.0(x) Mild mental retardation, _____

318.0(x) Moderate mental retardation, _____
318.1(x) Severe mental retardation, _____

318.2(x) Profound mental retardation, _____
319.0(x) Unspecified mental retardation, _____

Attention deficit disorder
314.01 with hyperactivity
314.00 without hyperactivity
314.80 residual type

Conduct disorder
312.00 undersocialized, aggressive
312.10 undersocialized, nonaggressive
312.23 socialized, aggressive
312.21 socialized, nonaggressive
312.90 atypical

Anxiety disorders of childhood or adolescence
309.21 Separation anxiety disorder
313.21 Avoidant disorder of childhood or adolescence
313.00 Overanxious disorder

Other disorders of infancy, childhood, or adolescence
313.89 Reactive attachment disorder of infancy

313.22 Schizoid disorder of childhood or adolescence
313.23 Elective mutism
313.81 Oppositional disorder
313.82 Identity disorder

Eating disorders
307.10 Anorexia nervosa
307.51 Bulimia
307.52 Pica
307.53 Rumination disorder of infancy
307.50 Atypical eating disorder

Stereotyped movement disorders
307.21 Transient tic disorder
307.22 Chronic motor tic disorder
307.23 Tourette's disorder
307.20 Atypical tic disorder
307.30 Atypical stereotyped movement disorder

Other disorders with physical manifestations
307.00 Stuttering
307.60 Functional enuresis
307.70 Functional encopresis
307.46 Sleepwalking disorder
307.49 Sleep terror disorder

Pervasive developmental disorders
Code in fifth digit: 0 = full syndrome present, 1 = residual state.
299.0x Infantile autism, _____
299.9x Childhood onset pervasive developmental disorder, _____
299.8x Atypical, _____

Specific developmental disorders
Note: These are coded on Axis II.
315.00 Developmental reading disorder
315.10 Developmental arithmetic disorder
315.31 Developmental language disorder

Table 1-4. DSM-III Classifications (continued) .

315.39 Developmental articulation disorder
315.50 Mixed specific developmental disorder
315.90 Atypical specific developmental disorder

ORGANIC MENTAL DISORDERS

Section 1. Organic mental disorders whose etiology or pathophysiological process is listed below (taken from the mental disorders section of ICD-9-CM)

Senile and presenile dementias arising in the senium and presenium
   Primary degenerative dementia, senile onset,
290.30 with delirium
290.20 with delusions
290.21 with depression
290.00 uncomplicated
Code in fifth digit: 0 = uncomplicated, 1 = with delirium, 2 = with delusions, 3 = with depression.
290.1x Primary degenerative dementia, presenile onset, _____
290.4x Multi-infarct dementia, _____

Substance-induced
   Alcohol
303.00 intoxication
291.40 idiosyncratic intoxication
291.80 withdrawal
291.00 withdrawal delirium
291.30 hallucinosis
291.10 amnestic disorder
Code severity of dementia in fifth digit: 1 = mild, 2 = moderate, 3 = severe, 0 = unspecified.
291.2x Dementia associated with alcoholism, _____
   Barbiturate or similarly acting sedative or hypnotic
305.40 intoxication (327.00)
292.00 withdrawal (327.01)

292.00 withdrawal delirium (327.02)
292.83 amnestic disorder (327.04)
   Opioid
305.50 intoxication (327.10)
292.00 withdrawal (327.11)
   Cocaine
305.60 intoxication (327.20)
   Amphetamine or similarly acting sympathomimetic
305.70 intoxication (327.30)
292.81 delirium (327.32)
292.11 delusional disorder (327.35)
292.00 withdrawal (327.31)
   Phencyclidine (PCP) or similarly acting arylcyclohexylamine
305.90 intoxication (327.40)
292.81 delirium (327.42)
292.90 mixed organic mental disorder (327.49)
   Hallucinogen
305.30 hallucinosis (327.56)
292.11 delusional disorder (327.55)
292.84 affective disorder (327.57)
   Cannabis
305.20 intoxication (327.60)
292.11 delusional disorder (327.65)
   Tobacco
292.00 withdrawal (327.71)
   Caffeine
305.90 intoxication (327.80)
   Other or unspecified substance
305.90 intoxication (327.90)
292.00 withdrawal (327.91)
292.81 delirium (327.92)
292.82 dementia (327.93)
292.83 amnestic disorder (327.94)
292.11 delusional disorder (327.95)
292.12 hallucinosis (327.96)
292.84 affective disorder (327.97)
292.89 personality disorder (327.98)
292.90 atypical or mixed organic mental disorder (327.99)

Section 2. Organic brain syndromes whose etiology or pathophysiological process is either noted as an addi-

Table 1-4. DSM-III Classifications (continued) .

tional diagnosis from outside the mental disorders section of ICD-9-CM or is unknown.

293.00 Delirium
294.10 Dementia
294.00 Amnestic syndrome
293.81 Organic delusional syndrome
293.82 Organic hallucinosis
293.83 Organic affective syndrome
310.10 Organic personality syndrome
294.80 Atypical or mixed organic brain syndrome

SUBSTANCE USE DISORDERS

Code in fifth digit: 1 = continuous, 2 = episodic, 3 = in remission, 0 = unspecified.

305.0x Alcohol abuse, _____
303.9x Alcohol dependence (Alcoholism), _____
305.4x Barbiturate or similarly acting sedative or hypnotic abuse, _____
304.1x Barbiturate or similarly acting sedative or hypnotic dependence, _____
305.5x Opioid abuse, _____
304.0x Opioid dependence, _____
305.6x Cocaine abuse, _____
305.7x Amphetamine or similarly acting sympathomimetic abuse, _____
304.4x Amphetamine or similarly acting sympathomimetic dependence, _____
305.9x Phencyclidine (PCP) or similarly acting arylcyclohexylamine abuse, _____ (328.4x)
305.3x Hallucinogen abuse, _____
305.2x Cannabis abuse, _____
304.3x Cannabis dependence, _____
305.1x Tobacco dependence, _____
305.9x Other, mixed, or unspecified substance abuse, _____
304.6x Other specified substance dependence, _____

304.9x Unspecified substance dependence, _____
304.7x Dependence on combination of opioid and other non-alcoholic substance, _____
304.8x Dependence on combination of substances, excluding opioids and alcohol, _____

SCHIZOPHRENIC DISORDERS

Code in fifth digit: 1 = subchronic, 2 = chronic, 3 = subchronic with acute exacerbation, 4 = chronic with acute exacerbation, 5 = in remission, 0 = unspecified.

Schizophrenia
295.1x disorganized, _____
295.2x catatonic, _____
295.3x paranoid, _____
295.9x undifferentiated, _____
295.6x residual, _____

PARANOID DISORDERS

297.10 Paranoia
297.30 Shared paranoid disorder
298.30 Acute paranoid disorder
297.90 Atypical paranoid disorder

PSYCHOTIC DISORDERS NOT ELSEWHERE CLASSIFIED

295.40 Schizophreniform disorder
298.80 Brief reactive psychosis
295.70 Schizoaffective disorder
298.90 Atypical psychosis

NEUROTIC DISORDERS

These are included in Affective, Anxiety, Somatoform, Dissociative, and Psychosexual Disorders. In order to facilitate the identification of the categories that in DSM-II were grouped together in the class of Neuroses, the DSM-II terms are included separately in parentheses after the corresponding categories. These DSM-II terms are included in

Table 1-4. DSM-III Classifications (continued) **.**

ICD-9-CM and therefore are acceptable as alternatives to the recommended DSM-III terms that precede them.

AFFECTIVE DISORDERS
Major affective disorders
Code major depressive episode in fifth digit: 6 = in remission, 4 = with psychotic features (the unofficial non-ICD-9-CM fifth digit 7 may be used instead to indicate that the psychotic features are mood-incongruent), 3 = with melancholia, 2 = without melancholia, 0 = unspecified.
Code manic episode in fifth digit: 6 = in remission, 4 = with psychotic features (the unofficial non-ICD-9-CM fifth digit 7 may be used instead to indicate that the psychotic features are mood-incongruent), 2 = without psychotic features, 0 = unspecified.
    Bipolar disorder,
296.6x mixed, _____
296.4x manic, _____
296.5x depressed, _____
    Major depression,
296.2x single episode, _____
296.3x recurrent, _____

Other specific affective disorders
301.13 Cyclothymic disorder
300.40 Dysthymic disorder (or Depressive neurosis)

Atypical affective disorders
296.70 Atypical bipolar disorder
296.82 Atypical depression

ANXIETY DISORDERS
    Phobic disorders (or Phobic neuroses)
300.21 Agoraphobia with panic attacks
300.22 Agoraphobia without panic attacks
300.23 Social phobia
300.29 Simple phobia
    Anxiety states (or Anxiety neuroses)
300.01 Panic disorder
300.02 Generalized anxiety disorder
300.30 Obsessive compulsive disorder (or Obsessive compulsive neurosis)
    Post-traumatic stress disorder
308.30 acute
309.81 chronic or delayed
300.00 Atypical anxiety disorder

SOMATOFORM DISORDERS
300.81 Somatization disorder
300.11 Conversion disorder (or Hysterical neurosis, conversion type)
307.80 Psychogenic pain disorder
300.70 Hypochondriasis (or Hypochondriacal neurosis)
300.71 Atypical somatoform disorder

DISSOCIATIVE DISORDERS (OR HYSTERICAL NEUROSES, DISSOCIATIVE TYPE)
300.12 Psychogenic amnesia
300.13 Psychogenic fugue
300.14 Multiple personality
300.60 Depersonalization disorder (or Depersonalization neurosis)
300.15 Atypical dissociative disorder

PSYCHOSEXUAL DISORDERS
Gender identity disorders
Indicate sexual history in the fifth digit of Transsexualism code: 1 = asexual, 2 = homosexual, 3 = heterosexual, 0 = unspecified.
302.5x Transsexualism, _____
302.60 Gender identity disorder of childhood
302.85 Atypical gender identity disorder
Paraphilias
302.81 Fetishism
302.30 Transvestism

Table 1-4. DSM-III Classifications (**continued**).

Paraphilias (continued)
302.10 Zoophilia
302.20 Pedophilia
302.40 Exhibitionism
302.82 Voyeurism
302.83 Sexual masochism
302.84 Sexual sadism
302.89 Atypical paraphilia

Psychosexual dysfunctions
302.71 Inhibited sexual desire
302.72 Inhibited sexual excitement
302.73 Inhibited female orgasm
302.74 Inhibited male orgasm
302.75 Premature ejaculation
302.76 Functional dyspareunia
306.51 Functional vaginismus
302.79 Atypical psychosexual
      dysfunction

Other psychosexual disorders
302.00 Ego-dystonic homosexuality
302.90 Psychosexual disorder not else-
      where classified

FACTITIOUS DISORDERS
300.16 Factitious disorder with psycho-
      logical symptoms
301.51 Chronic factitious disorder with
      physical symptoms
300.19 Atypical factitious disorder with
      physical symptoms

**DISORDERS OF IMPULSE
CONTROL NOT ELSEWHERE
CLASSIFIED**
312.31 Pathological gambling
312.32 Kleptomania
312.33 Pyromania
312.34 Intermittent explosive disorder
312.35 Isolated explosive disorder
312.39 Atypical impulse control disorder

ADJUSTMENT DISORDER
309.00 with depressed mood
309.24 with anxious mood
309.28 with fixed emotional features

309.30 with disturbance of conduct
309.40 with mixed disturbance of
      emotions and conduct
309.23 with work (or academic)
      inhibition
309.83 with withdrawal
309.90 with atypical features

**PSYCHOLOGICAL FACTORS
AFFECTING PHYSICAL
CONDITION**
Specify physical condition on Axis III.
316.00 Psychological factors affecting
      physical condition

PERSONALITY DISORDERS
Note: These are coded on Axis II.
301.00 Paranoid
301.20 Schizoid
301.22 Schizotypal
301.50 Histrionic
301.81 Narcissistic
301.70 Antisocial
301.83 Borderline
301.82 Avoidant
301.60 Dependent
301.40 Compulsive
301.84 Passive-aggressive
301.89 Atypical, mixed or other
      personality disorder

**V CODES FOR CONDITIONS
NOT ATTRIBUTABLE TO A
MENTAL DISORDER THAT
ARE A FOCUS OF ATTENTION
OR TREATMENT**
V65.20 Malingering
V62.89 Borderline intellectual
      functioning (V62.88)
V71.01 Adult antisocial behavior
V71.02 Childhood or adolescent
      antisocial behavior
V62.30 Academic problem
V62.20 Occupational problem

Table 1-4. DSM-III Classifications (**continued**).

V62.82 Uncomplicated bereavement	**ADDITIONAL CODES**
V15.81 Noncompliance with medical treatment	300.90 Unspecified mental disorder (nonpsychotic)
V62.89 Phase of life problem or other life circumstance problem	V71.07 No diagnosis or condition on Axis I
V61.10 Marital problem	799.91 Diagnosis or condition deferred on Axis I
V61.20 Parent-child problem	
V61.80 Other specified family circumstances	V71.08 No diagnosis on Axis II
	799.92 Diagnosis deferred on Axis II
V62.81 Other interpersonal problem	10A-7

American Psychiatric Association. Washington, D.C. Printed with permission.

Table 1-5. Diagnostic and Statistical Manual III.

Multiaxial Evaluation	
Axis I	Psychiatric diagnosis
Axis II	Personality disorders and specific developmental disorders
Axis III	Physical disorders and conditions
Axis IV	Severity of current psychosocial stressors
	(1) none
	(2) minimal
	(3) mild
	(4) moderate
	(5) severe
	(6) extreme
	(7) catastrophic
	(0) unspecific
Axis V	Highest level of adaptive functioning past year
	(1) superior
	(2) very good
	(3) good
	(4) fair
	(5) poor
	(6) very poor
	(7) grossly impaired
	(0) unspecified

circumstantiality—Pattern of speech that is indirect and delayed in reaching its goal.

clanging—A type of thinking in which the sound of a word, rather than its meaning, gives the direction to subsequent associations; punning and rhyming may substitute for logic, and language may become a senseless compulsion for word association, taking the place of communication.

cognitive—Refers to the mental process of comprehension, judgment, memory, and reasoning, as contrasted with emotional and volitional processes.

compulsion—An insistent, repetitive, intrusive, and unwanted urge to perform an act that is contrary to one's ordinary wishes or standards. Since it serves as a defensive substitute for still more unacceptable unconscious ideas and wishes, failure to perform the compulsive act leads to overt anxiety. Compulsions are obsessions that are still felt as impulses.

confabulation—Fabrication of stories in response to questions about situations or events that are not recalled.

coping mechanisms—Ways of adjusting to environmental stress without altering one's goals or purposes; includes both conscious and unconscious mechanisms.

decompensation—The deterioration of existing defenses, leading to an exacerbation of pathologic behavior.

delusion—A false belief firmly held despite incontrovertible and obvious proof or evidence to the contrary. Further, the belief is not one ordinarily accepted by other members of the person's culture or subculture.

depersonalization—Feelings of unreality or strangeness concerning either the environment, the self, or both.

derealization—A feeling of detachment from one's environment. May be accompanied by depersonalization.

developmental disability—A handicap or impairment, originating before the age of 18, which may be expected to continue indefinitely and constitutes a substantial impairment. The disability may be attributable to mental retardation, cerebral palsy, epilepsy, or other neurologic conditions and may include autism.

disorientation—Loss of awareness of the position of the self in relation to space, time, or other persons; confusion.

distractibility—Inability to maintain attention; shifting from one area or topic to another with minimal provocation. Distractibility may be a manifestation of organic impairment or it may be a part of a functional disorder such as anxiety states, mania, or schizophrenia.

ego-dystonic—Aspects of a person's behavior, thoughts, and attitudes viewed as repugnant or inconsistent with the total personality.

ego-syntonic—Aspects of a person's behavior, thoughts, and attitudes viewed as acceptable and consistent with the total personality.

euphoria—An exaggerated feeling of physical and emotional well-being, usually of psychologic origin. Also seen in organic mental disorders and in toxic and drug-induced states.

factitious disorders—Characterized by physical or psychologic symptoms that are under voluntary control.

flattened affect—Displaying an abnormally small range of emotional expression.

flight of ideas—Verbal skipping from one idea to another. The ideas appear to be continuous but are fragmentary and determined by chance or temporal associations. Sometimes seen in bipolar disorder.

formication—The tactile hallucination or illusion that insects are crawling on the body or under the skin.

grief—Normal, appropriate emotional response to an external and consciously recognized loss; it is usually time-limited and gradually subsides. To be distinguished from depression.

hallucination—A sensory perception in the absence of an actual external stimulus. May occur in any of the senses.

hypnagogic—Related to the semiconscious state immediately preceding sleep; may include hallucinations, which are of no pathologic significance.

illusion—A misperception of a real external stimulus. Example: the rustling of leaves is heard as the sound of voices.

insight—Self-understanding; the extent of a person's understanding of the origin, nature, and mechanisms of attitudes and behavior.

labile affect—Rapidly shifting emotions, seen in extreme form in brain syndromes.

la belle indifference—Literally, "beautiful indifference." Seen in certain patients with conversion disorders who show an inappropriate lack of concern about their disabilities.

learning disability—A syndrome affecting school age children of normal or above normal intelligence characterized by specific difficulties in learning to read (dyslexia), write (dysgraphia), and calculate (dyscalculia). The disorder is believed to be related to slow developmental progression of perceptual motor skills.

loosening of associations—A disturbance of thinking in which ideas shift from one subject to another in an oblique or unrelated manner. The speaker is unaware of the disturbance. When loosening of associations is severe, speech may be incoherent.

magical thinking—A conviction that thinking equates with doing. Occurs in dreams, in children, in primitive peoples, and in patients under a variety of conditions. Characterized by lack of realistic relationship between cause and effect.

mood—A pervasive and sustained emotion that in the extreme markedly colors one's perception of the world. Common examples of mood include depression, elation, and anger.

neologism—In psychiatry, a new word or condensed combination of several words coined by a person to express a highly complex idea not readily understood by others; seen in schizophrenia and organic mental disorders.

neurotic disorder—A mental disorder in which the predominant disturbance is a distressing symptom or group of symptoms which one considers unacceptable and alien to one's personality. There is no marked loss of reality testing;

behavior does not actively violate gross social norms although it may be quite disabling. The disturbance is relatively enduring or recurrent without treatment and is not limited to a mild transitory reaction to stress. There is no demonstrable organic etiology.

obsession—A persistent, unwanted idea or impulse that cannot be eliminated by logic or reasoning.

orientation—Awareness of one's self in relation to time, place, and person.

perseveration—Tendency to emit the same verbal or motor response again and again to varied stimuli.

phobia—An obsessive, persistent, unrealistic, intense fear of an object or situation. The fear is believed to arise through the displacing of an internal (unconscious) conflict to an external object symbolically related to the conflict.

psychophysiologic disorders—A group of disorders characterized by physical symptoms that are affected by emotional factors and that involve a single organ system, usually under autonomic nervous system control. Symptoms are caused by physiologic changes that normally accompany certain emotional states, but in these disorders the changes are more intense and sustained. Frequently called psychosomatic disorders, these disorders are usually named and classified according to the organ system involved (e.g., gastrointestinal, respiratory).

psychosis—A major mental disorder of organic or emotional origin in which a person's ability to think, respond emotionally, remember, communicate, interpret reality, and behave appropriately is impaired so as to interfere grossly with the capacity to meet the ordinary demands of life. Often characterized by regressive behavior, inappropriate mood, diminished impulse control, and such abnormal mental content as delusions and hallucinations. The term is applicable to conditions having a wide range of severity and duration.

reality testing—The ability to evaluate the external world objectively and to differentiate adequately between it and the internal world. Falsification of reality, as with massive denial or projection, indicates a severe disturbance of ego functioning and/or the perceptual and memory processes upon which it is partly based.

secondary gain—The external gain derived from any illness, such as personal attention and service, monetary gains, disability benefits, and release from unpleasant responsibility.

sensorium—Synonymous with consciousness. Includes the special sensory perceptive powers and their central correlation and integration in the brain. A clear sensorium conveys the presence of a reasonably accurate memory together with orientation for time.

thought disorder—A disturbance of speech, communication, or content of thought, such as delusions, ideas of reference, poverty of thought, flight of ideas, perseveration, loosening of associations, etc. A thought disorder can be caused by a functional emotional disorder or an organic condition. A formal thought disorder is a disturbance in the form of thought rather than the content of thought, e.g., loosening of associations.

unconscious—That part of the mind or mental functioning of which the content is only rarely subject to awareness. It is a repository for data that have never been conscious (primary repression) or that may have become conscious briefly and later repressed (secondary repression).

verbigeration—Stereotyped and seemingly meaningless repetition of words or sentences.

*Psychological Defense Mechanisms**
(Unconscious strategies to reduce subjective stress)

acting out—Expression of conflicts or feelings in actions rather than words.

compensation—Attempts to make up for real or imagined deficiencies.

conversion—Focus placed on a variety of somatic symptoms rather than on the actual distressing feelings or events.

denial—A disavowing of intolerable thoughts or feelings.

displacement—Transferring of an emotion from its original object to a more acceptable substitute.

dissociation—Emotional significance and emotions are separated and detached from an idea, situation, or object.

idealization—Overestimating an admired aspect or attribute of another person.

identification—Unconsciously patterning or modeling after another person.

incorporation—A primitive mechanism where aspects of another person are taken in and become part of psychic life.

introjection—Hated or loved external objects are taken within oneself symbolically.

projection—Emotionally unacceptable feelings or ideas are rejected and attributed to others.

rationalization—Providing excuses to justify otherwise intolerable feelings, motives or behavior.

reaction formation—Attitudes and behaviors presented are the opposite of those actually felt.

regression—Return to a more infantile pattern of reacting.

sublimation—Instinctual drives, consciously unacceptable, are channeled into personally and socially acceptable channels.

substitution—Unattainable or unacceptable goal, emotion, or object is replaced by one that is more attainable or acceptable.

symbolization—A related idea or object represents in disguised form the emotional feelings vested in the initial idea or object.

---

*Adapted from Frazier, SH et al. (eds): *A Psychiatric Glossary*, 5th ed. Washington, D.C. American Psychiatric Association, 1980. Printed with permission.

undoing—An unacceptable completed act is symbolically and often repetitiously acted out in reverse in the hope of relieving anxiety.

II

DIAGNOSTIC AND TREATMENT STRATEGIES

2

Diagnosis and Treatment of Acute Psychotic Disorders

PATRICK T. DONLON, M.D.

Acute psychotic disorders are commonly seen in clinical practice, and their origin may be either organic or functional. These disorders have had increased frequency in recent years with greater availability of substances which produce toxic CNS effects. A dysphoric affect and a general state of excitement are often associated with acute psychosis because the individual experiences subjective distress during the breakdown of reality testing and the loss of control over cognitive processes. As might be expected, the patient is at high risk for injury to himself or to others, in addition to being unable to care for his personal needs and responsibilities. For these reasons acute psychotic disorders are psychiatric-medical emergencies requiring immediate evaluation and treatment.

A proper diagnosis is important so the correct treatment may be offered. However, diagnosis may be problematic, especially with the patient who is

31

uncooperative or who presents with a limited history. A precise diagnosis is nonetheless important to predict the course and prognosis more accurately, to provide proper treatment, to avoid adverse effects from incorrect treatments and possible stigmatization, and to ensure proper data collection. This chapter reviews the common acute psychotic disorders and their differential diagnosis. A six-phase scheme for assisting proper diagnosis is presented, followed by practical guidelines for treatment strategies.

COMMON CLINICAL DISORDERS

Biological Disorders

Acute Organic Brain Syndrome (Acute OBS). Delirium or acute OBS is the clinical, psychological and behavioral manifestation associated with a wide range of acute biologic disorders which affect normal brain functioning. Common causes of OBS include:

- Metabolic disorders (diabetes, malnutrition, renal and hepatic failure, thyroid disease)
- Infections
- Cardiovascular disorders (abnormalities, spasms, occlusion, hemorrhage, hypertension)
- Intoxication (drugs, pollutants, solvents, various chemicals)
- Drug withdrawal (alcohol, sedative-hypnotic, minor tranquilizers)
- Postoperative complications (electrolyte imbalance, anesthesia, blood loss)
- Convulsive disorders
- Severe physical exhaustion
- Trauma (concussion, contusion, hematoma)
- Neoplasm (primary or metastatic lesion of CNS)
- Collagen and immunologic disorders (lupus, immunologic reaction to exogenous substances)
- Degenerative diseases (multiple sclerosis)
- Environmental (sensory stimulation, deprivation)
- Sleep deprivation

Acute OBS occurs more frequently with the aged and those in ill health or on medication. The etiology is either gross brain pathology or underlying metabolic or biochemical abnormality.

Distinguishing between psychotic OBS and functional psychosis normally is not difficult because organic states can be distinguished by history, specific clinical signs and laboratory studies. Acute OBS is characterized by disorientation, an attention defect, sensorium changes, and progressive impairment of intellectual functions, especially recent memory. The clinical picture may also include restlessness, perplexity, agitation, affectual lability, anxiety, visual hallucinations, impaired judgment, and perceptual distortions. The symptoms often become worse in the evening and with heavy sensory input. When symptoms are mild, the picture is one of mild confusion and is labelled nonpsychotic OBS. When severe and psychotic ideation or hyperactivity are present, the term psychotic OBS is used. Acute OBS refers to reversible cases and chronic OBS to irreversible (and often progressive) cases. An EEG can be used to detect delirium. The extent of the diagnostic work-up depends on clinical data and laboratory findings.

The treatment of choice for OBS is correction of the underlying medical or neurological condition. Other concurrent measures are helpful in patient management. These include good nursing care and a calm and supportive approach. Because a new environment may be disruptive and disorienting, it is helpful to add familiar objects (pictures, appliances, furniture) from the home to the hospital room. A night light and frequent visits by family members and friends are similarly helpful. Because both psychotropic and non-psychotropic drugs may often precipitate or increase symptoms, it is important to start with the smallest effective dose of an agent, if one is indicated, and closely monitor the response. Also, it is best to avoid agents with high anticholinergic or cardiovascular lability, because they increase the risk for adverse effects.

Amphetamine Toxicity. Amphetamines have few clinical indications but they are widely abused as CNS stimulants. They normally are taken orally or intravenously and often in combination with a barbiturate. No specific personality type appears at higher risk for abuse, although some individuals will self-administer the drug to treat a depressed state, to produce a greater alerting or stimulating effect, or to force weight reduction. Newly-presenting patients who are a higher risk for CNS stimulant abuse include poly-drug abusers, those chronically depressed, paramedical and medical personnel, long-distance truck drivers, and possibly athletes.

The course of amphetamine toxicity is self-limiting once the abuse is discontinued, and the paranoid ideation and increased psychomotor activity begin to abate within two or three days. Unlike most other drug-related psychiatric disorders, withdrawal psychosis is not associated with abrupt abstinence. However, abrupt withdrawal normally is followed by marked drowsiness, irritability, hypersomnolence and moderate to severe depression, which may be associated with suicidal ideation.

The diagnosis is normally made by a historical review, clinical signs and symptoms and laboratory confirmation. The clinical picture of amphetamine toxicity closely mimics that of paranoid schizophrenia and mania. There may be considerable emaciation due to the anorexic effect. However, in many chronic abusers with tolerance, the physical signs may be minimal. The signs and symptoms of sympathomimetic intoxication shown here* list the wide variety of

---

*From: Slaby AE, Lieb J, Tancredi LR: *Handbook of Psychiatric Emergencies*, 2nd ed. Flushing, New York. Medical Examiners Publication Co., Inc., 1981. Reprinted by permission.

undesirable effects that may occur with a single administration, but more commonly they present insidiously with chronic administration. They include:

Symptoms	Signs
Euphoria	Dilated but reactive pupils
Hyperarousal	Tachycardia
Grandiosity	Elevated temperature
Irritability	Elevated blood pressure (both tachycardia and elevated blood pressure may be absent in chronic users)
Loquacity sometimes to the extent of pressured speech	Dry mouth
Emotional lability	Perspiration or chills
Hypervigilance	Nausea and vomiting
Anorexia	Psychomotor excitement
Aggressiveness and hostility	Tremulousness
Anxiety	Hyperactive reflexes
Panic	Furtive glancing about the room
Resistance to fatigue	Malnutrition (especially apparent after prolonged intravenous use of large doses)
Restless wakefulness (Insomnia)	Repetitious compulsive behavior
Changes in body image	Stereotypic movements may cause ulcers on the tongue and lips
Chronic muscular tension	Teeth may be worn from bruxism
Severe abdominal pain sometimes mimicking an acute abdomen	Needle marks on the arm if the drug is taken intravenously
Impaired judgment	Cardiac arrhythmias and subdural and subarachnoid hemorrhage are occasional complications of the elevated blood pressure and tachycardia
Interference with social and occupational functioning	Skin flushing
Chest pain	Cutaneous abscesses and excoriation

If stimulant abuse is suspected, amphetamines are most frequently implicated. However, acute psychotic reactions and paranoid ideation may be associated with nonamphetamine CNS stimulants, such as methylphenidate (Ritalin®), phenmetrazine (Preludin®), diethylpropion (Tenuate®, Tepanil®) and cocaine.

Treatment is directed at reducing the toxic effects and managing the behavioral disturbances. Patients with needle tracks from injections require even closer medical screening as infections occur commonly in this population. Lavage or induction of vomiting is indicated for large oral dosages. Hospitalization may not be indicated for the less ill patient, especially if adequate care can be provided at home and neuroleptics are not required. Usually within 24 hours of the last dose, hypersomnolence will appear and persist up to 72 hours. The more belligerent patient normally responds best to reduced stimuli, as in a quiet room, but may require restraining initially. The patient's vital signs require frequent monitoring. On rare occasions, hyperthermia with possible convulsions and hypertension will present; both suggest life-threatening toxicity and require special medical attention. The duration of the amphetamine reaction can be reduced through hydration and acidification of the urine to increase excretion. Also, neuroleptics will antagonize the toxic effects of amphetamines. Chlorpromazine is the agent of choice if adrenergic changes are present. Because many amphetamine abusers also abuse sedative-hypnotics, it is important to evaluate the patient for other habituation and withdrawal symptoms. The post-amphetamine depressed state can be treated with tricyclic antidepressants (TCAs), which may also reduce the likelihood of further amphetamine abuse.

CNS Depressant Withdrawal Syndromes. Central nervous system depressants are common agents of abuse and include barbiturates, nonbarbiturate sedative-hypnotics, and antianxiety agents. Pentobarbital, secobarbital, methaqualone, and glutethimide are most commonly abused, while meprobamate and the benzodiazepines are the least frequently abused.

Two patterns of abuse have been identified. First are the middle to upper-class women in the 30 to 50-year-age group who were initially prescribed sleeping pills for insomnia. Later, as tolerance develops, they increase the dosage (often without their physician's knowledge) and take extra daytime doses for the control of anxiety. Often "doctor-shopping" then occurs to maintain their increasing needs as physical dependency and tolerance develop. In contrast to these habitual abusers are the predominantly youthful males who episodically abuse the CNS depressants seeking "highs." This latter group often concurrently abuses opiates and amphetamines and may prefer IV to oral administration. These patients are at a higher risk for multiple addictions and medical complications from contaminated needles and syringes (infections, allergy, etc.). Occasionally, a person who was hospitalized for an unrelated illness may experience withdrawal because he was removed from his drug source.

Addiction normally requires several months of progressive abuse. The tolerance is due both to CNS tolerance and to the increased liver destruction by the agent. The severity and onset of the withdrawal syndrome depend on the agent, extent of abuse, and individual susceptibility. Withdrawal occurs with abrupt drug discontinuation or reduction. Individuals who abuse 1,500 mg daily (or equivalent) of a short-acting barbiturate have a marked physical dependency and abrupt withdrawal can be life-threatening. In one study all subjects taking 800 mg or more of pentobarbital or secobarbital reportedly developed weakness, tremors, and anxiety upon withdrawal. Seventy-five percent of these patients showed convulsions and 60 percent a picture similar to delirium tremens.

It is important to establish by an historical analysis the degree and type of abuse and when the agent was last taken. This history often requires confirmation from peers, a period of observation, plus administration of the pentobarbital test dose to establish the degree of tolerance (Table 2-1). Drug intoxication and withdrawal signs and symptoms are nonspecific for the various CNS depressants and are similar to those of alcohol as shown below:

Intoxication	*Withdrawal*	
Mental confusion	Insomnia	Postural hypotension
Intellectual impairment	Anorexia	Muscle twitching
Personality changes	Restlessness, irritability	Fever
Motor incoordination	Sweating	Psychosis
Aggression/euphoria	Shaking	Hallucinations
Stuporous, drowsy	Anxious, apprehensive	Coma
Course nystagmus	Nausea, vomiting	Seizures
Slurring of speech		
Ataxia		

An EEG is helpful in distinguishing intoxication from withdrawal, and the abstinence syndrome must be distinguished from other psychotic states. Unfortunately, the patient may present an unreliable drug history or become abusive or demanding. It is important to explain the evaluative and treatment programs in detail to ensure greater cooperation.

Table 2-1. Pentobarbital Test Dose.

1. Give 200 mg of pentobarbital orally on empty stomach to sober patient in bed.
2. One hour later observe for signs of intoxication and estimate the amount of barbiturate needed initially to manage patient.

Patient's Condition	Degree of Tolerance Indicated	Estimated 24-hour Barbiturate Requirement
Asleep but arousable.	None.	None.
Drowsy, slurred speech, course nystagmus, Rombergism.	Definite tolerance.	500–600 mg.
Comfortable, steady state, only fine lateral nystagmus.	Marked tolerance.	800 mg.
No signs of drug effect, perhaps sign of abstinence persisting.	Extreme tolerance.	1000–2000 mg or more.

3. If signs of abstinence persist, another 200 mg test dose is given.

From: Ewing, JA, Bakewell, WE: Diagnosis and management of depressant drug dependence. *Am J Psychiatry* 123:909-917, 1967. Printed with permission.

Most patients in withdrawal require hospitalization. They should be treated with the agent of abuse or pentobarbital (cross-tolerance) and given a divided 24-hour dosage sufficient to produce a mild intoxicated state. Neuroleptics are contraindicated and phenytoin is not effective for preventing withdrawal seizures. Some recommend gradual medical withdrawal using pentobarbital and substituting 30 mg for every 100 mg of pentobarbital. With pentobarbital substitution, the dosage is gradually reduced on a 10 percent/day basis, thereby keeping the patient mildly intoxicated. Even though major withdrawal symptoms are avoided by this method, the patient often complains of some subjective distress, and feelings of anxiety, irritability, and insomnia may persist for months. Following withdrawal the patient is again at high risk for abusing CNS depressants and alcohol.

Medical withdrawal is only one phase of the treatment program. Intense patient motivation is required for continued abstinence. Depending on the individual case, removal from stress or peer pressure, psychotherapy rehabilitation, and antidepressant medication may all be helpful treatments.

Chronic Alcoholism. Alcoholism is the most ignored public health problem in America and it affects some 5-10 percent of the adult population. The vast majority of alcoholics are working males who deny their addiction despite placing undue hardship on their financial resources and family members. No personality type is more susceptible to alcoholism, and little is known about the natural history of the spontaneous remission rate. Etiologies are incompletely understood but genetic and cultural influences are seemingly important. Alcohol may be initially abused to alleviate tension resulting from poorly developed coping skills or environmental stresses, or as a self-administered attempt to reduce symptoms associated with a life crisis, major affective state, or developing psychosis. As the illness progresses, continued abuse also prevents the appearance of distressing withdrawal symptoms.

The diagnosis of alcoholism may be difficult to establish with the denying or uncooperative patient. Most alcoholics, like sedative-hypnotic addicts, offer a conservative estimate of their abuse, and the clinical signs of alcoholism may be absent in the younger drinker. In such cases, an added history should be obtained from the patient's friends and relatives. Alcoholics also are at higher risk for poly-drug abuse, physical trauma and underlying medical disorders. Finally, it is common for unsuspected alcoholics to experience withdrawal symptoms a few days after being hospitalized for an unrelated illness.

Six forms of psychosis may be associated with alcohol abuse, and the three most commonly seen in the differential diagnosis of acute psychosis are described in more detail below. Pathological intoxication can be ruled out early by history, signs and symptoms of acute CNS intoxication, odor of alcohol, and toxicology determination. Korsakoff's psychosis is associated with chronic alcoholism and is mainly the result of nutritional deficiency, especially thiamine and niacin. The clinical features include amnesia, confabulation or falsification of memory, disorientation, and peripheral neuropathy. Wernicke's syndrome is diagnosed when prominent eye signs (oculomotor palsy to ophthalmoplegia) are present in combination with the confusional state.

Alcoholic Paranoia. Paranoid ideation may be associated with a long history of alcoholism. This occurs most frequently with males and in those who have immature sexual relationships premorbidly. The clinical picture is characterized by denial, blaming, intense jealousy and concerns of infidelity, suspiciousness, distrust, anger and panic. These individuals are a higher risk for assaultive and suicidal behavior. The treatment includes neuroleptics, psychotherapy, abstinence, and rehabilitation.

Acute Alcoholic Hallucinosis. This syndrome may occur either during heavy abuse or during withdrawal and is characterized by a paranoid psychosis, a clear sensorium, and an appropriate orientation. It normally occurs in males between ages 30 and 50. Clinical phenomena are usually auditory hallucinations and delusions of persecution. Sexual concerns are often paramount. With males the theme is often homosexuality, and for females promiscuity. The illness may closely mimic paranoid schizophrenia and the usual course runs five days to a month. During this period the dysphoric mood is often accompanied by anger and depression. Suicide attempts are common. Treatment includes hospitalization and adequate nutrition. Low dosage neuroleptics are the agents of choice and abstinence should be encouraged.

Acute Withdrawal Syndrome. The withdrawal syndrome invariably occurs following an absolute or relative abstinence from alcohol in individuals with severe and sustained alcoholism. Its onset normally occurs within 24 hours of abstinence. Following is a brief description of three types of withdrawal symptoms:

1. *Mild Withdrawal Symptoms.*
   Irritability, malaise, GI symptoms (especially nausea and vomiting), startle, and disordered sensory perceptions are common. When hallucinations are present, their duration is normally brief. Medical treatment is typically not required, but benzodiazepines may reduce symptoms.
2. *Seizures ("Rum Fits").*
   Seizures, if present, normally occur 12 to 48 hours following cessation of drinking and are associated with an abnormal EEG. Seizures are "grand mal" in form and may occur individually, in clusters, or occasionally as status epilepticus. These seizures must be distinguished from those resulting from acute trauma or a seizure disorder worsened by alcohol intake. Treatment is supportive, but anticonvulsants are required if status epilepticus appears.
3. *Delirium Tremens.*
   This acute psychotic state normally occurs two to 10 days following absti- nence and may last from hours to several days. The clinical course and

presentation may be complicated by a number of medical problems (e.g., pneumonia, head trauma, dehydration). The delirium is normally preceded by the milder withdrawal symptoms listed above and ends with a prolonged sleep. The clinical picture is one of excitability, dysphoria, marked attention defect, increased motor activity, visual hallucinations, illusions, and delusions. Physical signs are multiple and include dilated pupils, coarse tremor, muscle irritability, and changes in vital signs.

The mortality rate is up to 15 percent and usually is secondary to hyperthermia and circulatory collapse. The primary treatment aims are to correct for dehydration and electrolyte imbalance and to anticipate and treat shock and hyperthermia should they develop. Nutritional needs require attention. A variety of agents, predominantly CNS depressants (e.g., benzodiazepines), have been used with some benefit in treating delirium tremens.

Phencyclidine. Phencyclidine (PCP) has become a common agent of abuse and may reach the popularity that LSD had a decade ago. It is abused by both sexes of all personality types and mostly by adolescents and young adults. The effects of the drug are dependent not only on the dosage, kinetics, and biologic sensitivity, but also on where the drug is taken and on the expectations and emotional response of the individual. Many of these effects are distressing to the novice. However, the popularity of the drug suggests that the chronic abuser finds it enjoyable. The agent also has marked physiological and psychological effects which may be life-threatening.

The pharmacologic classification of PCP is unclear and the agent has stimulant, depressant, hallucinogenic, and analgesic properties which are partially dose related. It has no medical use in humans but is marketed as an anesthetic and tranquilizer for animals. Because it is easy and inexpensive to manufacture, a black-market atmosphere has been created by unauthorized labs and dealers with little concern for purity and quality control of its street preparations. PCP may be sold as a granular powder ("angel dust") or in combination with various other agents. Furthermore, there are some 30 other chemical analogs which may be substituted and produce similar clinical features. PCP is commonly smoked or snorted, but some may take it orally, or, less frequently, intravenously. The desired effects normally last four to six hours, but residual effects may persist and these are the ones normally seen clinically. Tolerance and habituation may occur, but there are no withdrawal symptoms from chronic abuse.

The diagnosis may be missed if PCP is not suspected in acute intoxicated and psychotic states. The features of low dosage (mild) and high dosage (severe) intoxification include the following:

Low Dosage	High Dosage
Agitation and excitement	Respiratory depression
Ataxia and gross incoordination	Convulsions

Low Dosage (continued)	*High Dosage* (continued)
Catatonic features	Coma
Mutism	Hyperthermia
Horizontal and vertical nystagmus	Hypertension
Increased tolerance for pain	Generalized anesthesia
Flushing	Decerebrate positioning
Diaphoresis	Muscular rigidity
	Flushing
	Diaphoresis

Intoxication may be associated with coma, seizures, or a psychotic state associated with severe depression, paranoia, or violence that places the individual at a risk for harm to self or others.

The difference between a PCP-induced state and other drug-induced (LSD, amphetamine, CNS depressants, opiates) intoxicated states is the presence of ataxia, vertical and horizontal nystagmus, assaultiveness or catatonic staring, and generalized anesthesia for PCP. Furthermore, a urine or blood sample may document the presence of PCP. The psychotic state can be distinguished from acute schizophrenia and mania by history, clinical signs, and a vascillating clinical course.

The initial management of the patient depends on the degree of intoxication and disordered behavior. For persistent and severe effects, hospitalization and intensive medical and psychiatric treatments are indicated. Because no specific antidote is available, the severely intoxicated patient requires life-support measures when medical complications (e.g., respiratory depression, convulsions, coma, hyperthermia or hypertension) are present. Gastric lavage and acidification (ammonium chloride, ascorbic acid) of the urine will prevent reabsorption and increase urinary excretion of PCP, respectively. Severe behavioral changes may present initially as the intoxication state resolves. At times the patient may be seriously depressed, paranoid or belligerent, increasing the risk of harm to self or others. The nursing staff may find the patient most difficult to manage due to the psychotic state and the increased tolerance for pain. Physical restraints and placement in an isolated environment with reduced stimuli are helpful. The period of continued intoxication can be documented by the presence of nystagmus and ataxia. Then neuroleptics can be more safely administered without potentiation of the PCP anticholinergic effects. Even then the psychosis may only gradually remit and residual cognitive changes similar to those found in chronic schizophrenia may persist.

Central Anticholinergic Toxicity. Anticholinergic psychotic states are common toxic states associated with a wide variety of prescribed or over-the-counter (OTC) preparations with anticholinergic effects. Among the many agents that have substantial central and peripheral anticholinergic effects are the phenothiazine neuroleptics (especially thioridazine and chlorpromazine), the

TCAs (especially amitriptyline and doxepin), the antiparkinsonians, the antihistamines (diphenhydramine, promethazine), and the antispasmodic drugs. The OTC preparations include Compoz®, Sleep-Eze®, and Sominex®.

The diagnosis may be initially mistaken with iatrogenic disorders, and the dosage increased as the anticholinergic effects are interpreted as evidence of psychotic deterioration. Also, many patients who take OTC preparations may fail to inform their physician.

The signs and symptoms of anticholinergic toxicity* are listed as:

Central	*Peripheral*
Confusion	Fever
Disorientation	Flushed skin
Short-term memory loss	Dry mucous membrane
Hallucinations	Dilated, poorly reactive pupils
visual (auditory, tactile)	Blurred vision and photophobia
Dysarthria	(cycloplegia)
Ataxia	Nausea and vomiting
Coma	Abdominal distention
Euphoria	Constipation
Decreased anxiety	Urinary urgency and hesitancy
Fatigue	Cardiac arrhythmias
Insomnia	Burning mouth
Agitation and restlessness	Trouble swallowing
Inappropriate affect	Thirst

Some patients may be extremely psychotic. The greatest risk of toxicity is found in patients on higher dosages of anticholinergic drugs, alone or in combination, and especially the elderly and those with underlying medical problems. Finally, when the agent is taken in overdosage it can produce significant peripheral toxicity, including abnormalities in cardiac conduction and rhythm requiring ICU monitoring.

The correct diagnosis normally is not difficult to confirm once it is considered. The peripheral and central manifestations are unique from the other disorders and toxicologic screening helps identify the offending agent(s). In confusing cases, physostigmine may be used to reduce the toxic effects and establish the diagnosis.

Treatment includes the discontinuation of the offending agents. Neuroleptics should not be given due to their anticholinergic properties. The patient should have initial and repeated monitoring of vital signs, pupil size, bowel sounds, urinary output and mental status. Physostigmine 2 mg IM may be given at one to

---

*From: Dysken MW, et al: Anticholinergic psychosis. *Psychiatric Annals* 8:30-42, 1978. Printed with permission.

two hourly intervals until the clinical status improves or cholinergic toxicity presents. In cases of cholinergic excess, atropine sulfate should be given.

Functional Disorders

Schizophrenia, Paranoid Disorders, Affective Disorders. These psychotic states are described in Chapters 3, 4, and 5, respectively.

Borderline Personality Decompensation. The diagnosis and treatment of the borderline personality has received considerable publicity in recent years and with DSM-III is incorporated as a diagnostic classification. The borderline personality is a stable personality disorder and is not a prodromal for schizophrenia or other psychotic disorders. Nonetheless, the borderline person may have a definite underlying impairment in reality testing which may become psychotic in proportion, especially during periods of emotional stress or a breakdown in emotional support or environmental structure.

The borderline personality often comes from a disordered family background, with a heavy exposure to stress as a child. He may go on to function adequately socially and occupationally, especially if outside assistance is available. However, his relationships often are superficial, infantile, and dependent. Subjectively, these patients are relatively anhedonic, with anger, loneliness and anxiety being prominent affects. Their self-identify is poorly developed, resulting in inconsistent and often unpredictable emotional responses. Behavior often is impulsive and rage episodes are common. The end result is often maladaptive behavior with broken emotional ties, suicidal attempts, substance abuse, promiscuity, and incarcerations. A transient psychotic episode with shifting clinical features may appear and be associated with a thinking disorder mimicking brief schizophrenia. Delusions and hallucinations normally do not present, but looseness of associations and paranoid ideation are common. These gross psychotic features normally last only a few days and are not associated with cognitive residual. Borderline decompensation may also be precipitated by psychedelic or sympathomimetic drug use.

The differential diagnosis is mostly with schizophrenia, affective disorders and severe character disorders. The borderline patient who is frequently seen at the clinic will often have numerous past psychiatric diagnoses and variable clinical presentations. Diagnosis is best established by history, transient nature of the psychosis, and superficial involvement in social relationships by the borderline individual.

Treatment consists of identifying stresses, providing structure, and reducing acute symptoms through reassurance and pharmacologic management. Brief hospitalization may be required to reduce symptoms and the risk of impulsive behavior. Pharmacologic management is less effective with long-term management. Here psychotherapy and long-term structure may be helpful.

Severe Character Disorders. These nonpsychotic individuals have severe and chronic personality disturbances which greatly interfere with their social and occupational adjustments. As with the borderline personality, they often have a disorganized family background with an early exposure to emotional stress and inconsistent parenting leading to the development of poor coping skills. In contrast, however, the person with a character disorder experiences much less emotional distress but has a greater tendency to treat himself with alcohol or drugs or act out behaviorally during periods of stress. This response leads to an immature and impulsive behavior and a lack of commitment or responsibility. Much of his behavior is motivated by short-term symptom relief at the expense of long-term, more adaptive behaviors.

Patients presenting as psychiatric emergencies can be divided into three crisis categories. First are the acute situational crises which may be associated with a flooding of behavioral symptoms, including dysphoria and assaultive behaviors. These symptoms, which may be severe, normally subside rapidly without treatment. Second, a crisis can also be triggered by the effects of acute or chronic alcohol or drug abuse. The third instance occurs when the patient feigns mental symptoms to avoid criminal charges or wishes to be diagnosed as disabled to obtain permanent public funding.

The most common differential diagnosis is with schizophrenia which can be incorrectly diagnosed if the symptom picture and low socioeconomic functioning are confused with an acute and residual thinking disturbance of schizophrenia. The differential is most problematic in the characterologic patient with chronic substance abuse who has developed a secondary thinking disorder.

Most somatic treatments, including neuroleptics, have limited efficacy. Some patients benefit from low dosages of the more sedating TCAs. A sedative-hypnotic should be administered with extreme caution due to the potential of possible abuse. Lithium carbonate may be helpful for those patients with histories of spontaneously explosive and assaultive behavior. Psychotherapy and rehabilitation can assist only the more motivated patient.

Hysterical Psychosis. Hysterical psychosis is an acute psychotic reaction that often occurs when a person undergoes profoundly distressing events or circumstances. They occur much more frequently in young adult females and especially those with a hysterical-type personality. This premorbid personality is characterized by excitability, emotional instability, over-reactivity, and self-dramatization which is always attention-seeking and commonly seductive.

The acute episode normally lasts a few days and seldom more than a week or two. The onset is typically dramatic and the course very brief. These psychotic episodes have been labelled "24-hour schizophrenia," but this form of psychosis is probably unrelated to schizophrenia. Recovery is complete and there is no residual.

The differential diagnosis deals predominately with acute schizophrenia, mania, and drug-induced psychotic states. Hysteria can be distinguished by identifying the premorbid adjustment, stresses, course, and negative physical and laboratory findings. Clinical manifestations include dysphoria, delusions, hallucinations, depersonalization, and grossly unusual behavior which often has strong histrionic or attention-drawing features. A wide variety of forms may persist and mimic several clinical syndromes, including seizure disorders, paralysis, and catatonia. Related forms of hysterical psychosis include amnesia, somnambulism, fugue, and multiple personality.

Treatment is mainly supportive and includes a brief separation from the trauma-producing environment. Often family members and friends will rally additional support which helps to reduce acute symptoms. The psychotic features will remit without medication although sedative-hypnotics and neuroleptics will reduce symptoms and perhaps shorten the course. With further remission, medication normally is not indicated. Psychotherapy, including marital and family therapy, is then the treatment of course.

Catatonic Disorders. The chief characteristic of catatonia is a marked psychomotor disturbance which may appear in four clinical forms: stupor, rigidity, excitement, and waxy flexibility. Mutism is common although the patient is often highly aware of ongoing conversation. Often there is a rapid switching between the extremes of stupor and excitement, resulting in unpredictable behavior.

At one time catatonia presentations were very common, but now they have become relatively rare. Many of these patients, despite their external immobility, are in a state of extreme emotional distress. Tachycardia, systolic hypertension, and dilated pupils are common. The catatonic patient, especially in a stuporous phase, may also be highly suggestible and demonstrate automatic obedience, echolalia, echopraxia, and waxy flexibility. Many patients seemingly have reduced response to painful stimuli as they seldom complain, even in retrospect, of pain associated with prolonged posturing.

That catatonia may occur in schizophrenia is well known, but it may also occur with other illnesses, particularly affective disorders, organic states, drug (including neuroleptic and PCP) toxicity, and hysteria. Intravenous amytal can help with the differential diagnosis. With schizophrenia the administration of the drug often briefly clears the catatonic features while revealing the thinking disorder; with depression or hysteria a mood or affect disturbance may present, and the organic patient often becomes sleepy or gets more confused.

PCP toxicity often involves a variety of catatonic manifestations, and patients on neuroleptic drugs may develop behavioral toxicity, akinesia, rigidity, and akathisia which resemble retarded or excited forms of catatonia. Here the treatment is a reduction and not an increase of medication.

Much of the behavior in catatonia is purposeless and results from idiosyncratic internal stimuli. Therefore, the patient needs ongoing supervision or the illness might become a medical emergency due to the risk of exhaustion, dehydration, hyperpyrexia and the possibility of injury to self or others. Psychiatric treatment depends on the underlying etiology. Catatonia normally is associated with a relatively good prognosis, but this is dependent on the diagnosis, premorbid adjustment, and availability for early treatment.

DIFFERENTIAL DIAGNOSIS

Diagnosis in psychiatry is complicated by the absence of pathognomonic biologic signs for the functional disorders and by the mimicking ability of the various psychotic disorders in general. Other problems include:

- Shortcomings with diagnostic criteria
- Diagnostic bias
- Early presentation of illness
- Poorly trained staff
- Masking effects of drug treatment
- Poor cooperation of patient
- Incomplete histories
- Clinical states mimicking each other

Unless the diagnosis is readily apparent through history or clear-cut clinical signs, it is best to begin with the provisional diagnosis of "acute psychotic reaction of unknown etiology." This diagnosis is preferred to the probable biasing of future treatment by an incorrect diagnosis and better allows for the objective gathering of additional clinical data. DSM-III supports this diagnostic position. According to DSM-III, acute psychotic reactions resembling schizophrenia are called "brief psychotic reactions" when the florid psychotic symptoms are present for less than fourteen days. In addition, the diagnostic term "schizophreniform" is used for schizophrenic-like illnesses which last between two weeks and six months. Such a system of separating the more benign and brief psychotic episodes from the more chronic and malignant ones allows for more precision in outlining prognosis and treatment strategies.

To be more precise in diagnosis, we have found it advantageous to compile data from a six-phase diagnostic scheme to establish the definitive diagnosis more accurately. Information gathered from each scheme can provide evidence for or against a particular diagnosis.

Delineation From Other Disorders. The functional disorders must first be separated from the biologically-induced acute psychotic states, and the primary from the secondary disorders. A tentative diagnosis can be established by a careful history and a mental status examination, a physical exam, a family history, and a laboratory determination. A history of, physical findings of, and clinical evidence of sensorium changes, disorientation, and memory impairment suggest organic states. Illicit and iatrogenic drug toxicity is common and can be diagnosed by history, clinical findings, and laboratory tests. Amphetamine abuse can produce a paranoid psychotic state or mania in manic-depressive patients. Similarly, persistent psychedelic drug abuse can produce marked behavioral changes or schizophrenic-like psychotic features.

Medical conditions may also mimic affective disorders or schizophrenias, and treatment should be directed at the underlying disorder. For depression, these conditions include endocrine disturbances, such as hypothyroidism and Cushing's syndrome, carcinoma of the lung or head of the pancreas, and diseases of the CNS. Depression is also commonly associated with viral diseases, such as mononucleosis, influenza, and infectious hepatitis. Finally, some medications may produce depression. This list includes reserpine, contraceptive hormones, corticosteroids, alcohol, and other CNS depressants.

Mania may be mimicked by hyperthyroidism and diseases of the CNS. Drug administration or abuse may produce a manic-like state. The list includes amphetamines, steroids, and antidepressant drug toxicity.

Schizophrenia may be mimicked by sympathomimetic agents, psychedelics, and steroids. Furthermore, a large variety of biologic disorders which affect the CNS may produce a picture similar to acute schizophrenia.

Clinical Description. The course and distinguishing features of acute psychotic features have been discussed above. A comprehensive history and a period of evaluation are necessary to collect this important information. Family, friends, and past medical records often can add worthwhile historical data.

Laboratory Studies. Laboratory evaluations are extremely helpful in more accurately establishing the correct diagnosis and in separating biologic from functional disorders. More extensive evaluation tests or procedures (e.g., LP, CT scan) can be added to the routine ones (CBC, UA, chemistry profile, VDRL) if indicated. Psychological testing normally is not helpful in establishing the etiologies or the prognosis of acute psychotic disorders, but can provide information on the form and content of an illness.

Response to Treatment. The information on the patient's response to past treatments is useful in both establishing diagnosis and initiating present treatment. This data is also important in documenting whether the patient is toxic from current drug adverse effects and in assessing the possible interactional drug effects.

Family Studies. No particular pattern of family conflict or interaction has been found to characterize any of the acute psychotic disorders. Nonetheless, there is an increased familial incidence of schizophrenia, affective disorders, and alcoholism in individuals with these respective illnesses. Thus, the presence or absence of a particular familial disorder is helpful in establishing a diagnosis.

Follow-up. A clinical follow-up is important in documenting the course and confirming a correct diagnosis because patients are often seen early in their illness, may be misdiagnosed, or the clinical features may be particularly masked by treatment. Initially, only a tentative diagnosis should be given. Later the diagnosis can be confirmed or changed as further data become available.

EVALUATING THE ACUTE PSYCHOTIC PATIENT

Most diagnoses in medicine are made by history and confirmed by physical exam findings and laboratory tests. This is normally not the case in acute psychotics because histories may be unreliable and the patient's cooperation poor. Yet, a physical exam and laboratory determinations may be most helpful in establishing the diagnosis, especially with the biologic disorders. In summary, the initial steps to be followed for evaluation and treatment are:

1. Obtain preliminary history.
2. Evaluate clinical and medical status of patient.
3. Explain treatment approach to patient and his escorts and answer questions.
4. Provide emergency medical treatment if indicated.
5. Obtain routine laboratory tests (CBC, UA, Chem panel, VDRL, toxicology). Obtain more extensive tests or procedures if indicated.
6. Evaluate risk of injury to self or others.
7. Isolate, seclude, and restrain if necessary.
8. Contact family, friends, prior treatment facilities to solicit additional history.
9. Use neuroleptics (preferably IM) if psychotic features are catastrophic and agents not contraindicated.
10. Observe patient for a few hours to monitor course and treatment response. Outline treatment program (hospital, drug treatment, home, follow-up plans, etc.).

The initial goals are obtaining a history, providing safety to patient and others, providing a period of observation, establishing the need for hospitalization, and initiating treatment. Indications for hospitalization include:

Protective-Custodial
- Safeguarding the patient's life and reputation.
- Safeguarding the community from the patient's behavior.
- Removing the patient from a noxious environment.

Diagnostic
- Closer observation.
- Availability of specialized procedures.

Therapeutic
- Motivation of the patient and family to:
    Accept and support therapy.
    Make necessary life changes.
- Pharmacotherapy
    Administration of medication schedules too complex to be carried out at home.
    Rapid initiation of potentially toxic medication schedules that require careful observation.
- Special therapy not feasible outside the hospital (ETC, involuntary observation and treatment, etc.).

Unnecessary hospitalization, nonetheless, can be avoided by making the best use of the observation period in the psychiatric emergency area by initiating early treatment and by assessing the social support system. Many patients will have a rapid symptom reduction allowing for early release. This is especially true when the illness is not life-threatening, when friends and family members can provide adequate care outside of the hospital, and when comprehensive follow-up care is available.

EMERGENCY TREATMENT CONSIDERATIONS

General Considerations

Many non-drug techniques are effective in reducing acute psychotic symptoms. These range from emotional support and reassurance to a quiet, protective environment, to physical restraint and protective custody for the most belligerent. The treatment plan should be explained to the patient step-by-step to allay fears and gain greater cooperation. If clinical status allows, it is helpful to withhold medications.

Medical

Biologic Disorders. The treatment of patients with medical disorders producing psychotic features should be directed at the underlying disturbance. For example, patients who are toxic from PCP or amphetamines should be given acidifying agents to increase urinary excretion. Addicts should be placed on a mildly intoxicating daily dosage and slowly withdrawn medically. Finally, alcoholics with hallucinosis and paranoia may be helped by low-dose neuroleptics and steps taken to prevent and minimize dangerous effects associated with withdrawal.

Neuroleptics, except for the amphetamine psychosis, should be used with reservation with the biologically-induced psychotic states, for they may potentiate the psychosis as with the delirious, psychedelic and anticholinergic toxic patient, or mask important clinical signs.

Functional Disorders. Neuroleptics are the treatment of choice for acute functional psychotic disorders. This applies not only to the schizophrenic and paranoid patient but also to the manic and psychotic depressed. The latter two can be best managed by lithium and antidepressants, respectively. Neuroleptics often are not necessary for hysterical-psychotics, severe character disorder, or decompensated-borderline patients as the psychotic symptoms normally are brief with spontaneous remission, and neuroleptics are less well tolerated. Table 2-2 lists indications for neuroleptics.

Repeat dosages of IM neuroleptics (2.5 to 10 mg haloperidol) can rapidly reduce the signs and symptoms of acute functional psychosis. Normally one to four injections are necessary. Often there is reduction in the core psychotic manifestations (hallucinations, delusions, cognitive disorganization) as well as

Table 2-2. Indications for Neuroleptics.

Disorder	Indication	Comment
I. Psychosis		
A. Functional		
1. Schizophrenia	Drug of choice.	Therapeutic; Prophylactic.
2. Affective disorders		
A. Acute mania	As effective as lithium. More rapidly effective than lithium.	Lithium after acute treatment, no prophylactic value, higher risk for tardive dyskinesia.
B. Depression	Limited except for psychotic depressions (delusions, hallucinations, cognitive disorganization).	Potentiates TAD. May use in combination for agitation.
3. Paranoid disorders	May be helpful.	Rapport and trust important.
B. Organic		
1. Psychedelics (LSD, PCP, etc.)	Withhold initially, use benzodiazepines and sedative-hypnotics for symptom relief.	May potentiate psychosis.
2. Atropine-like	Withhold initially, Physostigmine.	Supportive nursing care.
3. Delirium	Hold neuroleptics.	Treatment dependent on etiology.
4. Chronic OBS (Diffuse organic brain disease)	Low dosage may be helpful.	Possible paradoxical or potentiated OBS effects. Higher risk adverse effects.
II. Borderline Personality	Acute symptom relief.	No prophylactic value, long-term supportive psychotherapy.
III. Neurotic Disorders	Limited.	Patients dislike adverse effects, anxiolytic agents.
IV. Personality Disorders	Limited. Acute symptom reduction.	No prophylactic value, potentiates CNS depressants.
V. Sleep Disorders	Not generally recommended.	Reduces REM.
VI. Hypochondriacal States	Only when associated with psychosis.	Adverse effects may increase hypochondriasis.

the dysphoric mood and belligerent attitude within a few hours. With potent neuroleptics there is normally a calming effect without sedation in contrast to chlorpromazine where sedation and hypotension are more common. Intramuscular medication begins acting faster than oral preparations allowing for faster initial symptom reduction. Once acute symptoms have responded to IM neuroleptics, the patient can be switched to oral neuroleptics if continued administration is indicated. More on neuroleptics will follow in Chapter 3.

Comprehensive Care

Nearly all active psychotic patients require continued medical and supportive care throughout the remainder of the illness and convalescent periods. The exact long-term treatment goals vary and depend on the etiology, severity and format of the illness and the aspiration of the patient. Comprehensive treatment plans (drug treatment, psychotherapy, rehabilitation, etc.) are necessary to reduce residual effects and insure optimal functioning.

CASE HISTORY I

Mary is a 22-year-old maritally-separated college student who recently left school and returned to her parents' home. Her parents were concerned with her changing behavior and reduced all-around performance. Her physician knew her well as he had provided her medical care for 12 years.

According to her parents, Mary had changed drastically. Two years ago, she was more vivacious and spoke of dropping enrollment for a new career. Then came a very unexpected marriage which ended after several weeks. Since then Mary had withdrawn more and seemed to have lost interest in most everything. Her parents really became alarmed when they visited her during her quarterly break and found that she was not attending classes. She also smiled inappropriately, seemed unusually preoccupied, and at times made unusual and even bizarre comments. Her parents wondered if she had been abusing drugs, but Mary did not indicate that she had.

On evaluation it was apparent that Mary was psychotic, but it was concluded that she could be treated as an outpatient because the family could provide supportive care. The physical examination was unremarkable. Also, there was no evidence for depression and her affect was flat. Auditory hallucinations, looseness of association and delusions were present. The course and clinical features favored the diagnosis of schizophrenia.

Mary was started on 5 mg of fluphenazine daily which was increased to 15 mg over the next two weeks. The medication was well tolerated. Benztropine mesylate 1 mg was also given twice daily and increased to 2 mg twice daily when akathisia presented. Nonetheless, the akathisia did continue until the fluphenazine was reduced to 10 mg daily two days later.

The psychotic symptoms slowly began to remit during the first week of treatment, and the parents commented that Mary was becoming her old self.

The treatment plan is to maintain Mary on a maintenance dosage of a neuroleptic for three months and then provide a trial period off the medication. She will live with her family and perhaps return to a job she formerly held in the community. She will require long-term follow-up due to the risk of relapse.

CASE HISTORY II

Michael, a 25-year-old unemployed male, was brought to the emergency room by police. According to neighbors he had barricaded himself in his home three days earlier. He refused to answer his phone and mentioned that he feared others wanted to kill him. In recent days he had been seen frequently gazing out of the windows and parading about his home late in the evening.

On initial evaluation he was extremely hostile and shouted obscenities. He denied being ill. He demonstrated increased psychomotor activity, a great deal of irritability, and refused to cooperate with the forced evaluation. His presentation was guarded, suspicious and aloof. He appeared to have strong feelings of persecution. Family members were contacted and they reported a recent history of heavy drug abuse, especially amphetamines. Michael refused to talk with them, saying that they wished him dead.

A physical examination revealed a slender and somewhat emaciated man with needle tracks on his arms, tachycardia, and mydriasis. Toxicologic reports revealed a toxic dosage of dextroamphetamine and a trace of pentobarbital. The clinical diagnosis of amphetamine toxicity was made.

Michael was isolated in a room to reduce sensory input and was given 5 mg of IM haloperidol. No further medications were given as his level of irritability rapidly subsided. He was kept in observation for 24 hours. It was observed that he spent much of his time sleeping. By the third day his paranoid psychosis had subsided, and he was released to follow-up care. Depression and further amphetamine abuse appeared possible.

SUGGESTED READING

Bourne, PG (ed): *Acute Drug-Abuse Emergencies—A Treatment Manual.* New York, Academic Press, 1976

Shader RI (ed): *Manual of Psychiatric Therapeutics.* Practical Psychopharmacology and Psychiatry. Boston, Little, Brown and Co., 1975

Slaby AE, Tancredi LR: *Handbook of Psychiatric Emergencies: A Guide for Emergencies in Psychiatry.* Flushing, N.Y., Medical Examination Publishing Co., Inc. 1975

Swonger AK, Constantine LL: *Drugs and Therapy: A Psychotherapist's Handbook of Psychotropic Drugs.* Boston, Little, Brown, and Co., 1976

Woodruff Jr RA, Goodwin DW, Guze SB: *Psychiatric Diagnosis.* New York, Oxford University Press, 1974

3

The Schizophrenias: Medical Diagnosis and Treatment

PATRICK T. DONLON, M.D.

The occurrence of schizophrenia has probably remained constant over the past 100 years and still affects approximately one percent of the adult population.[1] Although the incidence of the illness remains unaltered, the treatment of schizophrenia has changed dramatically. Until the middle 1950's the treatment was primarily supportive and custodial, but with the introduction of neuroleptics, ambulatory treatment became possible. Neuroleptics, though not curative, greatly reduce the signs and symptoms and modify the course of schizophrenia, allowing most patients to function on an ambulatory basis. Some patients may recover completely and may not require continued care, but most patients require close monitoring for years. The following review offers the primary physician practical guidelines for the differential diagnosis and medical management of the schizophrenic patient.

DIAGNOSIS

The schizophrenias represent a clinical syndrome of poorly understood etiologies. Schizophrenic individuals are a seemingly heterogeneous population, all having a relatively similar end-state. No pathognomonic biologic signs have been identified, and the thought disorder remains the unique diagnostic sign. Thus, the schizophrenias remain classified as "functional psychoses."

Early Signs

Nevertheless, there are some vague signs of a predisposition toward schizophrenia. A schizophrenic person often has a family history of schizophrenia and chronic family communication disturbances. As children, many pre-schizophrenic individuals have asocial development, poor peer relationships, and emotional eccentricity leading to scapegoating.[2] Neurologic soft signs and ill health are frequently present. Among adolescents, unsocialized aggressiveness in males and over-inhibited hyperconformity in females may prevail.[3]

Psychotic Decompensation

Although psychosis may present at any age, the highest risk is with young adults. Emotional and biological events may antecede psychotic decompensation in the vulnerable individual. Frequently, a personal or family emotional crisis will precede the onset of symptoms, although a direct causal relationship between emotional stress and psychosis remains unclear.[4] Often the stress represents an actual or fantasized loss (death, separation, etc.)[5] or a failure in reaching an important goal or mastering a developmental stage.[6] Medical procedures, such as childbirth and surgery, may immediately predate decompensation; drug abuse or administration (sympathomimetics, hallucinogens) may also precipitate schizophrenia in those perhaps biologically predisposed.

Unfortunately, it remains impossible to predict which individuals will ultimately develop schizophrenia. No valid biologic marker or clinical profile has yet been identified. Thus the premorbid characteristics are usually documented retrospectively and treatment is predominantly *ipso facto* rather than preventative.

The signs and symptoms of schizophrenic decompensation may present insidiously or acutely. Although acute symptoms may appear within hours, a careful history usually reveals that psychotic symptoms have been developing for days or weeks. Some of the symptoms are: cognitive and perceptual changes, anxiety and depression, somatic preoccupation, emotional and behavioral changes, physiologic response to stress and social withdrawal. The somatic complaints may be vague or may represent developing psychophysiologic symptoms, and are often diagnosed as neurasthenia, neurosis, or malingering.

With the transition to the overt psychotic phase, reality testing breaks down and thinking processes become uncontrollable, leading to the cognitive and perceptual disorganization typically found in schizophrenia.[7] Because this process is subjectively distressing, it often is associated with autonomic signs of mydriasis, tachycardia, increased systolic blood pressure, and sweating. Notably, once the illness has fully developed, the schizophrenic individual is less likely than the non-schizophrenic individual to have psychosomatic illnesses.[8] Somatic delusions and preoccupations, nonetheless, may remain and make the diagnosis of developing medical problems more difficult. Once the psychotic disorder has fully developed, the individual can no longer discriminate between psychopathological and more normal phenomena, emotions, and thoughts. By this time the individual appears less subjectively distressed. Cardinal clinical features are the overall bizarreness, the idiosyncratic interpretation of events, and the marked fragmentation in thinking processes. As time passes most individuals demonstrate improvement but waxing and waning often occur. A characteristic of schizophrenia is that some residual tends to remain. Not all acute patients move into the chronic stabilized phase, and the long-term course cannot be accurately predicted from early presenting features.

Schizophrenia Diagnosis

The diagnosis of schizophrenia should be made only when psychosis presents. There is no exact diagnostic scheme, and the diagnosis rests on the clinical evaluation of the course and symptomatology. The diagnostic system of Bleuler[9] and Schneider[10] is listed below.

Bleuler's Primary and Secondary Symptoms*
Primary Symptoms: Bleuler's 4 A's, which may not be evident early in the disorder:

1. Disturbances in *affect,* either inappropriate or flattened
2. *Loose associations,* wandering from topic to topic with little relevancy
3. *Autistic* thinking, or involvement in fantasy material, often with complete absorption in ideas of reference to self
4. *Ambivalence,* often not quickly apparent but characterized by conflicting and simultaneous positive and negative feelings toward another person

Secondary Symptoms:
1. Erratic behavior, often day-night reversal
2. Anhedonia, or inability to experience gratification from immersion in life experiences
3. Anger and frustration, often in reaction to inability to function
4. Dependence, a part of the boundary problem and the reality problem of being unable to handle the exigencies of life
5. Depression, with occasional suicide attempts
6. Pathologic coping devices, or attempts to "explain" what is happening (e.g., delusions, hallucinations, preoccupations, and depersonalizations)
7. "Boundary" problems, or inability to separate oneself (both self and body) as a distinct entity from others

---

*Brophy JM: The Schizophrenias. In *Current Medical Diagnosis and Treatment.* Krupp MA, Chatton MS (eds). Los Altos, CA: Lange Medical Publications, 1976, p. 620. Printed with permission.

8. Feelings of enhanced or muted sensory awareness
9. Reports of "racing thoughts"
10. Mental exhaustion
11. Deficits in focusing attention and concentration
12. Disturbances in speech perception and word meanings

Schneider's First-Rank Symptoms:
1. Hears voices speaking his thoughts aloud
2. Experiences himself as the subject of hallucinatory voices, arguments or discussions
3. Hears hallucinatory voices describing his activity as it takes place
4. Experiences delusional percept
5. Experiences somatic passivity
6. Experiences thought insertion
7. Experiences thought withdrawal
8. Experiences thought broadcast
9. Experiences externally controlled or imposed affect
10. Experiences externally controlled or imposed impulses
11. Experiences externally controlled or imposed motor activity

According to Bleuler, the four A's are characteristic of schizophrenia and are present under no other conditions. Schneider concludes the same about his first rank symptoms. The secondary symptoms of Bleuler are frequently seen with other psychotic disorders but may be absent in schizophrenia. Although the primary-care physician will find these schemes useful, recent study has documented that both of them are not unique for schizophrenia and neither has prognostic value.[3]

DSM-III offers some advantage over previous classification. Here duration of psychosis enters into the diagnostic scheme allowing for greater homogeneity. With this scheme, schizophrenia can only be diagnosed if overt features (including prodromal and residual) are present for six months and before the age of 45. Mimicking syndromes lasting less than 14 days and those lasting between 14 days and 6 months are called "brief psychotic reaction" and "schizophreniform" psychosis respectively.

DSM-III Diagnosis of Schizophrenia

Diagnostic Criteria
Characteristic symptoms (at least 1 of the following during the acute phase):
Characteristic Delusions
1. Delusions of being controlled
2. Thought broadcasting
3. Thought insertion
4. Thought withdrawal
5. Other bizarre delusions

6. Somatic, grandiose, religious, nihilistic or other delusions without persecutory or jealous content
7. Delusions of any type if accompanied by hallucinations of any type

Characteristic Hallucinations

8. Auditory hallucinations with either running, connecting or multiple voices conversing with each other
9. Auditory hallucinations with no apparent relation to depression or elation

Other Characteristic Symptoms

10. Either incoherence, derailment, marked illogicality, or marked poverty of content—if accompanied by affect disturbance, delusions, hallucinations or disorganized or catatonic behavior

Acute symptoms must be disabling (e.g., work, social relations, self-care).

Chronicity: Symptoms must be present for at least 6 months, prodromal deterioration must be present and residual must occur.

Schizophrenia Types

Schizophrenia is divided into various clinical types. These types are distinguished by presenting form, course, and age of onset. Such typing is of limited value to the physician because many patients present with mixed symptoms and the form may change with subsequent exacerbations. Nevertheless, correctly diagnosing a type facilitates treatment and helps to insure as quick a remission as possible.

All eleven types listed in DSM-II involve a pathology of the total personality, manifested as disorganized and illogical thinking, inadequate or inappropriate emotional responses to people or events, heightened emotional sensitivity, impaired volition and judgment, idiosyncratic belief systems (e.g., delusions) and perceptual distortions (illusions and hallucinations). In contrast to other psychotic disorders, residual and a tendency towards deterioration are common.

The *simple* type is characterized chiefly by a slow and insidious onset plus emotional detachment and apathy. The *hebephrenic* type is associated with the fragmentation of thinking processes, silliness, and regressive mannerisms in behavior. The *catatonic* type consists of two subtypes: excited and withdrawn. The *excited* subtype is associated with excessive and sometimes violent motor behavior and emotions; the *withdrawn* subtype, with stupor, mutism, negativism, and waxy flexibility. The *paranoid* type is characterized primarily by the presence of grandiose and persecutory delusions, often associated with hallucinations. Excessive religiosity, blaming, aggressiveness and hostile behavior are also common. However, personality disorganization is less common with this type than with the hebephrenic and catatonic ones.

Besides the simple, hebephrenic, catatonic and paranoid types, there are seven additional types. The *acute schizophrenic* type is associated with excitement, dysphoria, confusion, perplexity, and emotional turmoil. The *latent* type includes patients with nonpsychotic schizophrenic symptoms, and the *residual* type refers to the post-psychotic period when psychotic symptoms are no longer present. The *schizo-affective* type is a mixture of schizophrenic symptoms and elation or depression. In the childhood type, symptoms appear before puberty and include atypical behavior, inability to distinguish self from the environment, and delayed or uneven personality development. The *chronic undifferentiated* type is a mixture of schizophrenic symptoms that cannot be classified under other types. The *other and unspecified* type includes any type of schizophrenia not previously described.

The catatonic and hebephrenic types are seen less often now than a half century ago, in contrast to the paranoid form which is more frequently diagnosed. Furthermore, the acute and chronic undifferentiated types are commonly diagnosed today because the symptoms picture is often mixed. DMS-III lists five types of schizophrenia: disorganized, catatonic, paranoid, undifferentiated, and residual.

Differential Diagnosis

The differential diagnosis between schizophrenia and other disorders which may mask schizophrenia is shown below:

Schizophrenic-like (Secondary) Psychosis Associated With:
Central Nervous System Disorders
  Huntington's chorea
  Temporal lobe disorders
  Multiple sclerosis
  Systemic lupus erythematosus
  Neoplasm
  Luetic disease
Metabolic, Endocrine, Nutritional Disorders
  Porphyria
  Thyrotoxicosis
  Myxedema
  Addison's disease
  Cushing's syndrome
  Hypoparathyroidism
  Pituitary dysfunction
  Pernicious anemia
  Folic acid deficiency
  Pellagra
  Folate deficiency
  Alcoholic hallucinosis and paranoia
Drug Toxicity
  Sympathomimetics—e.g., amphetamines, methylphenidate, levodopa, diethylpropion
  Anti-inflammatory agents—e.g., steroids, phenylbutazone, indomethacin
  Disulfiram

Chronic bromism

Hallucinogenic agents (psychedelics, ketamine, phencyclidine)

Tricyclic antidepressants and monoamine oxidase inhibitors

Anticholinergic agents — e.g., antiparkinsonian drugs, belladonna and atropine-like agents.

Other Organic Psychotic Disorders

Other Functional Disorders

Affective disorders

Hysterical reactions

Borderline syndromes

Severe characterologic disturbances

Ganser syndrome

Nonspecific psychosis

Malingerers

Differential diagnosis was discussed in detail in Chapter 2. The diagnosis, however, may be difficult to establish in the acute psychotic patient. Thus the provisional diagnosis of "acute psychosis" should be given until the course further unfolds. The most common differential diagnosis is affective disorders (withdrawn depressive, agitated manics) or drug toxicity (amphetamines, hallucinogens, corticosteroids). The physician should obtain a complete longitudinal history and observe the patient for some period before making the diagnosis. A physical examination and indicated laboratory tests (chemistries, drug screens, etc.) should be obtained prior to initiating treatment. Unless the patient is experiencing catastrophic symptoms where rapid symptom relief is necessary, drug treatment should be withheld pending adequate documentation of the diagnosis.

PROGNOSIS

Prognosis varies widely although, in general, it ranges from fair to guarded. Langfeldt proposed a reactive-vs-process classification to separate more precisely the schizophrenic-like illnesses from true schizophrenia.[11] As the name implies a "reactive" patient's illness is an acute reaction against an identifiable stress. Reactive patients have a better prognosis, tending to have a family history unlike most true schizophrenics and a better premorbid social and occupational adjustment. Indeed, many of these patients will recover completely without medical intervention, although neuroleptics normally hasten the recovery. In contrast, the process group, with its guarded prognosis, has a seemingly greater biologic predisposition, more premorbid cognitive and affectual impairment, and an insidious onset. Without medication many of this group will deteriorate so drastically that they will require custodial care. Their response to neuroleptics may range from marked improvement to a marginally functioning, stable, chronic state.

The risk of personality deterioration increases with each schizophrenic relapse. Although the distinction between these two classes is not clear cut, it provides the physician with some sense of the course of the illness. With DSM-III and with the requirement of 6 months of psychopathology before the diagnosis of schizophrenia may be made, newly diagnosed patients will fit predominantly into the process and poor-prognosis end of the spectrum.

TREATMENT

General Considerations

A relationship based on trust is important for the development of any long-term, doctor-patient relationship, but especially with patients who exhibit schizophrenic symptoms because they have heightened emotional sensitivity and greater reliance on the physician's guidance. To establish the diagnosis and monitor the response to treatment, the physician must encourage the patient to discuss fears and anxieties openly. Such a relationship will help the physician prevent a patient in remission from decompensating. Physical findings and laboratory tests are of limited value. Careful clinical observation is essential.

Occasionally, nonpsychotic young adults will present with developing psychopathology. If the symptom picture includes cognitive disorganization, obsessive rumination, depression and anxiety, and reduced or inappropriate socio-occupational functioning, the possibility of schizophrenia must be considered, especially if there is no history of drug abuse or clinical or laboratory evidence of organicity. In most cases the illness will not progress to overt psychosis if the physician administers neuroleptics and directive and supportive care promptly. Seldom is hospitalization required, but the patient will benefit from a few days of medical leave from work.

Patients who suffer acute decompensation are often escorted to the doctor's office or hospital by friends or occasionally law enforcement officials. Patients typically have difficulty presenting a valid history, so this information should be gathered from others. The patient requires a regular medical workup to establish the differential diagnosis. Psychological testing, especially the MMPI and the Rorschach and thematic apperception tests, is helpful in establishing the diagnosis. Psychiatric consultation or patient referral may be indicated for patients who present with complex diagnostic or treatment problems. When made, the reasons for the referral should be openly discussed with the patient prior to making the referral appointment. Working with family members early and engaging them in the treatment and rehabilitation programs is helpful. The families' guilt feelings must be dealt with early. There is little evidence which suggests that faulty parenting causes schizophrenia. It is helpful to explain to the patient and family the nature of the illness and the need for immediate treatment.

Past familiarity with the patient is useful in outlining and implementing a treatment program, including establishing medication dosage schedules. The new patient can be safely started on low doses of any neuroleptic, and the dosage can be adjusted depending on clinical response. If the patient is to be followed as an outpatient, family members or friends must provide supportive care, and the patient should be seen regularly by his physician until the symptoms subside.

The decision to hospitalize should be carefully weighed and depends on the nature and severity of symptoms, the availability of a social support system (interested family and friends), the past familiarity with the patient, his response to neuroleptics or other medications, and the risk of the patient harming himself or others. Most patients who lack catastrophic developing symptoms or who have partially recovered can be treated on an ambulatory basis. In contrast, acute schizophrenia is a medical emergency and the patient must therefore receive vigorous and immediate treatment.[12]

The decision to discharge from the hospital is based on a significant reduction of symptoms which allows outpatient management and the development of sufficient rapport with the patient and his family to insure continuity of care.

Most patients will require long-term management and maintenance neuroleptics. Once symptoms have remitted the patient should be encouraged to resume pre-psychotic occupational and social responsibilities, but on a gradual basis. Patients with limited premorbid adaptability and those with significant post-psychotic residuals require referral to various community agencies and vocational rehabilitation centers for rehabilitative care.

The rehabilitation plan should be realistic for the patient, and positive behavioral and rehabilitative goals should be outlined with a tentative time schedule for completion. A "push program" may be realistic for some patients but just the opposite of what is required for others. The overall treatment emphasis should be toward producing symptom remission and improving the patient's socially-adaptive functioning.

Neuroleptic Agents

Neuroleptics are a group of antipsychotic drugs which currently include the phenothiazines, thioxanthenes, butyrophenones, dihydroindolones and diabenzoxazepines (Table 3-1). They vary greatly in potency, and, in general, the more potent agents are the least sedating. Like neuroleptics, the rauwolfia alkaloids (reserpines) also have antipsychotic effects, but they are seldom used today because of their delayed onset of action, reduced efficacy and greater adverse lability. Most neuroleptics (except thioridazine) are available in both parenteral and oral dosage forms, and fluphenazine has a long-acting injectable form. When administering neuroleptic drugs, the following points should be taken into consideration:

1. Are neuroleptics indicated? If so, are there any contraindications, such as comatosed states, presence of large amounts of CNS depressants (alcohol, barbiturates, narcotics, etc.), bone marrow depression and perhaps first trimester pregnancy?

Table 3-1. Major Tranquilizers (Neuroleptics).

Generic Name	Trade Name	Chlorpromazine Dose Ratio	Expert Dose Range
Phenothiazines			
A. Aliphatic	Thorazine	1:1	15–1500
Chlorpromazine	Chlor-PZ		
B. Piperidine			
Mesoridazine	Serentil	1:2	75–400
Piperacetazine	Quide	1:3	20–160
Thioridazine	Mellaril	1:1	150–800
C. Piperazine			
Butaperazine	Repoise	1:8	25–110
Fluphenazine	Prolixin	1:50	3–45
	Permitil		
Perphenazine	Trilafon	1:10	12–60
Prochlorperazine	Compazine	1:6	25–150
Trifluoperazine	Stelazine	1:20	10–40
Thioxanthenes			
Chlorprothixene	Taractan	1:1	40–600
Thiothixene	Navane	1:20	10–60
Butyrophenones			
Haloperidol	Haldol	1:50	2–16
Dihydroindolones			
Molindone	Moban	1:15	50–225
Dibenzoxazepines			
Loxapine	Loxitane	1:10	50–250
	Daxolin		

2. Comprehensive drug and medical history is essential for best selecting neuroleptic agent and initial dosage.
3. Injectable neuroleptics are highly effective for rapidly reducing agitation and catastrophic psychotic symptoms.
4. Identifying target symptoms is helpful for monitoring response to therapy.
5. Avoid combination and psychotropic polypharmacy whenever possible.
6. Give the drug a chance to work in therapeutic dosages before switching to or adding another.
7. Dosages can normally be consolidated to single daily bedtime dose.
8. Adverse effects may be multiple and subjectively annoying. They may be minimized or prevented through agent selection and dosage schedule, thus increasing comfort and drug compliance.

9. Avoid underdosing. Higher dosages may be indicated initially for treating acute or severe symptoms.
10. Don't overdose. Maintenance dosage should be the minimal dosage required to maintain symptom relief and minimize side effects. Consider discontinuing drug treatment if symptoms come on acutely and are now absent. Maintenance therapy is not always indicated.
11. The relapse rate is nonetheless high in patients following neuroleptic discontinuation. Patients should be followed closely and neuroleptics readministered if psychotic symptoms reappear.
12. Consider long-acting depot neuroleptics for patients who take medication irregularly. They greatly reduce the relapse rate.
13. Most patients on maintenance neuroleptics do not require antiparkinsonian drugs.
14. The treatment program must be highly individualized. Most patients require long-term neuroleptic and rehabilitative care and a trusting, supportive doctor-patient relationship.

Acute Schizophrenic Decompensation. Neuroleptics and supportive care are the treatments of choice for acute schizophrenic decompensation. Brief hospitalization is often indicated. The dosage requirements for neuroleptics, however, vary greatly and should be individualized and dependent on response to previous neuroleptic trials, body weight, age, and severity of symptoms. In general, an agent like chlorpromazine 50-100 mg or fluphenazine 5 mg should be given initially and repeated every 4-6 hours as indicated. Older patients and those at risk for adverse effects should be given lower dosages. Sedation may be a welcome adverse effect because it provides for needed rest and sleep.

For the patient requiring medication yet refusing oral ingestion, parenteral medication is indicated. Injectable neuroleptics (e.g., haloperidol 2.5-5 mg) are highly effective for rapidly reducing psychotic excitement and cognitive disorganization when given on an hourly basis until the desired response occurs. By adjusting the dosage to maximize efficacy, the oral daily dose can be established after a few days of treatment. Prophylactic antiparkinsonian agents (benztropine mesylate, trihexyphenidyl) will reduce the risk of extrapyramidal symptoms (EPS), but they will also reduce resorption of oral medication and therefore reduce the efficacy of neuroleptics.

Maintenance Therapy for the Chronic Patient. When symptoms have subsided the dosage can be reduced slowly to a maintenance level, which is often one-half to one-third of the daily dosage for acute symptoms. Depot fluphenazines (fluphenazine enanthate and decanoate) should be considered for patients who take medications irregularly, a practice which places them at a high risk for psychotic decompensation. These injections are normally well tolerated and can be given on an every one-to-four-week basis.

Neuroleptic withdrawal should be considered for patients who have recovered well on low dosage treatment. Nonetheless, these patients must be closely monitored because approximately 40 percent of them will decompensate within six months.[13,14] Therefore, it is important that the clinician be familiar with the early signs and symptoms of decompensation so that treatment can be reinitiated. This list includes cognitive disorganization, perceptual distortions, disturbed sleep and dreams, panic, and depression. Normally treatment includes re-administering neuroleptic medication or increasing the dosage as well as evaluating the environmental stresses.

Schizophrenic people may also have periods of depression. Normally, they are reactive in origin, mild, and transient. A more severe and sustained depression may occur especially during the immediate post-psychotic period. The depression may be masked by the flattened affect, overall reduced social activity in the schizophrenic person, and reduction in insomnia due to the sedating effects of neuroleptics. Nonetheless, depression can be identified through the patient's reports and evidence of pessimism, low self-esteem, helplessness and hopelessness. The severity of the depression is a good general indication of the risk of suicide. However, occasionally suicide may occur unpredictably and not be associated with a depressed mood. This is especially true of patients responding to auditory hallucinations and delusions. Depressed schizophrenic patients should be followed more closely. It is helpful to discuss treatment plans and observation with those who are close to the patient and to discuss his concerns openly with the patient. Brief hospitalization may be required, but this is normally not necessary if rapport and a social-support system are available. Antidepressant drugs are often helpful, but they should be initially prescribed in low dosages because the patient may be highly sensitive to low dosages and may even experience psychotic decompensation on higher dosages. For the latter reason, stimulants, such as amphetamines and methylphenidate, are not recommended.

Adverse Effects of Neuroleptics

None of the neuroleptic agents produce true physical dependency, although withdrawal symptoms may develop with rapid discontinuation (headache, insomnia, nausea, vomiting).[15] Though neuroleptics have a wide range of safety, adverse effects are multiple and often annoying. Most of the adverse effects are dose-related and represent a pharmacologic extension of the drug actions. Tolerance to neuroleptic adverse effects often develops with continued administration. The elderly and those in ill health or with CNS impairment are at a higher risk and should be monitored at low dose neuroleptic medication before the dosage is increased.

Because of their distressing nature and the reduced drug compliance associated with them, adverse effects should be prevented or minimized through agent selection, dosage schedule, and contra-active treatment.

Neuroleptic-induced extrapyramidal symptoms (EPS) are common during neuroleptic administration, and tardive dyskinesia (TD) may persist following neuroleptic discontinuation. Because EPS occur commonly and may be difficult to diagnose and manage clinically, they are discussed more fully in a separate chapter (12). Pseudoparkinsonism, akathisia and dystonic reactions are a function of biological sensitivity, molecular structure, dose, age, sex and duration of administration. They are more commonly associated with the more potent neuroleptics and higher dosages. Dystonic reactions present more commonly in young adult males, akathisia and pseudoparkinsonism in older females. Approximately 50 percent of the patients started on neuroleptics will require contra-active antiparkinsonian (AP) drugs in contrast to 20 percent on maintenance neuroleptics. Contra-active treatment for these three EPS is AP drugs, reduction in neuroleptic dosage, or substitution of a less potent neuroleptic. Levodopa is not recommended as it may exacerbate the schizophrenic symptoms. Treatment of TD remains unknown, but it may possibly be prevented through conservative dosages of neuroleptics. Adverse effects are common. In general, they are well tolerated and subside with continued treatment and dosage reduction. The list includes:

Type	Comment
Anticholinergic	
Dry mouth, blurred vision, nasal congestion, constipation, urinary retention, may aggravate glaucoma, paralytic ilius	Dose related Tolerance develops
Tachycardia	
Inhibition of ejaculation and impotence	Mostly with thioridazine
Central Nervous System	
Seizures (rare)	Dose related
Sedation	Dose related—tolerance develops
Hypothermia	
Behavioral toxicity	Reduce dose
Toxic delirium	Dose related Mostly with aged
Cardiovascular	
Orthostatic hypotension	Mostly with chlorpromazine and thioridazine
Allergic	
Agranulocytosis (rare)	Occurs first three months of treatment
Eosinophilia	Benign—occurs early in treatment
Contact dermatitis	
Photosensitivity	Occurs mostly with chlorpromazine

Type *(continued)*	**Comment** *(continued)*
Endocrine and Metabolic	
Weight gain	
Edema	
Gynecomastia, galactorrhea	
Menstrual irregularities	
Death	
"Sudden onset"	Not proven
Neuroleptic overdose (rare)	May occur mostly with thioridazine and mesoridazine

Toxicity may develop. This includes agranulocytosis and cholestatic jaundice, but both are rare and normally occur within the first three months of neuroleptic administration. Thus, neuroleptic toxicity should be considered in the differential diagnosis of patients who develop these disorders during the initial neuroleptic period. Eye and skin changes are dose related with chlorpromazine and thioridazine. EKG changes are associated with thioridazine and mesoridazine administration and are reversible with drug termination. TD is associated with long-term neuroleptic administration but may manifest after months of therapy.

An overdose of neuroleptics may be lethal. It is associated with sedation, hypotension, EPS effects, hypothermia, grand mal seizures and cardiac-conduction disturbances. Gastric lavage, even hours later, can be effective in removing significant amounts of the drug. Hypotension can be reversed with the use of norepinephrine or isoproterenol. Epinephrine should never be used since this agent stimulates beta as well as alpha adrenergic receptors, and, since neuroleptics block the alpha receptors, epinephrine may lead to a further reduction of blood pressure.

Comprehensive Care

The primary care physician can and should oversee the comprehensive treatment of his schizophrenic patients in all phases of the illness. Besides providing ongoing care the physician must be acquainted with the various available community services (e.g., vocational rehabilitation, sheltered workshops, rehabilitation centers) and make the appropriate referrals. As several agencies may be involved in some aspect of the treatment program, it is important that the treatment plan be communicated and integrated to reduce redundancy.

The final treatment for schizophrenia remains undiscovered and therefore, despite recent advances, schizophrenia is often associated with some chronic functional limitations. Nonetheless, the schizophrenic patient appreciates the empathy and continued concern of the family physician who assumes the responsibility for his long-term management.

REFERENCES

1. Goldhamer H, Marshall AW: *Psychosis and Civilization: Two Studies in the Frequency of Mental Illness.* New York, Free Press of Glencoe (Macmillan), 1953
2. Klein DF, Davis JM: *Diagnosis and Drug Treatment of Psychiatric Disorders.* Baltimore, Williams & Wilkins Co., 1969
3. Mosher LR, Gunderson JG, Buchanan S: Special Report: Schizophrenia, 1972. *Schizophr Bull,* No. 7:12-52, Winter 1973
4. Jacobs S, Myers J: Recent life events and acute schizophrenic psychosis: A controlled study. *J Nerv Ment Dis* 162:75-87, 1976
5. Kris AO: Cast studies in chronic hospitalization for functional psychosis. *Arch Gen Psychiatry* 26:326-333, 1972
6. Bowers M: *Retreat from Sanity.* New York, Human Science Press, 1974
7. Donlon PT, Blacker KH: Clinical recognition of early schizophrenia decompensation. *Dis Nerv System* 36:323-327, 1975
8. Pedder JR: Psychosomatic disease and psychoses. *J Psychosom Res* 13:339-346, 1969
9. Bleuler E: *Dementia Praecox or The Group of Schizophrenias.* New York, International Universities Press, Inc., 1950
10. Schneider K: Primäre und sekundäre symptome bei schizophrenie. *Fortschr Neurol Psychiatry* 25:487, 1957
11. Langfeldt G: *The Schizophreniform States.* London, Oxford University Press, 1939
12. Anderson WH, Kuehnle JC: Strategies for the treatment of acute psychosis. *JAMA* 229:1884-1889, 1974
13. Gardos G, Cole JO: Maintenance antipsychotic therapy: Is the cure worse than the disease? *Am J Psychiatry* 133:32-36, 1976
14. Davis JM: Overview: Maintenance therapy in psychiatry: I. Schizophrenia. *Am J Psychiatry* 132:1237-1245, 1975
15. Lacoursiere RB, Spohn HE, Thompson K: Medical effects of abrupt neuroleptic withdrawal. *Compr Psychiatry* 17:285-294, 1976

4

Paranoid Conditions

PATRICK T. DONLON, M.D.

Paranoid conditions include a broad spectrum of clinical disorders ranging from the aloof, suspicious, nonpsychotic individual to the frank, well-systematized, psychotic individual with paranoia. Although their incidence is unknown, these conditions, with the exception of paranoia, are common. They differ from primary affective disorders because they do not involve periodic mood shifts; however, many paranoid patients are intermittently or chronically depressed. And in contrast to schizophrenia, paranoid conditions are not associated with hallucinations, cognitive disorganizations, or emotional deterioration.

Separating paranoid conditions into primary and secondary illnesses, and each of these into nonpsychotic and psychotic, is a useful distinction. Primary illnesses have no underlying associated psychiatric or medical disturbance, and the cause of the illness is considered functional. Secondary illnesses involve an underlying disturbance, and the paranoid signs and symptoms normally remit when it is treated or subsides.

CLINICAL FEATURES

The term "paranoid" was used loosely until the current century and often referred to any psychotic or delusional behavior. In 1863 Kahlbaumn narrowed the term to grandiose or persecutory delusions. Then Krapelin (1896) gave the terms "paranoia" and "paranoid personality" their current precise definition by outlining their clinical features, course, and differential diagnosis. He also divided paranoid delusions into persecutory, grandiose, jealous, and erotomanic categories.

69

The common clinical features of paranoid conditions include:

1. Feelings of distrust, suspiciousness, jealousy, irritability, inferiority and inadequacy.
2. Themes of power, control, vulnerability, retaliation and litigation.
3. Patients clinically are socially aloof, hypervigilant, hypersensitive, guarded, emotionally cold, humorless and noncooperative.
4. Often experience ideas of reference and influence, feelings of passivity, thought insertion and broadcast.
5. Lack psychological sophistication. Tend to deny self-involvement and blame others.
6. Emotions and behavior are consistent with the biased belief system.
7. Delusions normally develop insidiously and may take four forms: persecution, grandiosity, jealousy, and erotomania.
8. Orderly and clear thinking is normally maintained although delusions may vary in degree of logic, pervasiveness, and systematization.
9. Absence of major mood disorders (depression, mania), schizophrenia (hallucination, cognitive disorganization, deterioration) and organic mental disorders.
10. Seldom voluntarily request treatment.

The differential diagnosis of clinical disorders associated with paranoid features includes:

Primary Disorder

Nonpsychotic
- Paranoid personality—This personality type is lifelong and normally does not progress to psychosis. These individuals have a pervasive and unwarranted suspicion and mistrust of others. Despite their hypersensitivity, aloofness, and tendency to blame and find fault in others, they may marry and often have respectable employment records.
- Paranoid state—Many apparently "normal" individuals will develop paranoid symptoms during periods of emotional stress. Often the symptoms come acutely but are seldom chronic. If severe and associated with impaired reality testing, they are considered psychotic.

Psychotic
Here the spectrum ranges from the rare paranoia where the delusional system is systematized and logical and sociability is well maintained to (but excluding) paranoid schizophrenia where delusions are more pervasive, transient, and illogical. Primary paranoid disorders lie in between. The clinical features of each are outlined in Table 4-1.
- Paranoia—Here the paranoid delusional system develops insidiously and becomes fixed. However, thinking remains clear and orderly, and early in

Table 4-1. Differential Diagnosis—Psychotic Paranoid Conditions and Paranoid Schizophrenia.

	Paranoia	*Paranoid Dis-orders (States)*	*Paranoid Schizophrenia*
Delusions	Yes	Yes	Yes
Content	Persecutory Grandiose	Persecutory Grandiose Erotic Jealous	Persecutory Grandiose
Pervasive	No	Moderate	Marked
Systematized	Yes	Moderate	No
Course	Content fixed	Content transient	Content changeable
Hallucinations	No	Occasionally	Yes
Cognitive Disorganization	No	Occasionally	Yes
Sociability	Maintained	Moderate Impaired	Poor
Affect	Appropriate	Moderate Impaired	Inappropriate
Reality Testing	Intact	Moderate Impaired	Poor
Psychological Deterioration	No	Moderate	Yes

the course it may be difficult to establish if the individual is delusional or merely has a gift of special insight. In this extremely rare clinical condition the often elaborate delusional system is a logical extension of a psychotically held belief and not a misinterpretation of actual events.

- Paranoid disorders—Paranoid disorders share some of the features of "mild" paranoid schizophrenia, a fact which suggests a continuum between the two. The fact that some patients with paranoid disorders later develop frank paranoid schizophrenic symptoms further supports the likelihood of a close relationship between the two.

Secondary Disorders

There is a wide variety of psychiatric and biologic disorders which are associated with paranoid features, and the symptoms may be either nonpsychotic or psychotic in severity. Paranoid features are considered nonpsychotic if they are mild, and psychotic if they are severe and incapacitating, especially if they are associated with delusions, hallucinations and breakdown in reality testing.

Paranoid ideation is common with both severe depression and mania. It also commonly occurs with early dementia, alcoholism ("alcoholic paranoia"), and metabolic disorders. Amphetamine and psychedelic drug abuse are invariably associated with paranoid ideation which may be psychotic in severity and mimic acute paranoid schizophrenia. Other organic disorders such as alcoholism, metabolic disorders (e.g., myxoedema, Cushing's syndrome), and organic brain disease (e.g., pre-senile and senile dementia) may also be associated with paranoid ideation. Many individuals with secondary paranoid conditions show no paranoid features in their premorbid state. However, the person who is aloof and suspicious may be at a higher risk.

ETIOLOGY

Familial and biologic studies have failed to show a genetic or organic basis for primary paranoid conditions and their origin is considered functional. Despite this it is well known that CNS stimulants (e.g., amphetamines) are commonly associated with paranoid ideation.

Many paranoid individuals are raised in hostile environments which lead to early feelings of distrust and suspicion. Initially, the individual experiences an uncomfortable state similar to anxiety when in the presence of others. This state normally increases when the individual senses danger which leads to greater aloofness and suspiciousness. Later if persecutory delusions develop, the now-psychotic individual may feel subjectively relieved. For as the plot and names reveal themselves, the person feels better prepared to defend himself. An important characteristic of the paranoid is his denial of many unacceptable feelings (anger, sexuality) and deep concerns (feelings of inadequacy, inferiority), and his blaming of these on others. Thus, paranoid persons tend to find the same faults in others that they cannot admit to themselves. Consequently, they conclude that they are the victims of others' transgressions which they may use as evidence to support their own sense of superiority (grandiosity).

Paranoid ideation is traditionally separated into four types. They may occur separately or in combination.

Persecution. This is the most common clinical form and is a highly distressing state. Here the individual is convinced of being persecuted and develops a series of tactics to protect himself. Tragedy may occur if the paranoid attacks an innocent victim who he incorrectly judged was plotting against him. However, violence seldom occurs, because the paranoid more frequently flees than attacks his supposed persecutor.

Grandiosity (Megalomania). Grandiosity may be a highly gratifying subjective experience because it may be associated with messianic powers and identity. Not only does the megalomaniac feel in total control, but his feelings of vulnerability have dissipated. The grandiose individual feels so secure that he wants to inform others of his special attributes. But when challenged by them, he often becomes more persistent and irritable and may even become violent.

Jealousy. Pathologic jealousy is more severe and persistent than normal jealousy. Normally, it is associated with some objective external reason but with misinterpretation of the facts and overreaction.

Erotomania. This exaggerated sexual interest is found more commonly in females. Often the love relationship is with a prominent figure who may not know the person exists. The recipient is frequently flooded with romantic letters or phone calls which may be very annoying if not embarrassing.

TREATMENT

Paranoid conditions are among the most difficult of psychiatric disturbances to treat. First, they are associated with denial, and the individual does not consider himself ill. Second, because distrust and suspicion are so high, the individual is highly threatened by personal contact such as that required in ongoing treatment. Finally, primary paranoid delusions, when present even in a motivated patient, are relatively resistant to psychiatric and somatic therapies.

The initial treatment plan is threefold: evaluate safety, provide symptom remission, and establish rapport. Because many paranoid individuals will be brought to treatment involuntarily, it is important to evaluate the circumstances which prompted the evaluation so that the safety of both the individual and society can be accurately assessed. If the threat of violence is present, hospitalization and even incarceration may be necessary. Injectible neuroleptics are highly effective in rapidly calming the belligerent patient.

Early symptom remission is important. If the symptoms are mild and the patient is voluntary, aggressive treatment should not be required. Often the patient will agree to a trial on a low dose neuroleptic to control distressing feelings. Not only will the drug provide relief, but it will also prove to the doubting patient that treatment can be effective, proof that will increase compliance with maintenance drugs and follow-up care. If psychiatric referral is indicated, the physician should clearly explain his reasons to the patient. If the symptoms are marked, hospitalization can occasionally be avoided if the symptoms subside rapidly, if a social-support system is available, if there is no past history of violence, and if the patient has a history of reliably following through with treatment recommendations.

Rapport normally develops better with voluntary patients or with those who initially present with medical concerns. However, forcing the patient into initial involuntary treatment does not always interfere with the development of rapport. This is especially true if the patient has experienced adequate symptom remission to appraise realistically the circumstances indicating treatment. It is important that the physician be honest and straightforward during visits because the patient is expecting deceit and fears confinement. Focusing on the patient's emotional response to his environment is also helpful. However, confronting delusions directly is usually not beneficial and may even increase agitation.

Long-term management of psychotic paranoid conditions consists primarily of medication and psychotherapy. Changes in employment and living arrangements seldom have long-term value because the same problems will invariably surface later. Low dosage neuroleptic treatment normally is the agent of choice. The goal of psychotherapy is to help the individual better understand the deep-seated fears that he cannot tolerate in himself and consequently blames on others or identifies with them.

5

Diagnosis and Treatment of Primary Affective Disorders by the Family Physician

PATRICK T. DONLON, M.D.

Depression is an extremely common disorder which most people experience sometime during their lives. Normally, it is related to life events (e.g., loss, disappointments) and is usually self-limiting. The clinical picture is similar to that of grief with the exception that the loss may be more symbolic than real. Depression also normally lasts longer and has more symptoms, including loss of self-esteem, thoughts of self-harm and, at times, a fear of losing one's mind. Most depressed individuals do not initially seek medical advice but instead choose to discuss their concerns with friends and family members. Only if symptoms persist or become severe will a physician be contacted. And then medication is seldom necessary for the mild and situationally depressed person. The treatment of choice is an open discussion of the circumstances precipitating the depression and of the steps needed for recovery. Some patients, especially those with underlying neurotic disorders, are candidates for psychotherapy.

These mild and reactive depressions, *Minor Affective Disorders*, must be distinguished from the severe ones because their natural history and treatment differ significantly. Recently, the term *Major Affective Disorders* has been used to separate these clinically significant mood states from the mild disorders. As shown in Figure 5-1, they are divided into *Primary (PAD)* and *Secondary Affective Disorders (SAD)* and the PAD are further divided into *Unipolar* and *Bipolar.* In both PAD and SAD the essential feature is either a depressed or elevated mood. PAD are normally episodic, without personality deterioration between attacks, and often occur in socially striving people. A unipolar affective disorder involves depression alone, whereas a bipolar disorder involves both depression and mania. Unipolar disorders are much more common than bipolar. Two additional distinctive forms of depression, delusional and atypical, must be separated also because they require special medical treatment. SAD are distinguished from PAD by underlying psychiatric (e.g., schizophrenia) or medical disorders (e.g., alcoholism, drug abuse, debilitating diseases) and where treatment is directed at the basic disturbance.

The following review offers the family physician practical guidelines for the differential diagnosis and medical management of patients with PAD.

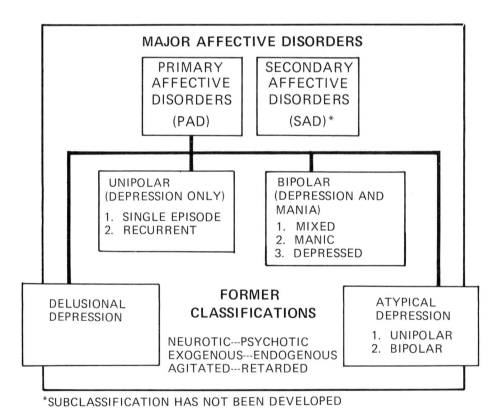

Figure 5-1. Major Affective Disorders.

DIAGNOSIS

Currently, there is much clinical, familial, biological, and pharmacological data for the unipolar-bipolar classification. Nonetheless, there are no known pathognomic biologic signs for either and the diagnosis of PAD remains clinical.

Unipolar (Depression Only)

Signs and Symptoms. The essential feature is either a depressive mood or a pervasive loss of interest or pleasure. Associated with the depressive syndrome is a wide spectrum of signs and symptoms which are divided into the following categories listed here:

Psychological and Cognitive
　Depressed mood
　Feelings of guilt, worthlessness, entrapment
　Tearfulness
　Loss of interest in activities
　Reduced sexual interest
　Hypochondriasis and somatic symptoms
　Helplessness and hopelessness
　Pessimism
　Indecisiveness
　Concentration disturbance
　Anxiety
　Suicidal ideation and attempts
　Paranoid ideation
　Increased obsessiveness
　Hallucinations and delusions (depressive content)

Physiologic (Vegetative)
　Diurnal variation
　Anorexia
　Weight loss
　Fatigue and lethargy
　Sleep disturbance (insomnia, hypersomnolence)
　Atropine-like effects (dry mouth, constipation, etc.)

Behavioral
　Psychomotor retardation
　Irritability
　Tension
　Agitation

Often, somatic symptoms (e.g., insomnia, anorexia, fatigue, bodily complaints) will bring the patient to the physician's attention, for some patients will not mention depression or suicidal rumination until questioned. Once the subject is approached, however, most of them willingly describe their symptoms in detail, volunteering their understanding of the possible origins. The diagnosis of the depression may be delayed unless it is included in the differential diagnosis of somatic complaints.

The global picture of sadness, gloom, and self-recrimination is most prominent clinically, and these signs are reflected in the patient's dress, mannerisms and comments. Pessimism, guilt, low self-esteem, and anxiety, which are invariably present, color the thought content and behavior. Diurnal variation and changes in drive, energy, sleep and appetite are also very common. Typically, the patient feels worse in the morning, with a lifting of mood as the day progresses. A reduced enthusiasm for life and energy are common. Sleeping becomes more difficult, and early-morning awakening is the most typical sleep disturbance. The patient's appetite is reduced, and there may be a substantial weight loss. Psychotic symptoms (e.g., hallucinations, delusions, cognitive disorganization, breakdown in reality testing) of a severity resembling schizophrenia may also be present. Even here depressive themes dominate. The treatment of choice for these patients is the use of TCAs unless psychotic or delusional features are present. Then a neuroleptic or ECT is indicated.

Some depressed patients may present with atypical symptoms. Here the symptoms may be associated with stress but their intensity may vary from day to day. The depression is often masked by phobic anxiety, hysterical features, and numerous somatic complaints. Vegetative symptoms occur less frequently. The patient's appetite may increase and his sleep remain undisturbed. Some of these patients respond better to monoamine oxidase inhibitors (MAOI) than to TCAs.

Natural History. No personality type is predisposed to depression. However, individuals who first become depressed (especially during their 4-6th decade) are often obsessional, rigid, and overconscientious and may lack drive and energy. The illness is often familial, but genetic studies fail to show strong hereditary influences. Females suffer from depression twice as often as men, with the mean age of onset about 40. Perhaps 10 percent of the population will experience at least one major depressive episode that requires medical treatment.

Depression normally begins insidiously, and the patient and his relatives have difficulty pinpointing the actual onset. The early symptoms are often associated with increased anxiety and exaggerated premorbid personality traits. The course is highly variable, with the risk of relapse remaining throughout life.

Depression may last days and even years (normally several months) and in some cases may be chronic. When the depression remits, the patient will usually return to the premorbid level of psychosocial functioning. The illness may be associated with increased suicidal ideation, increased alcohol and drug abuse along with impairment in occupational and social functioning. In fact, severely depressed patients may be totally debilitated by their illness and experience conceptual disorganization, delusions, and hallucinations. Indeed, they may be incorrectly diagnosed as schizophrenic or having organic brain syndrome.

The depressive syndrome may be modified somewhat by age and culture. In youths, negativism, antisocial behavior, school absenteeism, and sexual promiscuity may be associated with depression. In the elderly, cognitive symptoms may make the individual appear confused and pseudo-organic. However, in contrast to the true organic patient, the depressed patient often complains bitterly about his organic impairment. Cultural influences can also greatly modify the symptom picture. In some Asiatic countries, for example, cognitive and psychological features of depression may be absent or modified. Indeed, the clinical manifestations may be anorexia, catatonia, or somatization.

Bipolar (Depression and Mania)

Signs and Symptoms. Unlike unipolar disorders, bipolar disorders are characterized not only by depression but also by mania. Bipolar depression is similar clinically to unipolar depression with the following exceptions: psychomotor retardation is normally present instead of agitation, hypersomnolence may occur instead of insomnia, the duration is briefer and the onset and termination are more abrupt, and episodic mania is present.

There are interpersonal characteristics of the manic individual which are apparent clinically. These include an outgoing, confident and assertive behavior, an ability to manipulate and produce marked affectual changes in others, and an ability to project responsibility onto others and to test limits. In addition, there are the characteristic signs and symptoms of mania:

- Euphoria and expansiveness (may alternate with irritability and anger)
- Hyperactivity
- Flight of ideas (racing and jumping of thoughts)
- Excessive involvement in activities with increased sociability
- Distractability
- Circumstantiality
- Pressure of speech
- Impaired financial and business judgment
- Grandiosity with inflated self-esteem
- Increased energy with excessive involvement
- Increased sexuality
- Insomnia without apparent fatigue
- Hallucinations—visual or auditory (normally grandiose content)
- Delusions (normally grandiose or suspiciousness)
- Impaired judgment
- Shifts to depression

The diagnostic triad for mania is euphoria, hyperactivity, and pressure of speech. The euphoria may alter with irritability and anger, especially with patients brought involuntarily into treatment. These patients may even mimic the acute paranoid schizophrenic patient.

The increased psychomotor activity is characterized by enhanced physical and mental activity. The individual moves rapidly as he attempts to complete numerous tasks simultaneously. Distractions are common but fatigue is seldom mentioned. The pressure of speech is characterized by rapid speech and a jumping from one idea to another (flight of ideas).

Mania is a pleasurable state of feeling and most manic individuals do not consider themselves ill and have no insight into their illnesses. They become angered when others try to reason with them or control their behavior.

Natural History. Bipolar disorders have a high familial incidence, a fact which suggests genetic influences. The sex distribution is about equal. The lifetime prevalence is 0.5-1 percent. There is no single predisposing personality type, although some patients may be cyclothymic and many have high drive and energy. The mood changes may be preceded by life events, especially early in the illness. Typically beginning before age 30, the disorder is usually ushered in by an acute manic episode which may last a few days to months. Nearly all patients who present with mania will subsequently develop depression, unipolar mania being very rare. However, manic and depressive symptoms may be present in combination. The depressive episodes are usually longer than manic ones and the untreated depressions average about six months. As the number of previous cycles increases, the duration of the cycles decreases, for both depression and mania.

DIFFERENTIAL DIAGNOSIS

The PAD must be distinguished from SAD as well as other clinical disorders which may mask as affective states. Because the signs and symptoms of depression may suggest medical disorders, some medical workup is normally required to rule out underlying medical problems. The steps to reduce error in the differential diagnosis include:

1. Carefully evaluate and document presenting symptoms.
2. Obtain a complete longitudinal history and do a careful mental status examination.
3. Obtain a careful family history.
4. Use history, mental status, physical examination, laboratory and psychologic evaluations for differential diagnosis.
5. Follow sound diagnostic criteria guidelines.
6. If possible, observe patient without offering drug treatment to establish natural history.
7. Make only a tentative diagnosis based on phenomena, course, family history, and previous response to therapy.
8. Monitor response to treatment.
9. Continue to collect data and observation.
10. Be willing to change final diagnosis if suggested by new data.

Physical Disorders

Most patients with significant medical illnesses will be depressed especially early in their illness. Depressions are also common following major surgery, particularly lower abdominal operations, and very common following childbirth. Medical conditions may also present as depression. These conditions include endocrine disturbances such as hypothyroidism and Cushing's syndrome, carcinoma of the lung or the head of the pancreas, and diseases of the CNS, including early dementia. Depression is also commonly associated with viral diseases, such as mononucleosis, influenza, and infectious hepatitis. Finally, some medications may produce depression. This list includes reserpine, and other antihypertensives, contraceptive hormones, corticosteroids, alcohol, and other CNS depressants, plus stimulants and appetite suppressants.

Mania may be mimicked by hyperthyroidism and diseases of the CNS. Furthermore, drug administration or abuse may produce manic-like states. The drugs include amphetamines, steroids, and antidepressant drug toxicity.

Mental Disorders

Depression and psychosis are commonly seen in other disorders, predominately schizophrenia and borderline disorders. Because the clinical presentations may be similar, the differential diagnosis may be difficult at times. However, the age of onset, the longitudinal and present illness histories, and family history help to make the distinction. When psychotic symptoms (e.g., delusions, hallucinations) are secondary to depression, their content normally reflects the pessimistic and gloomy state. This is in contrast to schizophrenia where increased cognitive disorganization and bizarreness are present, and where greater debilitation and psychotic residual can be expected with chronicity. The borderline individual, like the schizophrenic, often functions marginally and has poor social relationships. In addition, the patient often experiences a chronic sense of emptiness and loneliness without prominent vegetative depressive symptoms. When under great stress, borderline patients may express a variety of behaviors, including agitation, increased depression, violence, or frank psychosis.

The conditions which most closely mimic mania are acute paranoid schizophrenia and stimulant drug abuse. Mania is characterized by an absence of drug abuse, adaptable premorbid adjustment, responsiveness to lithium, absence of residual from prior psychotic episodes, and a family history of bipolar illness.

TREATMENT (General Considerations)

Depression

The symptom complex in depression may be extremely distressing to the patient and may greatly increase the desire for treatment. Depressed patients respond best to an attitude of concern and empathy but not to a flood of sympathy. The patient should be encouraged to present his history in detail; additional data can be obtained by further questioning. With the suspicious or reticent patient, it may be necessary to obtain historical information from other family members.

It is important to assess the risk of suicide and the possibility of referral or hospitalization immediately. Suicide currently ranks as the tenth leading cause of death for all ages and is occurring with greater frequency in young adults, women, and Blacks. There are 25,000 certified cases of suicide in the United States each year and it is greatly under-reported. There are at least 25-30 attempts for each actual suicide. Hopelessness may be more closely related to suicide intent than depression. Nonetheless, 40 percent of those who commit suicide have a clear diagnosis of unipolar or bipolar PAD, and another 20 percent are chronic alcoholics. Retrospective studies show that up to 80 percent of suicide victims were depressed.

There remains the disturbing finding that 50 percent of those who commit suicide had been seen by their family physician the week preceding their deaths. Also, recently prescribed medications are often used in suicide. These facts suggest that depressed patients should be considered potential suicide candidates, and other factors listed here should be carefully assessed in evaluating that risk.

1. Closely related to depression and, in particular, hopelessness.
2. More likely when depression is lifting.
3. After hospital discharge.
4. Women attempt suicide 8 times more frequently than men, but men *commit* suicide approximately 3 times more frequently than women.
5. May occur at any age but is more common after 40 years of age.
6. Family history of suicide.
7. Past suicidal threats or gestures.
8. Exposure to violence (especially males).
9. Living alone.
10. Alcohol abuse.
11. Recent life crisis or important loss.
12. Disposing of valued possessions.
13. Schizophrenic and other psychotic individuals may unpredictably commit suicide.

Finally and despite folklore, those who speak of committing suicide may later do so. The risk of suicide, however, can be reduced by establishing rapport, telling the patient that he has a depressive illness, outlining the treatment program, and then following the patient regularly to evaluate progress, adjust medication and maintain interest. A trusting, positive doctor-patient relationship is most crucial, for drugs may relieve depression but the personal relationship is what prevents suicide. Therefore, drug treatment should never interfere with the doctor-patient relationship. If medications are used, the side effects and the lag period for response should be discussed. Most patients will experience some immediate relief from the sedative effect of the drugs plus the reassurance of being under medical care.

Supportive care, psychotherapy, and environmental manipulations are helpful to many depressed individuals. Because depression is normally disabling to some degree, the patient may need assistance in carrying out everyday responsibilities. Emotional support from peers and family members is helpful also. Most depressions, even those with a strong biological basis, can benefit from psychotherapy. Normally aggressive psychotherapy is of limited value in the severely depressed as lethargy may prevent full cooperation or guilt feelings may inadvertently increase. Psychotherapy becomes more productive as the depression lifts, and early therapy should be supportive. The effects of psychotherapy and TCA are distinct yet additive. TCAs reduce depressive symptoms and prevent relapse while psychotherapy affects interpersonal relationships and social effectiveness.

Environmental manipulations can include family meetings to correct detrimental attitudes, encouragement of the patient to move physically to a less noxious environment, and a leave of absence from work or school.

Most depressed patients do not require psychiatric referral. The exceptions are the problem or treatment-refractory cases, the suicidal patient, and those requiring hospitalization. When patients are referred, the indication should be discussed with them prior to making the referral. Hospitalization also is seldom required unless the patient is severely ill, is a high risk for suicide, requires close medical observation, or is in need of special hospital procedures like ECT.

Fortunately, depressed patients normally take their medications as recommended unless troublesome adverse effects present.

If provided an adequate dosage, approximately 70 percent will respond to a trial on TCA. Only ECT, which is 90-95 percent efficacious, is more effective. Patients refractory to TCA should be administered another TCA, an MAOI, or given ECT. Most delusional, depressed patients do not respond well to TCAs regardless of the dosage. These patients may do well if placed on neuroleptics, a neuroleptics-TCA combination therapy, or ECT. Finally, some patients with recurrent unipolar depressions may benefit from lithium.

Mania (or Mixed Manic-Depression)

In contrast to the depressed patient, the manic individual feels unusually good, and often finds total justification for his high energy level and behavior. The new patient seldom feels ill or seeks treatment. Much of the history must be obtained from others as the patient has few complaints other than the conservative attitude of others. Often family conflicts are monumental by this time because the manic's enthusiasm for life has led to marital strife, financial embarrassment and occupational setbacks. Family meetings are normally required.

Hospitalization is often indicated to place some control over the hyperactive manic and to initiate treatment. Neuroleptic medication will provide immediate symptom control, in contrast to lithium, and should be started immediately.

Lithium should be co-administered and the neuroleptic discontinued once manic symptoms are reduced. The physician should be prepared for frequent challenges by his initially dissatisfied patient, who dislikes being controlled and treated as if ill.

Later it is important to discuss the illness and treatment program in detail with the then-healthier patient. This will allow for greater participation and cooperation on the patient's part. Furthermore, if symptoms reappear later early treatment may be initiated by the patient.

Lithium is about 85-90 percent effective in preventing subsequent manic episodes in bipolar patients and also may prevent or reduce recurrent depression. Patients who do not respond to lithium should be considered for neuroleptic treatment or ECT. As mania is a periodic illness, remission may be spontaneous and occur without treatment.

MEDICAL TREATMENT

Antidepressants

There are two major groups in this category: TCAs and MAOIs. The MAOIs are seldom used today for they are less effective than TCAs and are associated with higher adverse lability. However, they may be effective for depressed patients with atypical features and those who do not respond to TCAs. As mentioned above, TCAs are most effective for non-delusional depressed patients and lithium is the treatment for bipolar manic patients. The following discussion will be limited to the TCAs. Currently available TCAs and recommended daily dosages are listed in Table 5-1.

The TCAs are similar pharmacologically to the neuroleptic agents although they rarely produce EPS. In addition, the TCAs are similar to each other in pharmacologic effects, onset of action, and adverse effects. Their potency is also similar with the exception of nortriptyline and protriptyline, which are more potent, and doxepin, which is somewhat less potent. Because there is a rather narrow margin of safety between therapeutic dosage and toxicity, patients will require close monitoring of medication. A tolerance will develop to the adverse effects but not to the agents themselves. Although TCAs are not addicting, some patients on prolonged treatment will experience mild withdrawal symptoms (nausea, headaches, and malaise) if the medication is rapidly discontinued.

TCAs have three clinically-important pharmacologic actions: sedation, anticholinergic effects, and an ability to block the "amine pump" for the aminergic neurotransmitters, such as norepinephrine and serotonin. Amitriptyline and doxepin are the most sedating and anticholinergic. Protriptyline is the least sedating, desipramine the least anticholinergic. Evidence is developing that some endogenously depressed patients suffer from a deficiency of noradrenergic transmission, while the others may suffer from a deficiency of serotonergic transmission. All TCAs equally block the amine pump with the exception of doxepin, which is much reduced. Tertiary amines (imipramine, amitriptyline)

Table 5-1. Antidepressant Agents.

Generic Name	Trade Name	Daily dosage (acute symptom control)	Daily dosage (maintenance)
1. Imipramine	Tofranil Imipramine pamoate Imavate SK-Pramine Presamine	150–300 mg	50–150 mg
2. Desipramine	Norpramin Pertofrane	150–300 mg	50–150 mg
3. Protriptyline	Vivactil	40–60 mg	20–30 mg
4. Amitriptyline	Elavil Amitril Endep	150–300 mg	50–150 mg
5. Nortriptyline	Rolavil Aventyl Pamelor	70–100 mg	20–60 mg
6. Doxepin	Sinequan Adapin	150–300 mg	50–150 mg
7. Trimipramine maleate	Surmontil	150–300 mg	50–150 mg
8. Amoxapine	Asendin	200–400 mg	100–300 mg
9. Maprotiline	Ludiomil	150–300 mg	50–150 mg

more strongly inhibit uptake of serotonin. In contrast, the demethylated or secondary amines (desipramine, nortriptyline) more selectively block uptake of norepinephrine; thus there is some evidence for switching between the groups in the refractory patient.

There are several reasons why a patient may fail to respond to TCAs. First, incorrect diagnosis; second, the patient has received an inadequate trial or a nontherapeutic dose; third, the serum level may be in a nontherapeutic range. A laboratory determination is helpful here; fourth, the patient may benefit from a different TCA with a different mode of action on neurotransmitters; fifth, poor compliance.

Dosage Schedules

Before administering antidepressants, the following guidelines should be considered:

1. The patient-doctor relationship is extremely important. When both have a positive attitude towards treatment, the outcome is enhanced.
2. Are antidepressants indicated? They are little better than a placebo with

mild or reactive depressions. The patients who respond optimally are at least moderately depressed and associated with vegetative symptoms (anorexia, insomnia, etc.). The doctor must distinguish between primary and secondary depressive disorders.

3. Before initiating treatment insure that contraindications such as concomitant MAOI treatment, recovery from acute myocardial infarct, known hypersensitivity are absent and that there are no special reasons to take precautions (pregnancy, schizophrenia, epilepsy, presence of large amounts of CNS depressants).

4. A comprehensive drug and medical history is essential for selecting the best agent and initial dosage.

5. Be familiar with drug interactions. Avoid combination and psychotropic polypharmacy whenever possible.

6. Adverse effects are multiple, annoying, and dose related. Start with a low divided dosage (e.g., imipramine 25 mg twice daily). A tolerance to adverse effects normally develops rapidly and therefore dosage can be increased.

7. Drug selection should reflect the adverse effect profile of agent, and the history of past response to TCAs. There is clinical value in giving a more sedating agent (e.g., amitriptyline) to the agitated patient and a less sedating agent (e.g., imipramine) to the psychomotor-retarded patient. Desipramine has relatively low anticholinergic effects, making it an agent of choice if atropine-like effects are of concern.

8. Therapeutic response may not present for three weeks. However, most patients report a reduction in anxiety and insomnia soon after treatment begins due to sedative effects.

9. Consolidate the dosage to a single bedtime dose. This increases compliance, aids sleeping, and reduces adverse effects.

10. Avoid underdosing. Daily dosages required for response vary widely. Most patients require 150-250 mg (or equivalent) of imipramine daily.

11. Don't overdose either. The elderly and those with underlying medical or neurologic disorders are at higher risk for adverse effects and toxicity and therefore should be treated with more conservative dosages.

12. Give the drug a chance to work in therapeutic dosages before switching to another.

13. Identifying and monitoring target symptoms are helpful in documenting progress.

14. After treatment response the dosage should be reduced to a maintenance level. Then the dosage should be gradually reduced. The total treatment period is normally 3-6 months. With a rapid drug termination, the patient may experience withdrawal symptoms or a "rebound" depression.

15. Perhaps 15 percent will require maintenance treatment to prevent symptom recurrence.

16. The efficacy of antidepressants in acute depression is about 70 percent. If there is no improvement after one month, reconsider the diagnosis and switch treatments (another antidepressant, ECT, MAOI, neuroleptic etc.).

Seldom is it necessary to give parenteral medication. Most patients tolerate a schedule beginning with a small, oral, divided dosage which is later consolidated to a single bedtime dose. Often there is a lag time of a few days to 3 weeks before response occurs. If the medication is well tolerated and the efficacy is delayed, the dosage should be increased up to 300 mg daily (or equivalent for protriptyline and nortriptyline). As long as the depression persists, the patients should remain on the lowest effective dosage. Some will require long-term maintenance therapy. The maintenance dosage is often one-third to one-half of that required for treatment of the acute episode.

Adverse Effects, Toxicity, Overdose

Adverse effects are multiple, and most represent extensions of known pharmacologic actions. But because they may be annoying, steps should be taken to minimize the effects and to increase comfort and drug compliance. Adverse effects, toxicity, and drug interactions are summarized as follows:

Type of Adverse Effects or Toxicity	*Comment*
C.N.S	
Sedation	Especially with amitriptyline and doxepin
Insomnia, restlessness, and agitation	Often early in treatment and transient
Toxic psychosis	Particularly in aged or those with underlying brain disease
Fine tremor	
Seizures	Especially those predisposed to epilepsy
Peripheral Anticholinergic Effects	
Dry mouth, constipation, pupillary dilation, blurred vision	Common but often transient
Urinary retention	Especially elderly
Paralytic ileus	Rare
Cardiovascular	
Tachycardia and orthostatic hypotension	Common especially early in treatment
Cardiac electrical conduction changes	Benign (?) in normal dosages

| *Type of Adverse*
Effects or Toxicity (continued) | *Comment* (continued) |

Miscellaneous

Mild cholestatic jaundice	Uncommon
Allergic skin reactions	
Agranulocytosis	Very rare
Mild withdrawal syndrome	Nausea, vomiting, headache

TCA drug interactions* are summarized in the following list:

TCA Drugs May Interact With	*Potential Result*
All neuroleptics, methylphenidate, morphine, and meperidine	Inhibition of metabolism of TCA in increased plasma levels and increased antidepressant efficacy or adverse effects of TCA.
Alcohol, barbiturates, meprobamate, glutethimide, chloral hydrate, anticonvulsants, smoking (?)	Induction of metabolism of TCA resulting in decreased plasma levels and decreased antidepressant efficacy or adverse effects of TCA.
Oral contraceptives and other estrogen preparations	May reduce plasma level of TCA and lessen antidepressant effect.
Piperidine and aliphatic phenothiazines, anticholinergics, especially antiparkinson drugs	Addictive anticholinergic effects.
Insulin	Reduces insulin requirements.
Acidifiers (NH_4Cl)	Antagonizes TCA effects.
Alkalinizers	Potentiates TCA effects.
Guanethidine (and guanethidinelike) antihypertensives	Reversal of hypotensive effect. Occurs less frequently with doxepin administration.
Monoamine oxidase inhibitors	Agitation, tremor, hypertensive crisis, hyperpyrenia
Sympathomimetics	Possible potentiation of effects of sympathomimetics in peripheral nervous system and CNS, hypertensive crisis.
Thyroid drugs	Perhaps increased efficacy of TCA in women, but risk of cardiovascular toxicity may be increased as well.

---

*Modified after: Ayd Jr. FJ: Psychotropic drug combinations: Good and bad. From: *Drugs in Combination with Other Therapies.* Greenblatt M (ed): New York, Grune and Stratton, 1975. Printed with permission.

TCA Drugs May Interact With (continued)	*Potential Result* (continued)
Meperidine	May enhance meperidine-induced respiratory depression.
Vasopressor	Marked increase in pressor response; circulatory effect may be enhanced.
Anticoagulants	May alter effects of anticoagulants.

The drug selection is often based on the adverse effect profile or past or family history of a positive response to a particular agent. For example, it is clinically sound to give a more sedating agent to an agitated depressed patient and a less sedating agent to a depressed patient with psychomotor retardation. Also, if a patient or family member has responded preferentially to an agent previously, it is best to initiate treatment with this agent.

Toxicity may occur but is uncommon in recommended dosages with healthy patients. These include cardiac arrhythmias and heart blocks, bone marrow depression, and obstructive type jaundice.

Overdoses, both accidental and deliberate, commonly occur with TCAs. One gram of imipramine or the equivalent is dangerous and potentially lethal. Overdosages are frequently taken in combination with alcohol and other agents, especially sedative-hypnotics, thus compounding the picture. The overdosage signs and symptoms for TCAs include ataxia, drowsiness, delirium, disorientation, and atropine-like effects. Neuromuscular irritability, seizures, coma with shock or acidosis may develop. Cardiac arrhythmias and rate disturbances are common and hypotension or hypertension may present. There is no specific antidote for overdose and the TCAs are not dialyzable. For treatment emesis and lavage are recommended. The management of cardiac problems may be difficult. Vitals should be watched and the cardiac function monitored. Shock, respiratory depression and acidosis should be treated, if present. Physostigmine (1-2 mg IM) is helpful in correcting the atropine-like and cardiac-rhythm disturbances. Lidocaine, propranolol, and phenytoin may be helpful but quinidine and procainamide are contraindicated. Other treatment is supportive.

Lithium

Lithium is the only true antimanic agent although neuroleptics (e.g., haloperidol 5-10 mg three times daily) are effective in controlling acute manic symptoms. Lithium is the agent of choice for acute mania and is also effective in preventing mania and even depression in bipolar patients. But it is not very effective in treating acute depression where TCAs are the agents of choice. There is a lag period of 4-10 days between starting lithium treatment and response. Therefore, lithium is often started in combination with a neuroleptic, which acts much faster.

Some manic patients may not respond to lithium. This is particularly true of subjects who swing frequently back and forth between mania and depression (above 4 cycles per year), those without a family history of bipolar illness and those with mixed manic-depressive or paranoid destructive presentations. These patients may require other treatments such as neuroleptics or ECT.

Dosage Schedule. Guidelines for lithium administration and the lithium pretreatment screening tests are presented here.

1. Lithium is the treatment of choice in bipolar affective disorders. Because the onset of clinical efficacy may be delayed several days, it is helpful to start neuroleptic treatment for acute symptom control.

2. Make sure of the absence of contraindications (significant renal or cardiovascular disease, severe debilitation or dehydration, sodium depletion, diuretic therapy, and possibly first trimester pregnancy).

3. Screening tests before lithium administration include a medical history, physical exam, evaluation of renal and cardiac status, CBC, and thyroid evaluation.

4. Identifying and monitoring target symptoms is a helpful way to document progress.

5. Lithium toxicity is closely related to serum lithium levels (above 2.0 mEq/L) but can occur at doses close to therapeutic (1.0-1.5 mEq/L) and even maintenance (0.6-1.2 mEq/L) levels.

6. Monitoring treatment response with clinical observations and repeat serum lithium levels. Total reliance should not be placed on serum levels alone.

7. Provided toxic symptoms are absent, lithium is normally well tolerated and many patients are totally free of adverse effects. Initial treatment may be associated nonetheless with a fine hand tremor, polyuria, polydipsia, and mild nausea. All may persist throughout treatment or be transient.

8. If a neuroleptic has been given in combination, it can be discontinued once the patient has stabilized on lithium.

9. Dosages must be individualized according to serum levels and response. However, 600 mg t.i.d. and 300 mg t.i.d. are therapeutic dosages for most patients during the acute and maintenance treatment periods respectively.

10. Normally only patients with frequent mood cycles require maintenance lithium. Medication can be restarted if indicated in patients with infrequent mood disturbances. Lithium should be discontinued in patients who develop lithium toxicity and in those with developing renal disease.

Lithium is available in 300 mg capsules, and most patients require about 600 mg three times daily for acute symptom control and 300 mg three times daily for maintenance. Corresponding serum levels are 1.0-1.5 mEq/L and 0.6-1.2 mEq/L respectively. The dosages are normally divided to reduce adverse effects which may occur after a consolidated dosage. Serum lithium levels should be drawn 8-12 hours after the last dose. Total reliance must not be placed on serum lithium values alone because clinical monitoring is essential to determine efficacy and toxicity.

Adverse Effects, Toxicity, Overdose

Adverse and toxic effects of lithium are as follows:

Initial Adverse Effects (benign)
GI (nausea, vomiting, anorexia, abdominal pain, diarrhea)
Mild hand tremor
Polydipsia, polyuria
Edema
Muscle weakness

Persistent Adverse Effects (benign)
Mild hand tremor
Polydipsia, polyuria
Weight gain
Leukocytosis
Metallic taste

Complications
Hypothyroidism and/or goiter
Nephrogenic diabetes insipidus
Renal interstitial damage
Hypercalcemia (?hyperparathyroidism)
Glycosuria
EKG/EEG changes
Folliculitis and other dermatological reactions

Intoxication Prodromal (1.6-2.0 mEq/L)
GI (nausea, vomiting, diarrhea)
Coarse hand tremor
Lethargy
Muscle weakness
Ataxia
Vertigo
Tinnitus
Hyperreflexia or muscle irritability
Muscle stiffness or rigidity

Toxicity (2.0 mEq/L or above)
Cardiovascular
Arrhythmias
Hypotension
Peripheral circulatory collapse

Toxicity (continued)
  Neuromuscular
    Muscular hyperirritability
    Fasciculations
    Clonic movements
  CNS
    Syncope
    Seizures
    Dysarthria
    Urinary and fecal incontinence
    Psychomotor retardation
    Restlessness
    Confusion
    Stupor
    Coma
    Death

Of special note is the development of hypothyroidism with or without a goiter, which may be mistaken for a recurrence of depression. A nephrogenic diabetes-insipidus-like syndrome may be distressing to the patient and a reason to discontinue lithium. Recent reports suggest that lithium therapy may produce renal interstitial damage in some patients. This should be suspected with the development of renal signs or symptoms and an increasing serum lithium level (despite fixed oral dosage) leading to lithium toxicity.

Lithium toxicity normally presents when the serum level is above 2.0 mEq/L and also reflects the lithium/sodium balance. The progression to toxicity normally is insidious but may be abrupt as that caused by an overdosage. This toxicity may be associated with decreased sodium intake (salt restrictions, influenza), or increased loss (diarrhea, dehydration, use of thiazide diuretics). Renal disease also affects the balance and these patients require very close monitoring if placed on lithium. There is no specific antidote to lithium toxicity.

Early symptoms can be treated by dosage reduction or brief termination as the biologic half life of lithium is 24 hours. The treatment goal of severe cases, as with overdosage, is rapidly to eliminate the drug from the body. The treatment consists of gastric lavage, correction of fluid and electrolyte balance, and regulation of renal function. Urea, mannitol, and aminophylline increase lithium excretion.

NEUROLEPTICS

Neuroleptics have been discussed in Chapter 3. Their role in PAD is limited primarily to the delusionally depressed or the acute manic patient. Neuroleptics should be discontinued once delusions or the more debilitating symptoms subside, and the patient should then be maintained on TCA or lithium respectively. Neuroleptics probably have limited prophylactic value in PAD.

ELECTROCONVULSIVE THERAPY (ECT)

Perhaps no somatic treatment in psychiatry is as controversial as ECT. The concern is not with efficacy in PAD where it is well documented for both mania and depression, but with administration in other clinical disorders where efficacy is more in question. In many states, legal guidelines now regulate the use of ECT. With the advent of effective drug treatment in PAD, as outlined above, ECT is now used sparingly and mostly with drug-refractory patients and those requiring rapid symptom remission.

Newer innovations with ECT have reduced risk of complications and adverse effects. This includes the now routine use of anesthesia, oxygenation, and muscle relaxation. Furthermore, unilateral placement of electrodes over the nondominant hemisphere results in considerably less memory impairment compared with bilateral electrode placement and without compromising efficacy.

COMPREHENSIVE CARE

Even though medication plays a decisive role in treating patients with major affective disorders, the patient-doctor relationship remains crucial and significantly affects the outcome. The treatment response is enhanced when the doctor is enthusiastic about the treatment and prognosis, and when the patient and his family appreciate whatever special interest can be directed towards them. Finally, affective disorders are severe mental illnesses which interfere with all areas of psycho-social-occupational functioning and may have grave consequences if untreated. Nonetheless, those properly treated are among the most rewarding patients in medicine because the normal response is a speedy recovery and bright prognosis.

SUGGESTED READING

Beck AT: *The Diagnosis and Management of Depression.* Philadelphia, Univ Penn Press, 1973

Bielski RJ, Friedel RO: Subtypes of depression-diagnosis and medical management. *West J Med* 126-347, 1977

Davies B: Diagnosis and treatment of anxiety and depression in general practice. *Drugs* 6:389, 1973

Hollister LE: Treatment of depression with drugs. *Ann Intern Med* 89:78, 1978

Jefferson JW: A review of the cardiovascular effects and toxicity of tricyclic antidepressants. *Psychosom Med* 37:160, 1975

Jefferson JW, Greist JH: *Primer of Lithium Therapy.* Baltimore, Williams and Wilkins, 1977

Maas JW: Clinical and biochemical heterogeneity of depressive disorders. *Ann Intern Med* 88:556, 1978

Whitlock FA, Evan LEJ: Drugs and depression. *Drugs* 15:53, 1978

Woodruff Jr. RA, Goodwin DW, Guze SB: *Psychiatric Diagnosis.* New York, Oxford Univ Press, 1973

6

Atypical Depressive Illness and Depressive Equivalents

ROBERT M. BITTLE, M.D.
PATRICK T. DONLON, M.D.

The depressive syndromes consist of a group of clinical conditions rather than a single illness. Etiologic theories range from exclusively genetic in origin to responses to life events, with the most accepted theory being a complex interaction between the biological and psychological systems.

Manifest depression is easy to recognize when it appears in the classic form. Clinical experience, however, demonstrates that serious depressions may also present in disguised or atypical forms. Again, proper and early diagnosis is essential since the symptoms may be distressing, disabling, and potentially life-threatening.

The understanding of atypical or masked (depressive equivalents) depressions and their relationship to affective illness has expanded in recent years due to an increased awareness of familial determinants and advances in genetic, longitudinal, pharmacologic, and biochemical studies. Currently, there is developing support for the concept of atypical depressions and depressive equivalents and their relationship to primary affective disorders.

This chapter provides an overview of the clinical features, natural history, differential diagnosis, and treatment of the atypical depressions.

CASE HISTORY

Mr. M. is a 41-year-old married man who was admitted to the University hospital in a comatose state following a suicide attempt by hanging. Four days later, when he was medically stable, he was transferred to the psychiatric unit. A careful history from the patient and his family provided the following data:

There were no previous significant medical illnesses or psychopathological states. He was a college graduate, a successful businessman, and there were no major recent life stresses. Family history documented that his mother had suffered from migraine headaches and that she had been treated medically for two serious depressive illnesses. Mr. M. had two sons, ages seven and ten years, and his wife enjoyed her role as a homemaker and mother. A single complaint was "strange" headaches, which had first presented some months previously, and which he had treated himself with over-the-counter analgesics and hypnotics. No other significant events or problem areas in his premorbid history were discovered.

The day of the suicide attempt seemed routine and uneventful. After returning home from work, Mr. M. told his wife he was going to shower. His wife heard the water running for a short time. After a few minutes of silence she heard a strange noise—a bathroom stool had fallen over. She hurried to the bathroom to investigate and was horrified to discover that her husband had hung himself, using a nylon clothesline.

Following transfer to the psychiatric unit, the severity of Mr. M's depression first became apparent. By this time his mood was depressed and many of the classic features of depression were more obvious. Yet somatic concerns, predominantly frequent headaches, were the only disturbances that the patient reported prior to his suicide attempt.

This history represents a case of atypical or masked depression. Other names for this presentation include depression without depression, thymopathic, or depressive equivalents. Atypical depressions are common and the clinical phenomena may vary widely. Yet despite variable symptom or phenomenologic masks, there is invariably found an underlying depressed mood with or without anxiety, or an inability to experience pleasure.

CLINICAL FEATURES

Contrasting features between classic clinical depression and atypical or masked depression are provided below.

Symptoms	Typical Depression	Atypical Depressions
Sleep	Insomnia	Hyperinsomnia/ Insomnia
Appetite	Decreased	Increased/decreased
Weight	Loss	Obesity/loss
Hostility	Self-deprecation	Irritability
Anxiety	Overshadowed by depression	Often prominent
Paranoid tendencies	Infrequent unless depression severe	Common
Impulsivity	Infrequent	Common
Suicidal predictability	Yes	No
Consistency of symptoms	Consistent	Inconsistent
Associated diseases	Uncommon	Common
Premorbid personality	Often obsessive	Often hysteroid
Family history	Common for depression	Less common for depression
Response to therapy	Good	Fair

The atypical depression may present as a variation of clinical depression but with greater affect and anxiety and fluctuation in course. Or it may present in a more masked form as a depressive equivalent where medical symptoms or disturbed behavior are the outstanding clinical features. Common presentations of atypical depression are:

1. Hyperactivity in children
2. Acting-out behavior (sociopathic, affective aggression), particularly in adolescents
3. Eating disorders
4. Substance and alcohol abuse
5. Hysteroid dysphoria syndrome
6. Phobic-anxiety syndrome
7. Migraine or cluster headaches
8. Psychosomatic disturbances
9. Chronic pain
10. Pseudodementia

With atypical depressions, vegetative signs (insomnia, anorexia, weight loss, fatigue) often fluctuate in course and intensity in contrast to clinical depressions where they are more persistent and tend to be progressive. Also, with atypical depressions impulsivity, anxiety, hysteroid and paranoid features are more common than with clinical depressions, but suicide predictability is more difficult. The atypically depressed patient often does not complain of depression and prefers to focus on other functional or somatic symptoms.

COMMON PRESENTATIONS FOR DEPRESSIVE EQUIVALENT STATES

Several well-defined clinical states may at times represent cases of masked depression. Some of the more common presentations are described below:

Hyperactivity in Childhood

Hyperactivity in childhood probably results from numerous etiological determinants and is characterized by distractibility, impulsivity, increased motor activity, and learning disorders. From longitudinal and family studies, it is now recognized that some of these children are experiencing early-onset affective disorders, particularly bipolar manic-depressive illness.

Adolescent Behavioral Disorders

Atypical forms of depression are extremely common during early and mid-adolescence. The most common form is that of behavioral disturbance. Patterns vary widely and include substance abuse, promiscuity, deterioration in academic and social performances, criminal activity, irritability, angry-hostile outbursts, and other self-defeating behaviors.

Eating Disorders

Depression may also be masked as eating disorders, and include both anorexia and obesity. Anorexic patients longitudinally often present with significant histories both pre- and postmorbidly for affective disorders. Mothers of these patients also frequently have histories of affective disorders.

Early onset obesity may have a distant relationship to depression. This is especially true if obesity is familial. In contrast is the obesity which occurs with adulthood and in association with distressing life events. Here underlying depressive states are often responsible.

Substance Abuse

Substance abuse leading to habituation and even addiction may result from the individual's attempt to modify distressing emotional states. CNS stimulants are often the agents of abuse for the depressed, and CNS depressants (ethyl alcohol, sedative-hypnotics) for the irritable, dysphoric, or manic individual. These pharmacologic effects may in turn greatly alter the clinical picture. CNS stimulant withdrawal and continued CNS depressant abuse may also pharmacologically produce a severe clinical depression.

Hysteroid Dysphoria Syndromes

These syndromes are usually seen in female patients with many hysterical features in addition to significant depressive and affective components. An unstable ambivalent relationship with males is common. A marked emotional lability and excessive overreaction to stress are central psychopathologic features.

Phobic-Anxiety Syndrome

This clinical syndrome is characterized by multiple phobias including a fear of open spaces (agoraphobia). Such phobic responses often produce anticipatory anxiety, free-floating anxiety and spontaneous panic attacks. Often the individual develops a life-style to avoid the phobic situations. In severe cases the illness may become disabling due to the severity of symptoms and the restrictions that the avoidance of the phobic object or situation places on everyday functioning.

Migraine and Cluster Headaches

A significant subgroup of patients experiencing migraine and cluster headaches seemingly have a disguised form of affective disorder. Evidence is again provided by longitudinal follow-up studies where recurrent depressions often are noted, a family history of affective disorder is present, and a positive response to antidepressant medication occurs.

Psychosomatic Disturbances

Affective illness may also present as single or multiple somatic concerns. The clinical picture may be highly variable. Nonetheless, presenting complaints commonly reflect the vegetative signs or symptoms of classic depression (insomnia, anorexia, weight loss, fatigue), psychophysiologic responses to stress (gastrointestinal, cardiovascular), conversion reactions (where emotional distress is converted into somatic complaints), and somatic delusions. In many of these cases, the patient prefers to focus on somatic complaints and the subsequent disability rather than distressing life events or mental discomfort. Recent research has demonstrated that serum glucose levels are significantly influenced by growth hormone which is secreted by the anterior pituitary gland. It has further been demonstrated that brain catecholamine levels influence the release of growth hormones. These data help clarify the relationship between primary affective disorders and borderline to frank hypoglycemic states found in affectively disordered individuals and their immediate families.

Chronic Pain Patients

These patients are often highly adaptable people who experience good general and mental health premorbidly. The onset of pain often is associated with an illness, injury, or surgical procedure. But the severity, persistence, and disability caused by the pain is often difficult to explain clinically. Typically, the patient becomes obsessed with his pain and subsequent disability and at the expense of focusing on troublesome life events. Many of these patients travel from physician to physician and receive trials on numerous medications and some receive unnecessary surgery. These patients often show significant depression when followed longitudinally and often there is a family history of depression.

Pseudodementia

Significantly depressed (and occasionally manic) patients frequently present with cognitive impairment and a presentation suggestive of diffuse organic brain disease (labile affect, impaired judgment, disorientation, memory impairment, concentration and comprehension disturbances). In contrast with the organically impaired, the depressed patient with pseudodementia normally complains bitterly about impaired cognitive functioning. Once the depression is treated or spontaneously remits, the pseudodementia disappears.

DIFFERENTIAL DIAGNOSIS

Assessment should include a complete psychiatric and medical history, family history, indicated laboratory and psychological tests, histories for proprietary and illicit substance abuse, physical examination and a period of observation. Atypical depression must be considered in patients with a fluctuating depressive mood disturbance with or without anxiety and in those where somatic or behavioral changes may represent a disguise for a depressive state. The diagnosis should be especially suspected in those with past mood disorders, concurrent distressing life events, and especially a family history of affective disorders, alcoholism, or sociopathic behavior. Other suggestive signs include substance abuse, "acting-out" behavior, and puzzling medical complaints.

The differential diagnosis includes medical disorders, organic brain disease, and schizophrenia. These normally can be excluded by history, physical and mental status examinations, and indicated laboratory tests. Also, primary and secondary affective disorders must be distinguished. Secondary affective disorders are altered mood responses to an illness or toxic manifestations from an illness or agents administered.

TREATMENT

Correct treatment depends on proper diagnosis. As the origins of depressions commonly result from an interaction between psychological events and biological factors, treatment approaches vary. A positive doctor-patient relationship is essential. Evaluation of life events is helpful and treatment may be exclusively psychotherapy. In other cases the patients may be physically removed from stressful events or antidepressant agents may be administered. Often all three approaches are consolidated into a single treatment plan.

Tricyclic antidepressants or TCAs are typically the agents of choice and they have been discussed in Chapter 5. Lithium therapy may be effective, especially if there is a family history of bipolar affective illness. Neuroleptics are indicated in low dosage if psychotic phenomena are present. The monoamine oxidase inhibitors or MAOI (see Table 6-1), particularly phenelzine, may be especially therapeutic with cases of hysteroid dysphoria, phobic anxiety, and other forms of atypical depression. Daily dosages of 30-40 mgs are often adequate but higher dosages may be necessary. The lag period for clinical response on a therapeutic dosage of an MAOI may be three to four weeks. Patients on an MAOI must be monitored carefully. Special precautions are indicated as some agents and foods must be avoided. The most serious adverse effect is hypertensive crisis and this occurs most commonly when an MAOI is taken in combination with a sympathomimetic agent or foods high in content with tryptamine or tyramine.

Table 6-1. Monoamine Oxidase Inhibitors.

Generic Name	Trade Name	Effective Dose Range
MAO Inhibitors		
Tranylcypromine*	Parnate	20–40
Isocarboxazid	Marplan	20–60
Phenelzine*	Nardil	45–75
Parhyline	Eutonyl	25–75
Nialamide	Niamid	150–225

Contraindications: Hypersensitivity, pheochromocytona, congestive heart failure, significant liver disease.

Restrictions with combination therapy: Sympathomimetic drugs (including methyldopa, levodopa, dopamine, amphetamines, epinephrine, and norepinephrine). Special caution with TCAs.

Special dietary restrictions: Foods with a higher concentration of tryptamine—containing substances or tyramine (pods of broad-leaf beans, aged cheese, beer, wines, pickled herring, chicken liver, yeast extract). Excessive amounts of caffeine and chocolate can also cause hypertensive reactions.

Common adverse effects: Dizziness, constipation, dry mouth, postural hypotension, drowsiness, weakness and fatigue, edema, gastrointestinal disturbances, tremors, twitching, and hyporeflexia.

*Approved for use as antidepressants in the United States.

SUGGESTED READING

Cantwell DP, Sturzenburger S, Burroughs J, et al: Anorexia nervosa: An affective disorder? *Arch Gen Psychiatry* 34:1087-1093, 1977

Klein DF, et al: *Diagnosis and Drug Treatment of Psychiatric Disorders: Adults and Children* 2nd ed. Baltimore, Williams and Wilkins, 1980, pp. 303-324

Lopez-Ibor JJ: Masked depressions. *Br J Psychiatry* 120:245-258, 1972

Manual of Psychiatric Therapeutics. Shader RI (ed). Boston, Little, Brown and Co., 1975, pp. 39-63, 281-293

Schaffer CB, Donlon PT, Bittle RM: Chronic pain and depressions: A clinical and family history survey. *Am J Psychiatry* 137:188-120, 1980

7

Anxiety and Related Disorders

DON A. ROCKWELL, M.D.

ANXIETY-OVERVIEW

Anxiety is a universal symptom. Everyone has had the experience of being "anxious" or "nervous." Unfortunately what everyone calls anxiety may reflect a variety of other affective states. A major task the clinician faces is to identify anxiety and separate it from fear, alarm, panic, dread, etc.—each of which relates to clinical anxiety in some diagnostically and therapeutically important way.

103

By definition anxiety is a disagreeable emotional state characterized by apprehension, tension, uneasiness and feelings of impending danger, is associated with autonomic nervous system discharge, and threatened behavioral discharge ("I feel like screaming"). Anxiety signals the presence of conflict or threat. It is different from fear in that there is no clear object or situation which would provoke fear. There also may be situations which would normally evoke mild fear but are responded to with major anxiety.

Anxiety/Fear

All of us experience anxiety at points in our lives. Anxiety and/or fear are, in fact, quite healthy and useful. Anxiety/fear in tolerable amounts increases one's capacity to cope with situations. Fear of failure of an exam, for example, makes one "anxious"—to use the patient's perspective. This anxiety motivates one to study. While this anxiety is in fact fear, clinicians often respond to the patient's subjective description of "anxious or nervous" and treat it as a disease rather than recognizing it as a healthy signal symptom. Further, our culture has pushed very hard to eliminate "feeling sad or nervous" as normal behavior. Often patients view "nervousness" as pathologic when, in fact, it is an appropriate healthy response. This is discussed further below.

Incidence

Anxiety is quite widespread. Five percent of primary care patients will have anxiety as a primary disease. Ten percent of "cardiac" patients are in fact suffering from an anxiety disorder. Most illnesses and all diseases are associated with fear/anxiety. The symptom of anxiety is especially widespread in late adolescence, youth and young adulthood. The symptom decreases with age. Anxiety appearing for the first time in the over 40-year-old patient is most likely to be associated with depression.

Symptoms and Signs

The patient's complaints can have a psychological, physiological or behavioral emphasis. Key symptoms include chronic nervousness, attacks of nervousness or panic, a sense of impending doom, apprehensiveness, unceasing worry, difficulty concentrating, fatigue, low blood sugar. Complaints from the systems review include shortness of breath, muscle aches or tension, headaches, sweating, chest pain or discomfort, paresthesias, trembling, palpitations, nausea, vomiting, lightheadedness, blurred vision, trouble breathing or swallowing, lump in the throat (globus hystericus) and so on. Often a positive review of systems tips one off to an anxiety disorder. The patient also reports trouble sleeping, weakness, fear of illness, fear of dying or death, fear of insanity, and irritability. The development of phobias is discussed below.

Signs revealed in the physical exam include hyperactivity, sweating, cold palms, hyperhidrosis, agitation, tremor, tachycardia, increased muscle tone and deep tendon reflexes, frequent sighing respiration, dry mouth, tics or grimaces, and pressured speech.

At the interactional level, the clinician often feels keyed up or anxious when with the clinically anxious patient. Behaviorally this may be noticed more as an urgency by the clinician to do something to or to "move" the patient.

DIFFERENTIAL DIAGNOSIS—THE ANXIETY DISORDERS

STEP I. Normal Versus Pathological Anxiety

Since patients will rarely differentiate fear from anxiety, it is useful to begin the differential on the basis of what patients typically present to the clinician. Thus nervousness or anxiety may mean either fear or anxiety in the clinical sense.

Normal Appropriate Anxiety/Post-Traumatic Stress Disorder. If the patient has encountered a recognizable stressor that would evoke distress in almost anyone (witnessing a fatal accident, involved in a tornado, etc.) his symptoms are a normal stress response syndrome.[1] They are likely to have recurrent intrusive thoughts, recollections, dreams or images of the event and/or the sudden reexperiencing of feelings or behavior as if the event were reoccurring. This is associated with a psychological defensive response character-ized by a "numbing" experience with diminished interest in activities or people and a sense of emotional construction or withdrawal. In addition these patients will develop two of the following symptoms:

- Hyperalertness or increased startle reaction
- Sleep disturbance
- Survivor guilt
- Concentration or memory impairment
- Avoidance of recollection of trauma
- Increased symptoms by exposure to trauma or symbolic trauma

The onset of this syndrome may be acute or delayed. The appropriate intervention is brief therapy, support and education.

Situational/Appropriate Fear. Is there a current situation that is fear evoking? If there is a distinct external danger (real or symbolic) present or threatening, then the patient needs to be educated about the appropriateness of the response (i.e., "it's normal to feel nervous when public speaking" . . . "on a date" . . . "before exams," . . .), its healthy signal nature ("it serves to get you to do your best job" . . . "it adds spice" . . . "it makes you study"), and that it will resolve itself without any pharmacologic intervention. The reassurance by the clinician is ample therapy for 99 percent of such patients.

Life Change Fear/Anxiety. As people pass through life's developmental phases, they are likely to be apprehensive about the next stages. Some of the future may be known and hence fearful, and some is unknown and hence anxious-making. Again, however, this is a normal response to life change. The clinician's responsibility in this situation is to understand the patient's current developmental stage and to help anticipate the next stage. Two examples illustrate this; first, the 17-year-old leaving for college is certainly likely to be anxious. The clinician should be sensitive to not only issues of separation, grief, and loss but also wish/fears of independence, sexuality, etc.; the second, the 39-year-old male needs the sensitive clinician to recognize the changes from stable 30's to mid-life crisis and on to more stable 40's. In these life changes, anxiety is a common complaint. Again, education, support, and reassurance may be the only necessary therapeutic maneuver.

Stressful Life Situations. A broader and in many ways more common difficulty relates to individuals whose lives are stress-filled *and* who experience this as stressful. Note that we are now separating these patients from those with a major past stress (post-traumatic stress syndrome), normative life crisis (life change), or an acute situational reaction (anxiety/fear). These are patients who describe their lives as stressful or hectic and who experience not so much pure anxiety but rather chronic "tension" or an "inability to relax" or "not enough time." Contemporary patients are increasingly willing to acknowledge the stressful nature of their lives and to be open to successful interventions for stress reduction while denying any psychological problems requiring psychotherapy. We offer these patients effective behavioral treatments for stress and anxiety without having to psychiatrically stigmatize them.

Over and above dealing with the patient's manifest symptomatology, we also may effectively be improving their physical health and reducing their risk of accidents. There is now clear evidence that chronic stress is an illness precipitant. High stress occupations (air traffic controllers, policepersons, etc.) are the clearest examples, but Holmes and Rahe[2] have adequately demonstrated the relationship between life change and both physical health and accidents. Selye[3] notes that much contemporary disease is disease of adaptation. It should be noted that neither Holmes-Rahe nor Selye propose the elimination of stress but rather fostering improved coping mechanisms. In point of fact, we now appreciate that any change is, at a physiologic level, "stressful" but few would choose to live a life without change. The question is how to improve coping in patients whose lives are filled with change—especially change that is irregularly irregular.

In recent years increased data has shown various ways that patients can either reduce stress or increase their capacity to cope. The Social Readjustment Scale developed by Holmes and Rahe (Table 7-1) can be used to make voluntary choices about life events. The obvious goal is to stabilize the number of life change units over time. Perhaps as important as the reduction in life change units over six months is the fact that the person has exerted control over the course of his/her life. Kobasa[4] has demonstrated clearly that control is a critical variable in health status. For patients the opportunity to *act* in some positive way is effective in dealing with stress.

We have used a variety of ways to help patients reassert control over their lives. First we ask individuals to order their priorities. This can be done on an hourly,

Table 7-1. Life Events and Weighted Values.

Life Event	Value	Life Event	Value
1. Death of spouse	100	22. Son or daughter leaving home	29
2. Divorce	73	23. Trouble with in-laws	29
3. Marital separation	65	24. Outstanding personal achievement	28
4. Jail term	63		
5. Death of close family member	63	25. Wife beginning or stopping work	26
6. Personal injury or illness	53	26. Beginning or ending school	26
7. Marriage	50	27. Revision of habits	24
8. Fired at work	47	28. Trouble with boss	23
9. Marital reconciliation	45	29. Change in work hours	20
10. Retirement	45	30. Change in residence	20
11. Change in health of family	44	31. Change in schools	20
12. Pregnancy	40	32. Change in recreation	19
13. Sex difficulties	39	33. Change in social activity	18
14. Gain of new family member	39	34. Mortgage less than $10,000	17
15. Change in financial state	38	35. Change in sleeping habits	16
16. Death of close friend	37	36. Change in number of family get-togethers	15
17. Change of work	36		
18. Change in number of arguments with spouse	35	37. Change in eating habits	15
19. Mortgage over $10,000	31	38. Vacation	13
20. Foreclosure of mortgage	30	39. Minor violations of law	11
21. Change of responsibility at work	29		

Source: Adapted from Holmes TH and Rahe RH: The social readjustment scale. *J Psychosom Res* 11:213, 1967.

daily or weekly basis with a more global annual review. Many people have not set immediate, medium, or life goals very clearly and thus operate without direction and are thus easily buffeted by external events. Ask people to sit down and decide where they are headed in a day, a week, a year or a lifetime. If you don't know where you're headed, you'll never know when you get there!

A second reminder to many people is to point out that they are not in a race. Many "A" type people need this reminder. The best way is often not the fastest way. One question useful to such people asks, "is this going to be important five years from now?" This longer time perspective allows many people to back away from tasks they view as stressful. Altering time perspectives can also be achieved by encouraging these driven individuals to involve themselves in a volunteer activity that will confront them with alternative time perspectives—activities that expose them to preschoolers or geriatric populations and programs such as suicide prevention, hospice or bereavement outreach can be enormously eye opening.

A third reminder that is useful to people is to get them to recognize that they are making numerous choices daily. Often people view themselves as helpless pawns without choice. Pointing out that they can make active choices rather than being passive victims may be useful. Teaching people to replace the words "I should do . . . " with "I want to do . . . " forces them to look at the myriad daily choices they are making. This leads people to say "I want to do . . . " or "I don't want to do . . . " instead of "I have to." The difference in psychological set is crucial. "Should" and "have to" imply that someone or something other than the self is responsible or in charge.

Relaxation Skills. The final major reminder that we give to people who perceive their lives as being stressful is that they need to learn how to relax. Relaxation is *not* the same as recreation. Although recreation may be a welcome change in a person's life, many recreational activities are, in fact, not only not relaxing but often as stressful or more stressful than routine activities. Watching one's weekend behavior often reveals that the recreational activities are in fact more stressful than the routine week experiences. Relaxation skills are not naturally or spontaneously practiced by most individuals. To get people to practice relaxation skills, we have found it useful to suggest the following things to stressed individuals. In a manner appropriate for them in the course of every single day, they are to "take some time out." They can call this mental health time, they can call it quiet time, but they need to take it. One of the ways of facilitating this is by finding a quiet space somewhere in the work environment where they can spend 20 minutes resetting their psychological and physiological thermostat back to normal away from the stresses of their work-a-day world. A second way of learning relaxation skills comes from what we have called and prescribed to patients as *creative regression.* Creative regression is essentially the play behavior of children in the three- to five-year-old range. This play tends to be fantasy play and not the typical competitive play that is characteristic of our particular culture. We've often recommended to patients that they spend time with three to five-year-olds participating with them in this fantasy play as an alternative way of getting out of the competitive mode of thinking and into a looser and freer style of being in the world.

Relaxation Techniques. Creative regression may not be acceptable to some patients. For those we recommend *progressive relaxation* or *autogenic training.* A variety of resources fostering these techniques are available in most communities. A number of paperbacks are available written in lay language that are useful for patients. Training courses or programs are often available through local colleges or mental health associations. Audiotapes and complete audiocassette programs make active practice much easier for the patients. The ideal is for the clinician to make tapes providing these instructions. This takes advantage of the already established therapeutic relationship and fosters a positive outcome. Commercial tapes are available.

An alternative to Benson's[5] relaxation techniques is *meditation.* The essence of meditation is a relaxed posture with a focus on "a word without meaning." Practice twice a day for 20 minutes has a variety of physiologic and psychologic benefits. Most communities have some form of meditation training available with Transcendental Meditation® being the most popular. It is important to reassure patients that the religious or metaphysical overlay is irrelevant to the positive benefits of medication.

Biofeedback may be more acceptable to patients who prefer a more scientific approach to learning relaxation skills. Biofeedback techniques can be learned in a fairly small number of sessions. A wide variety of techniques are used, all based on providing the subject with systematic information about some monitored physiologic process. Many health and mental health professionals are utilizing biofeedback and again, community resources need to be explored and utilized.

A final stress reducer and coping facilitator is good *cardiovascular conditioning.* Jogging, swimming or other cardiovascular conditioners have been proved to have valuable psychological and physical effects in reducing the perception of stress and in increasing coping capacities. We often inquire of anxious, depressed, or stressed patients whether they are interested in a prescription for the single most effective antianxiety and antidepressant agent known today.[6] We warn them of its "addiction" potential and then advise them that jogging for 20 to 40 minutes a day is the least expensive and most successful agent available.

The use of some or all of these techniques gives the body an opportunity to reset the thermostat to normal each day and avoids the cumulative effects of acute or chronic stress. This approach can be very useful in the primary prevention of both physical and mental illness for people whose lives are marked by change and adaptation.

STEP II. Primary Versus Secondary Clinical Anxiety

The next step in most clinical practice situations is to investigate whether this is an anxiety syndrome that is primary and functional in origin *or* secondary to some other process or disease. Again the usual practice would be to explore the secondary causes first since the usual primary care person will be more comfortable with exploring the more medical differential.

This differential tree has three major branches (Figure 7-1). First and most common is that the anxiety syndrome is a response to the patient's perceived threat of illness or potential surgery. Nearly all people perceive illness as a threat and react to it with anxiety/fear. This is *secondary anxiety* and is treated by information and therapeutic use of the doctor-patient relationship. The process of eliciting informed consent for treatment of the medical illness or injury can be a most effective "anxiolytic" agent.[7]

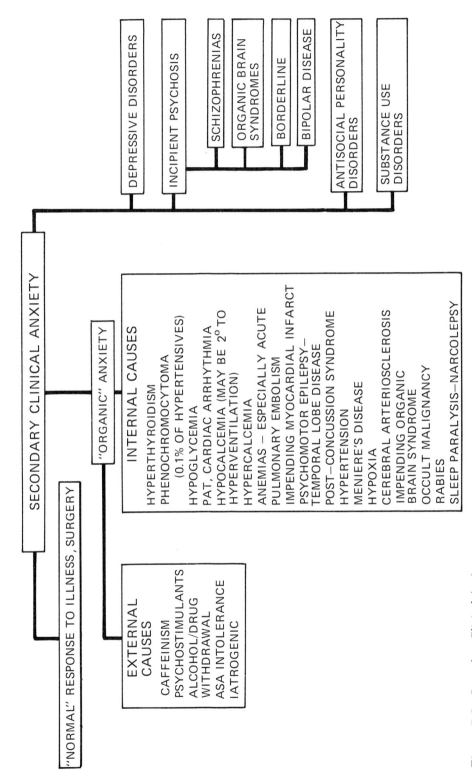

Figure 7-1. Secondary Clinical Anxiety.

The second major branch in this differential is what we call *organic* anxiety—anxiety stemming directly from an illness or drug. The etiology of this source of anxiety symptoms can be related to processes internal to the individual or as the result of external agents.

External Causes. Several comments about these are in order, however. Caffeinism—excessive coffee, cola, etc.—simulates anxiety neuroses. More than four cups a day (or its equivalent) causes symptoms in most people *and* is associated with a mild withdrawal when stopped. Psychostimulants continue to be widely abused. Most diet medications—prescription or over-the-counter—contain psychostimulant medications. Mild degrees of withdrawal from most psychoactive drugs may manifest as anxiety—including withdrawal from therapeutic levels of diazepam or reduction in "social use" of alcohol. Finally, physicians themselves have been iatrogenic anxiety generators. Vague, indefinite or jargon-filled communications often generate anxiety unnecessarily. Clear communication with an opportunity for the patient to feed back what he/she *heard* (as opposed to what you said) is the prophylaxis for this cause of anxiety.

Internal Causes. Most of these diseases or disturbances can be quickly confirmed or ruled out by history, physical exam, and laboratory tests. Several merit comment.

In the early phases of anemia, embolism, and infarct, anxiety may be the only early warning sign. In hospitalized patients, acute anxiety represents most commonly either a pulmonary embolism or an incipient toxic psychosis. In the elderly patient, consider an occult malignancy—especially of the pancreas—or impaired cerebral functioning. In younger persons, a new syndrome—a variant of narcolepsy—has been described in which sleep paralysis is experienced and is followed by a generalized anxiety syndrome. If early reports prove correct this could be a not uncommon problem.

The third "secondary" anxiety is *anxiety which is a symptom of psychiatric disease* other than the anxiety disorders. Many psychiatric disorders are associated with "classic" anxiety symptoms, *but* the treatment needs to be directed at the primary underlying process and not the anxiety symptoms. By far the most common psychiatric disorder with secondary anxiety is the depression disorders. Depressions of all types very frequently have associated anxiety symptoms. The major and serious error here is to treat the anxiety with anxiolytic agents. Minor tranquilizers have great potential for aggravating the depression and doing little for the secondary anxiety symptoms. *All* anxious patients should be queried about the presence of symptoms and signs of depression. If a depressive syndrome is present (unipolar or bipolar), then it is mandatory to treat the depression rather than the secondary anxiety.

The second group of psychiatric disorders that present with anxiety are incipient psychoses of all types. The early dissolution of defenses seen in the schizophrenias, early delirium or dementia, the borderline, or the bipolar psychotic leads first to the appearance of growing anxiety and only later to psychotic disorganization. There are two tipoffs to this source of anxiety. First, there well may be a prior history of a psychotic episode. Second, the quality of the anxiety is communicated persuasively to the clinician. One has the sense that the anxiety is out of the ordinary. The anxiety in these patients takes a rapid and malignant course. It may be difficult on the first visit with the patient to discern that this is a blossoming psychosis. A follow-up phone call or visit by the patient the subsequent day will reveal that support and reassurance have not caused a decrement in anxiety—so often seen in other secondary anxieties—but rather the patient feels less in control and more anxious. The signal to emergent intervention is an agitated, sleepless night by the patient. This often signals development of frank psychoses and will require emergent psychiatric intervention and often hospitalization.

The borderline patient may also present with anxiety as a primary complaint. The "borderline concept" is a controversial one. Many perceive it to be a schizophrenia-spectrum disease. It is important for primary care clinicians to recognize these very difficult patients. In addition to often presenting with pananxiety, they will have four or more of the following:[8]

- Magical thinking—"a sixth sense; others can feel my feelings"
- Ideas of reference
- Social isolation
- Recurrent illusions, depersonalization or derealization
- Odd speech—digressive, "off-target," vague or metaphorical yet without associative loosening
- Inadequate rapport established
- Suspiciousness
- Undue social anxiety or hypersensitivity

These patients will need referral to psychiatric care.

A final group with anxiety symptoms which mask or distract from the primary diagnosis is the antisocial or substance abusing patients.

The antisocial personality, contrary to belief, is often anxious. That anxiety waxes and wanes and rarely, except when confined involuntarily (as in prison), motivates the patient to change or exploration. The risk here is in providing antianxiety agents to patients with high potential for abuse or dependency and suicidal behavior. Behavioral techniques may be helpful for these patients.

The criteria for a diagnosis of an antisocial personality disorder are as follows:

History before age 15 of three or more of the following:
- Truancy (five days per year × two years)
- School expulsion or suspension
- Arrests or juvenile court referral
- Overnight runaway × two
- Persistent lying

- Repeated casual sex
- Substance abuse
- Thefts
- Vandalism
- School grades markedly below expectations
- Chronic rule violation
- Initiation of fights

Presence of four or more of the following after 18:
- Inability to sustain consistent work or appropriate social role behavior
- Failure to function in a responsible parent role
- Failure to accept social norms with respect to lawful behavior
- Failure to maintain enduring sexual relationship
- Repeated fights or assaults (including spouse or child beating)
- Failure to honor financial obligations
- Impulsivity and/or inability to plan ahead or consider consequences of behaviors
- Lying, "conning"
- Recklessness

Recognizing the antisocial personality early on will prevent being "conned" in a variety of ways.

Likewise the substance abusing patient may be anxious in a variety of ways. Withdrawal or even relatively small reductions in abuse may be followed by withdrawal anxiety. (See Substance Use Disorder, Chapter 8.) Alternatively the substance use disordered patient may manipulate and "con" in much the same way as the antisocial personality in order to achieve the drug prescription of his choice. The cautious clinician considers this possibility every time before reaching for a prescription pad. Both the antisocial personality and the substance use disordered patient seek magical relief from problems that cannot be magically solved and most especially not by medications.

STEP III. Primary Anxiety Disorders

The final step in working through the differential of the "nervous" patient is the differential of those experiencing *Anxiety Disorders.* In this differential we will consider the specific diagnosis and, in some cases, the specific treatment plan following diagnosis.

FREE-FLOATING ANXIETY

Generalized Anxiety Disorders (Anxiety Neurosis)

The patient will report chronic nervousness extending beyond a month with no evidence of depression or other psychiatric disorder. The patient will have symptoms in at least three of the following categories:[8]

- Motor tension: shakiness, jitters, jumpiness, "tense," muscle aches and pains, chronic or easy fatigability, trouble relaxing, restlessness, etc.
- Autonomic hyperactivity: sweating, racing or pounding heart, cold or clammy hands, dry mouth, light-headed or dizzy, "pins and needles" feelings, sighing respiration, lump in stomach or throat, "butterflies."
- Apprehensive expectation: anxiety, unceasing worry, sense of doom for self or others.
- Vigilance and scanning: hyperalert, distractible, trouble concentrating, trouble sleeping—especially falling asleep—feeling "on edge," irritable, impatient, wanting "to do something."

The treatment of this disease begins, in clinical practice, with its progressive recognition and definition. It will be unusual to work through a complete differential on the usual first visit. While coming to a conclusive diagnosis, nonspecific but effective treatment for anxiety takes place.

Nonspecific Treatment of Anxiety Disorders

The Doctor-Patient Relationship. The strength of a good doctor-patient relationship is a major force in alleviating anxiety symptoms, from whatever cause, and anxiety disorders. Serious, thoughtful, nonjudgmental consideration of the patient's complaints is, in and of itself, supportive and reassuring. Often the ventilation (catharsis) of complaints is sufficient to eliminate them or reduce their intensity to tolerable levels. Education of the patient about his symptoms, the diagnostic process, and the nonlethality of his disease changes overwhelming anxiety into tolerable worry. For most patients the fantasized problem or disease is much worse than the real one. It is important to recognize that "it's all in your head" applies to all illness. Just because it is "psychological" does not make it "not real."

Social Engineering. In initial contacts, "common sense" advice about home or work environment, life style decisions, and life priorities may facilitate the patient to take action to reduce overload in his life. "Taking a vacation" is effective not so much for the change of pace but because the patient reasserts control over his life. However, do not confuse "common sense" with psychotherapy. Doing counseling or psychotherapy with patients sometimes requires "uncommon sense" and counter-intuitive or paradoxical responses based on a thorough understanding of these patients and your own psychodynamics.

Physical Exercise. We have noted earlier that there is considerable evidence that repetitive cardiovascular conditioning exercise reduces anxiety significantly. The least expensive and most effective treatment for anxiety is a combination of running and fantasizing a positive scene for a total of 40 minutes a day.

Autohypnosis or Meditation. A variety of autohypnotic techniques for anxiety reduction are possible. Similarly any systematic investment of time and energy into a meditative technique will significantly reduce anxiety.

Specific Treatment of Anxiety Disorders

Behavior Modification. The relaxation techniques of Jacobson[8] can be taught to allow the patient to learn the relaxation response. Benson's book may be recommended to the patients or audiocassettes such as Biomonitoring Application[9] may be used. A competent behavior therapist may use some form of systematic desensitization process developed by Wolpe and Lazarus.[10] Flooding or implosion techniques have also been used for anxious patients.

Psychopharmacologic Treatment. Only after failure of the above methods— educative, nonspecific and specific—does one even consider a psychopharmacologic approach. Because psychopharmacologic approaches are so easily abused by doctor and patient alike we suggest several basic guidelines.

1. Specific diagnosis leads to specific treatment. Unless one has come to a criterion referenced diagnosis of a specific anxiety disorder then no pharmacologic treatment is indicated unless one chooses to do so on a placebo basis—a decision that needs to be conscious, and has ethical ramifications.
2. Any use of antianxiety agents is time limited (one to eight weeks), since failure to respond within eight weeks means no response is likely and persistent prescriptions beyond eight weeks for the responding patient needs very clear justification.
3. If a psychopharmacologic agent is to be used, it is to be used in adequate doses for adequate periods taken in a regular (not ad lib) divided dose schedule. This is mandatory (and sometimes diagnostic). All too often a homeopathic dose is used on an ad lib basis with inadequate results. Any agent prescribed must be taken on a rigid schedule to test its effectiveness. Anxiety is chronic and drug blood levels must be maintained if treatment is to be effective. The patient who fails to follow a serious drug regimen is communicating something either about the intensity of his symptoms (not as bad as we thought) or about the effectiveness of our communication (he doesn't understand the treatment program).
4. All antianxiety agents have abuse and dependency potential. The greatest abuse remains their use to subvert attention from other solvable problems. The prescription of chlordiazepoxide to a man "nervous" because of his job does nothing to alter the job situation. (See Chapter 8, Substance Use Disorders for other aspects of dependency.)

Psychotherapy/Counseling. While a treatment of choice for the clinically anxious patient who is unresponsive to nonspecific and specific treatment approaches, it is unlikely that the primary care clinician will have the time to undertake the specific psychotherapeutic work needed with these unresponsive patients. Having done all the specific and nonspecific things with a patient, a treatment failure should be referred (using the suggestions of Chapter 14) to a competent psychiatrist.

A Pharmacologic Approach to Anxiety Disorders

Our own approach is, therefore, a cautious one. In the process of evolving a diagnosis rely on educative and nonspecific treatments to reduce anxiety. Consider use of psychopharmacologic approaches only when *the patient* indicates that his level of dysfunction is intolerable. All too often a prescription is given out of the clinician's need rather than the patient's. The initial prescription is likely to be a non-"minor tranquilizer."

Three categories of drugs are possible:

1. *Sedative drugs:* It the patient tolerates sedation well (some will) and is a known reliable patient (low impulsivity, no depression, no prior dependency problems), prescribe phenobarbital. This is a very effective, very inexpensive treatment. Of course a discussion of the risks (drowsiness, synergistic effects with alcohol, etc.) is in order.

2. *Antihistamines:* Many antihistamines provide sedative and antianxiety effects, are inexpensive and relatively safe. As with the sedative drugs above, the focus is on breaking the anxious cycle, "taking the edge off," and encouraging several nights of restful sleep. Beyond this short interval these drugs are less and less useful, but with a sizeable number of patients this approach gets the job done with little expense and risk.

3. *Antipsychotic drugs:* The so-called "major tranquilizers" can be used with success in some anxious patients if used in low doses. They are especially effective in the following clinical situations:

   • Anxious elderly patients (especially when associated with irascibility and assaultiveness)
   • Highly anxious patients with high distractibility, racing thoughts, and thought blocking
   • Severely obsessional patients
   • Patients likely to abuse "minor tranquilizer" or sedative drugs
   • "Minor tranquilizer" treatment failures

The major problems with phenothiazines or butyrophenones is their atropine-like side effects and patient rejection. These drugs are, however, very safe drugs especially in low doses. Chlorpromazine (Thorazine) 10 to 25 mg t.i.d. or trifluoperazine (Stelazine) 2 mg q.d. or b.i.d. used over a two-week time period will reveal either effectiveness or treatment failure.

The most commonly used antianxiety agents are the "minor tranquilizers"— for the most part benzodiazepines. The most commonly used currently are diazepam (Valium) and chlordiazepoxide (Librium). Both relieve anxiety in association with both central nervous system depressant and muscle relaxant properties. Both drugs are widely used in treating alcohol or other depressant drug withdrawal but do, in and of themselves, have similar depressant dependency potential. Even at therapeutic levels (50 to 75 mg/d chlordiazepoxide, 10 to 30 mg/d diazepam), abrupt withdrawal is associated with mild withdrawal signs and symptoms—recrudescence of anxiety and sleep disturbance.

In prescribing the benzodiazepines, remember to prescribe an adequate dose, divided to maintain blood levels, over an adequate trial (four-to-six-weeks). Seventy-five percent of patients using this regimen should experience significant symptom reduction.

The major side effects of these drugs are:

- Drowsiness, ataxia, impaired fine motor performance
- Dependency
- Hypotension, skin rash, etc. (rarely)
- Paradoxical rage reaction
- Paradoxical increase in anxiety

The dosages are indicated in Table 7-2. The wise clinician picks one drug and knows it well. New agents will appear with enormous regularity. They will be successful initially because of a placebo or expectation effect. One might choose to take advantage of this or wait for thorough studies by recognized authorities (Hollister, Klein), to discover the real value. It's unlikely that any breakthrough miracle antianxiety drug will appear in the near future that does not have serious side effects. Propanediols (Meprobamate, Tybatran, etc.) are mentioned only to be thoroughly condemned as not only probably ineffective but dangerous in combination with alcohol. Propranolol has been used experimentally to treat the physiologic symptoms accompanying anxiety with some success. It is a drug with some risks and has not been FDA approved for use in anxiety as of this writing.

Panic Disorder

Panic Disorder is characterized by panic attacks—discrete periods of fear—and requires three attacks within a three-week period of time. These attacks are not associated with severe physical exertion, a life-threatening situation, or by confrontation with a phobic situation. In addition the patient describes:[7]

- Respiratory symptoms—such as shortness of breath, chest pain or discomfort, choking or smothering sensations, paresthesias
- Cardiovascular symptoms—palpitations, fear of heart attack, light-headedness or fainting, sweating
- Psychological symptoms—derealization, fear of dying, going crazy or losing control
- Other symptoms—hot or cold flashes, trembling or shaking

Table 7-2. Antianxiety Drugs.

Name		Manufacturer	Dose Range Mg/day	Addiction Potential	Duration of Action	Side Effects
Generic	Trade					
Propanediols						
Meprobamate	Equanil Miltown	Wyeth Wallace	400–1600	++++	S-1	1. Impaired performance
Tybamate	Tybatran Solacen	Robins	250–2000	?	?	2. Impaired judgment
Benzodiazepines						3. Drowsiness
Chlordiazepoxide	Librium	Roche	15–100	+	L	4. Dependency
Diazepam	Valium	Roche	6–40	++		5. Additive-synergestic effects
Oxazepam	Serax	Wyeth	30–120	+	S-1	lethargy
Clorazepate	Tranxene	Abbott	11.25–60	+	L	hangover
						skin eruptions
						nausea, vomiting
						paradoxical restlessness
						exacerbate OBS
						ataxia
						increased hostility
Antihistamines						
Hydroxyzine	Atarax Vistaril	Pfizer Roerig	30–200	0	?	Atropinism
Diphenhydramine	Benadryl	Parke-Davis	10–400	0	?	Atropinism

These panic attacks may precipitate abusive use of alcohol or drugs in an abortive attempt to relieve symptoms. Perhaps as many as 10 percent of symptomatic alcoholics suffer from panic disorder. The backgrounds of these individuals frequently reveal significant separation anxiety in childhood. The disorder may be precipitated by a sudden important loss (and thus be a variant of a grief reaction) or by patients with a recent or current endocrine imbalance. The disorder may generalize with increasing anticipatory anxiety and in some cases the development of phobic symptoms. The patient becomes phobic about travelling alone, being alone, or being in a place where escape would be difficult or help not available. This disorder has been successfully treated with imipramine—up to 250 mg daily, sometimes in combination with a benzodiazepine. The imipramine may also successfully reduce drug or alcohol use when it is initiated because of anticipatory anxiety. Note that this is a counter-intuitive treatment. It may be speculated that this disorder is really a depressive or grief state which manifests with primarily anxiety symptoms masking the more important depressive features.

Somatization Disorder

A third disorder with free-floating anxiety is the *Somatization Disorder.* Somatization disorder or Briquet's disease begins before the age of 30 and is a chronic illness in persons with a dramatic, complicated, or confusing medical history.[11] The pathognomonic sign is multiple physician contacts and multiple "to be R/O" diagnoses. The diagnosis should be made when, in the absence of medical explanation, the patient has symptoms (14 if female, 12 if male) from the following list of 37. A symptom must influence a person to take medicine, alter life patterns, or see a physician, to be counted as a symptom.

General

Sickly

Gastrointestinal

Abdominal pain
Vomiting spells
Bloating
Food intolerance
Diarrhea

Pain

Pain in back, joints, extremities, genital area, or urination

Conversion-Type

Difficulty swallowing
Loss of voice
Double vision
Blurred vision
Fainting or loss of consciousness
Memory loss
Seizures or convulsions
Trouble walking
Paralysis or weakness
Urinary retention

Psychosexual

Sexual indifference
Lack of sexual pleasure
Pain during intercourse

General (continued)	**Conversion-Type (continued)**
Gynecologic	*Cardiopulmonary*
Dysmenorrhea	Shortness of breath
Menstrual irregularity	Palpitations
Excessive bleeding	Chest pain
Hyperemesis gravidarum	Dizziness

These patients often report anxiety secondary to their major concerns. In addition many of their symptoms are those associated with classical anxiety. The rigid application of the above criteria—separating the anxiety disorder from the somatization disorder—leads to clear and quite different treatment courses. The anxiety disorder treatment has been described. The somatization disorder is managed as follows. The patient and family are told after a thorough exam that the patient has no life-threatening or severe illness but that he/she will have symptoms. The patient should be advised or cautioned against further medication or surgery. Only one clinician should care for the patient. The patient should be seen at regular intervals—prior to crises. The patient should not be told "nothing is wrong" since the patient is quite correct in knowing that, indeed, there is something wrong. The "wrong," however, is usually in terms of a paucity of positives in the patient's life. Setting limits on the patient's complaining by asking the patient to take a "vow of silence" about physical complaints to anyone else but you increases the patient's chances of having positive interactions with family and friends. Being clear and "grandfatherly" will reassure the patient. Knowing one's own limits in terms of tolerance for complaining or dependent patients is a mandatory prerequisite to treatment of this type patient. Medication—if used at all—should be framed paradoxically such as "I don't think this will work, but if you want to we can try . . . " and again the choice of medication is low dosage phenothiazine (25 mg of chlorpromazine or thioridazine).

Hyperventilation Syndrome

Finally under the free-floating anxiety disorders, we find the *Hyperventilation Syndrome.* Hyperventilation syndrome may occur in any anxiety disorder *and* most often occurs in young, otherwise healthy—psychiatrically speaking—persons making life changes. This acute symptom complex is an outgrowth of hyperventilation with an associated blowing off of CO_2. The symptoms that ensue include: feeling unable to catch one's breath, trouble breathing, palpitations, tachycardia, perspiring, pallor, sighing, and peripheral paresthesias, changes in consciousness, light-headedness and blurred vision. The common association the patient makes is to having "a heart attack." The treatment is symptomatic—rebreathing via a paper bag or anesthesia "bag"—and then educative. One explores the possibility of an infarct—usually ruled out by age and history—and having ruled out the possibility then explains the physiology to the patient including a demonstration with the patient of the induction of symptoms by asking him/her to hyperventilate. Then a supportive discussion of the anxiety inducing life changes which preceded the episode is usually sufficient to return the patient to his prior psychological homeostasis. Often the exploration will uncover some family dysfunction that may require referral for family counseling.

Where the anxiety is free-floating and evident, the patient is motivated to seek treatment since the experience of anxiety is psychologically painful. The concept of anxiety being "bound" as the result of psychological defenses is a useful one. The higher the degree of "binding" the more difficult the treatment of the patient by the nonspecialist. Most phobic disorders bind anxiety effectively, leaving only a displaced bolus of anxiety directed at some external situation.

PARTIALLY BOUND ANXIETY

Phobic Disorders

The essential characteristic of the *Phobic Disorder* is an irrational fear of something with an attendant desire to avoid the phobic stimulus. Irrational fears are not uncommon. The diagnosis is made when that fear is a significant source of distress or interferes with role functioning.

Agoraphobia—literally a fear of open spaces—is the most common phobia among those seeking treatment. The person has a marked fear of and thus avoids being alone in public places from which escape might be difficult or help not available in case of sudden incapacitation, e.g., crowds, tunnels, bridges, public transportation, etc. The treatment of simple agoraphobia is probably best accomplished through behaviorial techniques. Behavior therapists report high levels of success in the treatment of phobias. Alternatively insight-oriented psychotherapy has been used. The latter is unlikely to be used by the busy primary care clinician. The former may be available either because the clinician himself or herself has sought additional training in behavior therapy or has in his/her office a staff member with training. Referral to a competent behavior therapist is appropriate if it is not available "in house."

When panic attacks accompany the agoraphobia, then treat as above under panic disorders.

Social Phobia

Social Phobia is a fear and avoidance of situations where the individual may be exposed to the scrutiny of others and may perform in a way that will be embarrassing or humiliating. Again this diagnosis is made only if the symptom is above and beyond the usual fear—for example, of public speaking. Common social phobias include speaking or performing in public, using public lavatories, eating in public, writing in public, etc. Again the treatment of choice is behavioral.

Simple Phobias

Simple Phobias are specific phobias not covered by social or agoraphobia. These include fears of animals, snakes, closed spaces (claustrophobia), heights (acrophobia), disease or cancer. Rarely is there marked impairment and thus treatment is usually rarely sought. The individual adjusts his life to avoid the phobic stimulus. When treatment is indicated it is behavioral in nature and very successful with single simple phobias.

Obsessive-Compulsive Disorder

The second category of disorder, that in which anxiety is partially bound but with some "leakage," is *Obsessive-Compulsive Disorder.* Again the key to making the diagnosis rests with the patient having significant distress and/or interference with role functioning. The "O-C" style is clearly one campatible with or even successful in contemporary culture. The disorder usually begins in adolescence or early adulthood and follows a chronic course with some variation in symptomatology. It is often complicated by depressive features and abusive use of alcohol or antianxiety medications. The features are:

- Obsessions—persistent, intrusive thoughts that are repugnant or senseless but unable to be suppressed or ignored, and/or
- Compulsions—repetitive behaviors performed according to a certain program designed to produce or prevent future events but not connected in a realistic way, and done with a sense of desire to resist the compulsion but an inability to do so without great anxiety. No conscious pleasure is derived from the activity.

The obsessive-compulsive patient may be very seriously impaired by his/her symptoms. Again treatment is likely to be behavioral in nature initially, but subsequently may be insight oriented. In any case the impaired obsessive-compulsive will require referral. (See Chapter 14 for effective ways to make a referral).

BOUND ANXIETY (ANANXIOUS DISORDERS)

Finally we come to patients in which the anxiety is bound so tightly that no "leakage" occurs around the defense mechanisms. In these patients no anxiety or nervousness is noted, and the patient's focus may be quite far from the obvious problem or conflict. The bulk of these patients will require mental health referral. Initial diagnosis is often the responsibility of the primary care clinician.

We have already noted that some patients with phobic disorder or somatization disorder will have no anxiety at all. This is because their primary defense is effective and there is no overflow anxiety. However, the bulk of "ananxious" patients are suffering from other diagnoses.

Conversion Disorder

In *Conversion Disorder* a conflict is resolved or a need filled (primary gain) by the conversion of psychic distress into a physical symptom. Traditionally this symptom has been of the voluntary musculature or special senses, but in more recent times it has been broadened to include "a loss of or alteration in physical functioning suggesting a physical disorder" in the absence of a known physical disorder of pathophysiologic mechanism. The symptoms are psychologically precipitated since there is 1) evidence of a temporal relationship between a psychological event and onset of symptom—for example, an argument with her father enrages a young woman who immediately develops paralysis of her right arm, or 2) the symptom enables the person to avoid some situation noxious to them—for example, a man faced with laying off employees develops "loss of voice," or 3) the symptom enables the person to gain support which otherwise is absent (secondary gain)—for example, a young man who is unemployed and socially inept develops paralysis of the legs and receives sudden support from his extended family when they become frightened by his "illness."

These symptoms are *not* conscious *nor* under voluntary control (*Factitious Disorder or Malingering*). The differential between complex disease, conversion, factitious disease and malingering is a difficult one. Malingering is really a judgment and not a diagnosis. It is never useful to consider malingering until you have outside corroboration that the symptom is voluntary, conscious, *and* gainfully motivated. Factitious disorders are under voluntary control and are designed to simulate disease. Patients with factitious disease are uncommon and very complex. If the diagnosis is suspected, immediate consultation with a psychiatrist with a consultation-liaison hospital background is indicated before discussion with the patient of suspicion and certainly before a mental health referral is undertaken. The primary care physician may be able to do more, with consultative help, than a referral can accomplish. The separation of conversion from complex organic disease can be very difficult. Multisystem diseases, or early neurologic disease in particular, may start with conversion-like symptoms. Neuropsychiatric and in-depth neuropsychological consultation is warranted. Conversion symptoms occur in a wide variety of disorders—especially in somatization disorder or schizophrenia.

The treatment of conversion symptoms can usually be accomplished through suggestion, narcoanalysis, or hypnosis. Symptom removal, however, is not always sufficient *nor* diagnostic. Many organic lesions will improve under these same conditions. Treatment of the underlying conflicts or the dysfunctional system should be undertaken if immediate symptom resolution is followed by relapse or the appearance of new symptoms.

Psychogenic Pain Disorder

Chronic pain patients represent another complicated problem. The chronic pain patient has the same psychological precipitants for the pain that the conversion patient has for the conversion symptom. The patient experiences pain as the predominant feature. The pain presented is not consistent with the physical findings or known pathophysiology. There is usually no clear cut organic pathology.

These patients will often have a model for their pain syndrome in their background. The typical situation appears to be that a person with progressive role conflict or intrapsychic conflict experiences an accident, injury or illness that is ordinarily temporary but painful. The induction into the sick role meets both primary and secondary gain needs and the role becomes a permanent one. These patients are best managed by early referral to a regional interdisciplinary pain team for evaluation and active resocialization and vocational rehabilitation. Failure to do this results in a totally disabled chronic invalid who is miserable and makes others miserable (including the impotent physician).

Dissociative Disorders

The key element in these rare conditions is a sudden, temporary alteration in consciousness, identity or motor behavior usually precipitated by psychosocial stress.

Amnesia is the sudden inability to recall extensive important personal information not due to organic mental disorder. It may be circumscribed (a few hours after a major event), selective (failure to recall some but not all events of a time period), generalized (failure of recall of all previous life), or continuous (failure to recall events after a specific event up to the present). Termination of amnesia is usually rapid with suggestion, hypnosis or narcoanalysis and recurrence rare.

Fugue is sudden "flight" from one's home or work with no ability to recall one's past. This rare disorder occurs in the face of heavy alcohol use and is more common in wartime or following natural disasters. It typically is precipitated by severe psychosocial stress. It may be prolonged and a new identity may be assumed but recovery is usual and when it happens is rapid. Patients in fugue need psychiatric referral for treatment.

Multiple Personality—although widely described in the popular literature and media (*Sybil, The Three Faces of Eve*, etc.) this is a rare condition susceptible to manipulation by malingerers. The characteristic feature is the existence within an individual of two or more distinct personalities each of which is dominant at a particular time. These complex patients require referral to a psychiatrist experienced in such problems and, when legal issues are raised, to a forensic psychiatric expert.

Depersonalization is the experience of a strange alteration in the perception or experience of the self associated often with a sense of unreality, "in a dream-like," "out of the body," which is uncomfortable and recognized as unreal.

Depersonalization is quite common in adolescence and young adulthood. Mild depersonalization occurs in up to 70 percent of young adults. It is rare after 40. Immediate treatment is supportive and reassuring. However, the patient will have exacerbations and remissions. The anxiety may generalize and the symptom become disabling and cause impairment in functioning. Once this occurs referral to mental health professionals is in order.

REFERENCES

1. Horowitz M: *Stress Response Syndromes.* New York, Aronson, 1976
2. Holmes T, Rahe R: The social readjustment scale. *J. Psychosom Res* 11:213-218, 1967
3. Selye H: *The Stress of Life.* New York, McGraw-Hill, 1956
4. Kobasa S: Stressful life events, personality and health: An inquiry into hardiness. *J. Personal Soc Psychol* 37:1-11, 1979
5. Benson H: *The Relaxation Response.* New York, Morrow, 1975
6. Folkins C, Lynch S, Gardner M: Psychological fitness as a function of physical fitness. *Arch Phys Med Rehabil* 53:503-508, 1972
7. Rockwell D, Pepitone-Rockwell F: The emotional impact of surgery and the value of informed consent. *Med Clin North Amer* 63:1341-51, 1979
8. Jacobson E: *Progressive Relaxation.* Chicago, University of Chicago Press, 1938
9. Biomonitoring Application. 270 Madison Avenue, New York, N.Y. 10016
10. Wolpe J, Lazarus AA: *Behavior Therapy Techniques.* Oxford, Paragon, 1966
11. Guze S, Woodruff R, Clayton P: Hysteria: Studies of diagnosis, outcome and prevalence. *JAMA* 215:425-31, 1971

8

Substance Use Disorders

DON A. ROCKWELL, M.D.
MARK WILLENBRING, M.D.

127

William Osler in 1905 pointed out that "the desire to take a drug is one feature which distinguishes man, the animal, from his fellow creatures." This drug-taking penchant is pervasive (Table 8-1) in American culture and is associated with a series of problems—conceptual as well as clinical.

HISTORY OF THE CONCEPT

Ordinarily a medical concept requires little historical background. In the area of drugs, the development of the concept indicates the continuing evolution of attitudes about drugs and drug abuse. Because values and attitudes severely impinge on the diagnosis and treatment of drug-related problems, we find it useful to expose as far as possible latent values to the light of examination lest we fall into the trap of Alice's friends in Wonderland: "a word means what I say it means and . . ."

What are *substance use disorders*? Current definition divides them into two subdivisions.*

I. Substance Abuse
Minimal duration of use—one month
Social complication of use
Either psychological dependence or pathological pattern of use

II. Substance Dependence
All of above criteria for substance abuse
Tolerance or withdrawal

Notice that the word "drug" is no longer used. This is because definitions of "drug" are often value laden, situational, and transient. "Substance" is broader and more neutral in its value tone. The definition found above in DSM-III does not completely escape the value problems inherent in drug abuse or drug dependence, since social complications, psychological dependence, pathological patterns of use are subject to quite variable interpretations. As one example of these variable interpretations, note that a college student's "recreational use" of marijuana over a long period of time could meet his parents' (or physician's) definitions of "social complication" as he became less interested in his engineering major and his grades dropped; his insistence on continuing to smoke "nearly every day" can be construed as a pathological pattern of use. This student thus meets the criteria for substance abuse. Alternative explanations of this student's behavior in terms of changing psychological identity related to separation from parents, peer-group influences, and development of a different occupational goal might lead us to question the diagnosis of substance abuse.

Obviously in the extreme case we have no problem. In the more marginal case, the physician must be exquisitely aware that his/her own substance use and attitudes may distort his/her judgment or treatment of the problem. The clinician

---

*Diagnostic and Statistical Manual of Mental Disorders (DSM-III), 3rd ed. American Psychiatric Association, Washington, D.C., 1980.

Table 8-1. Drug Use.

	Percent Who Ever Used	Current Use*	Use on a Regular Basis**
Barbiturates	19.6%	2.8%	13.9%
Minor tranquilizers	19.4%	3.8%	19.3%
"Diet" pills	11.5%	1.6%	21.6%
Marijuana	10.5%	3.6%	33.8%
Hallucinogens	2.5%	0.4%	13.2%
Heroin	1.1%	0.3%	27.5%

*Required use six times a month.
**Percentage of those who have ever used who currently use on a regular basis.

who is a social drinker routinely discounts all drinking that is less than or equal to his/her own as normal—"what's ok for me must be ok." In fact, as we shall see, all substance use has some side effects, and there are no normal levels of use. Terms like "social" and "recreational" sometimes encourage denial in the user *and in his physician.*

Definitions of dependence are also vague. The ancients learned that ingesting certain naturally-occurring substances altered one's consciousness. Since that discovery, some people have become preoccupied with the phenomenon; what these people are called varies with the culture. A shaman using peyote is socially different, yet the same, as a "hip" user in a megalopolis.

Until quite recently, people differentiated addiction from habituation: addiction implied physiologic dependence, habituation a psychological dependence. This assumes that psychology and physiology are separate. In reality they are separated only artificially.

Current Definition

DSM-III groups substance use disorders together. The criteria for specific diagnosis will be discussed under the specific form of substance abuse or dependence. The general definitions of substance abuse and dependence are as follows:

Abuse

Duration: The substance must be continuously or episodically used for a minimum of one month.

Social Complications: Impairment in social, occupational, interpersonal, familial or other role functions or impairment in health are concomitants of substance abuse.

Psychological Dependence: The essence here is the urgency of drug use—a "drive" to use and a loss of control over use—sometimes in spite of repeated efforts to cut down or stop use.

Pathological Pattern of Use: Any of three patterns—daily intoxication, daily use, two or more episodes of complication—suggests pathologic use rather than "recreational" use.

Dependence

Dependence requires the characteristics of substance abuse plus either tolerance or withdrawal.

Tolerance: Tolerance to a drug's effects is a basic pharmacological-behavioral phenomenon common to dependency syndromes. A person headed for drug dependence starts to take a drug to achieve an effect such as induction of euphoria or reduction of anxiety. Through tolerance to effects, more of the drug is required to achieve the same effect. This occurs both because of altered drug metabolism and behavioral tolerance to effects. The person now finds that when he/she reduces use or stops using the drug, symptoms—at first subtle and later dramatic—occur. These symptoms are evidence of withdrawal. At this point the drug may be taken more to prevent these symptoms than to achieve the originally-sought special effect. Continued substance use is now required to feel "normal." Additionally and perhaps paradoxically, some substances induce "positive" feelings in low doses while at high doses they induce unpleasant feelings which may, in themselves, be addicting.

All drugs have various effects, and tolerance develops differentially among the effects. In this sense, what is an effect in one person may be a side effect in another. Cross-tolerance occurs when one drug induces tolerance to another drug in the same class.

Withdrawal: Withdrawal is a substance-specific syndrome that results when substance use is reduced or stopped. No specific syndrome of withdrawal has been identified from cannabis or hallucinogens. Withdrawal is evident following chronic intoxication with the following:

- Alcohol
- Barbiturate/sedative/depressants
- Opioids
- Psychostimulants

Definitional Complications

The issue of social complications is a complex one. Legal difficulties may be social complications, but they are subject to changes in law, enforcement and customs. Drug effects and effects of personality disorders are so intimately intertwined in some persons as to make differentiation an academic issue.

The issue of withdrawal likewise has situational meanings. There is clearly a chronic, albeit mild, intoxication from caffeine (coffee, cokes) and both tolerance and withdrawal, yet it is rarely considered a substance use disorder. Likewise, nicotine dependence or medically-prescribed "dependencies" are often viewed as non-pathologic.

Diagnosis

The diagnosis of substance use disorder can be used with any other diagnosis. One may find evidence for a coexistent psychotic or non-psychotic organic brain syndrome, functional psychosis, or other personality disorder. Other items likely to be found in these patients are sexual deviance, impaired energy level, antisocial acts and attitudes, interpersonal dependency, suicidal ideas and behavior, and depression.

Eliciting a straightforward admission of substance use is not common. The clinician must first consider the possibility of drug use and abuse in every patient. The "dope fiend" stereotype is as inaccurate for drug dependence as the "Bowery bum" is for alcohol dependence. The drug-dependent person is more likely to look like "the person next door" than "the hippie from Haight-Ashbury." There are no class, race, sex, or age boundaries.

Once considered, it is necessary to ask the right questions with a nonjudgmental attitude. Information about drug intake should be sought in several different ways. Clinicians and patients alike often ignore the fact that many medicines have dependency-producing potential. Inquire about routine ingestion of any agent—prescribed, over-the-counter, illicit—and about sleeping pills or potions, diet pills, pain killers, tranquilizers, and stimulants. Actual patterns of use are important. People rarely take medication in the way it is prescribed, and these variations may be important. Keep in mind that hospitalized patients often take drugs other than those prescribed. Any patient whose state of consciousness or behavior fluctuates inexplicably may be taking drugs. Inquiring about concern the patient may have about medications could uncover important information.

Staying in touch with the rapidly changing drug scene may facilitate asking the right questions in the right language. However, clinicians should not be seduced into using "street" language or assuming they or the patients know what the connection is between the street name of a drug and its actual composition. "Stuff" off the street often turns out to be quite different from what was represented at the time of sale.

SOME BASIC PSYCHOPHARMACOLOGY

Nonspecific Factors in Drug Response

The individual's set of expectations about a particular drug's effect can alter the effect. The now famous "banana" hoax of 1967 provides a good street example. Roast banana peels were touted to have psychedelic effects, and many young people had pleasant "trips" on bananas. Only later was it discovered that banana peels had no psychoactive properties.

Prior experience with a particular drug or drugs can alter response. Many first-time marijuana smokers experience little or no "high," while experienced users can get "high" on low-quality marijuana. Whether this is reverse tolerance or learning, prior experience alters response.

The setting in which the drug is taken can have an effect. Howard Becker[1] suggests that the paranoia associated with illicit drug use is more related to tension in the setting and genuine concern for discovery than to drug effects. Recent research on amphetamine psychosis confirms this; street users of amphetamines are markedly paranoid, while research subjects on amphetamines become grandiose. The setting and set thus alter delusional content and behavior. "Psychedelic effects" are seen less frequently in scientific studies of psychedelics, while psychotomimetic effects are seen more commonly. The sterile, objective laboratory alters the experience as much as a "hip" setting.

Personality factors interacting with pharmacological actions may influence the selection of a drug of choice for drug-dependent individuals as well as the response to drugs. It has been noted that preexisting psychopathology interacted with the setting in determining the extent of panic reaction in marijuana smokers. We know that people tend to be either sedation seekers or sedation avoiders. It is easier to become dependent on a class of drugs which meets such needs. In addition, it may be that these people are self-treating an underlying psychiatric illness, such as depression.

Drug dependence is rarely an individual problem. Often there exists a two-party or family system which in many ways encourages drug dependency. For every addict there may be an addictor—too often a physician.

Biological Predisposition to Substance Use Disorders

People seem to have differing inherent susceptibilities to drug dependence, which may reflect differing genetic and constitutional factors at birth. The only drug where this has been studied to any extent is alcohol. There has been a recent upsurge in interest about biological concomitants of alcoholism. According to Mendelson and Mello,[2] "alcoholism in the *biologic* parent appears to be a more reliable predictor of alcoholism in the children than any other environmental factor," including living with an alcoholic parent. There also appear to be racial differences in the effects of alcohol. For example, Asians tend to be more sensitive to the vasodilatation of alcohol, and this may reduce the rate of alcoholism in that culture. Early findings that American Indians metabolize alcohol differently, however, have since been disproved. A person with affective disorders, which clearly seem to have a genetic contribution, may be more prone to abuse drugs.

Intrapsychic Predisposition to Substance Use Disorders

No clear-cut constellation of intrapsychic conflicts is "causative" of drug dependence. In fact, it is not possible to give a clear picture or description of the drug-dependent individual. That is partly because of the difficulties presented by that kind of personality research and partly because drug dependence seems to cut across other diagnostic levels. Pihl and Spiers,[3] in an exhaustive review of the literature, concluded that the only commonality in the research is that drug abusers are "troubled individuals," who consistently show "rigidity;" hence " . . . all problems receive the same solution," which is drug use.

Alcoholism tends to be seen in a wide variety of people with differing make-up and a range of other problems. Alcoholism is a primary illness, which needs to be treated before other symptoms can be. Drug dependence can often be seen associated with depression, and depressed individuals may be at higher risk for developing drug dependence. Poly-drug abuse may be an attempt by a troubled individual to treat his/her own illness. Poly-drug abuse may also contribute to the development of severe pathology, such as psychosis. Drug dependence has been recognized for some time as a chronic form of suicide. It is useful to consider depressive individuals as being especially vulnerable to drug dependency problems. Equally important is the need to consider the coexistent depression and suicide potential of the dependent person. Frederick[4] makes the point that "addicts who are experiencing withdrawal at any stage, like depressives who are emerging from a depressive state, are in the period of greatest suicidal risk." Drug dependence is most likely to occur among individuals who lack the psychological resources needed to deal with minor conflicts or environmental stress. Adaptive capacity can be overwhelmed by either intrapsychic or environmental stress, and drugs may be used in an attempt to adjust. Reduced adaptive capacity may be the result of faulty parent-child relationships. Even a healthy adaptive capacity may be overwhelmed by a chronic psychotoxic environment such as a ghetto.

Substance Abuse as Dysfunctional Adaptation

Substance abuse can be symptomatic of social pathology. "Doing dope" is often a usual way of being-in-the-world in some subcultures. It is normative behavior in some urban and suburban ghettos. The drug of choice differs—heroin in Harlem, and pot and alcohol in San Mateo—but in each community it may represent social adaptation.

Sociocultural Predisposition to Drug Dependence

There are some currents in the mainstream of American society that promote drug dependence.

First is socialization into drug use: The acceptance of drugs to alleviate problems is very widespread and supported by our medical and clinical professions. Blum's work[5] indicates that 99 percent of the population use chemicals as "solutions to problems." Physicians support this, since taking medication for illness makes sense. This results in:

1. Medicines prescribed for illnesses which are not organic in origin. For example, minor tranquilizers or pep pills are used to treat the anxious or

tired housewife without considering the possibility that her exhaustion and nervousness may be appropriate responses to a situation which may have remedies other than drugs;

2. Increasing self-medication, evidenced by a booming trade in over-the-counter medications;

3. An orientation to medicine as the solution to all problems, including those that are non-medical.

We are a drug-taking culture. The line between legitimate use of a medication and the illegitimate use of drugs is increasingly fuzzy. The step from a pharmacological virgin to a street drug user is an immense one, but the step from abusive use of over-the-counter medicines or prescribed drugs by parents to abusive use of street drugs by their children is smaller.

A second characteristic of American society that contributes to drug abuse is its ambivalence about drugs. It is likely that our society's view of drugs will contribute to drug use problems, among them drug dependence, until we recognize that:

- Drugs per se are not the problem; that drug dependence is a characteristic of *people*, not drugs;
- *All* drugs have both attributes and liabilities;
- Education in drug use should be mandatory and preferably given in the home.

Once this is recognized, we may expect a reduction, though never an elimination, of drug problems. The same is true of alcohol.[6]

A third characteristic of contemporary society that contributes to drug dependence is an emphasis on "happiness" as a necessary and enduring state. People are made to believe that alternative states such as anxiety, depression, loneliness are unnatural and to be avoided. The media reinforce the idea that "pills solve problems," and that use of a drug (i.e., alcohol) changes who we are or how desirable we are.

The current emphasis on drug problems is misdirected in that there are no drug problems but rather a variety of people problems. Drugs are neither problematic nor problem free.

Socioeconomic Class

Drug dependence crosses all boundaries of class, race, and sex. The crass stereotype of the drug-dependent individual is most often a male, black, urban, ghetto dweller. This barely applies to heroin dependence and ignores the majority of drug-dependent individuals.

Interpersonal Factors

The family may contribute to substance use disorders. First, parental use patterns are important. While parental use of psychoactive drugs does not seem to influence adolescent drug use, parental use of alcohol is highly correlated with adolescent use of alcohol.

Second, drug use can serve a homeostatic, albeit pathologic, function within a troubled family system. This may include an individual protecting himself/herself from painful interactions within the family, protecting a poor marital relationship, or reducing anxiety within the family. The substance abuse may, by drawing attention to the abuser, deflect attention from other pathologic problems of the family system. The role of the "enabler" or "addictor," who covertly encourages substance abuse behavior in the significant other, is a well-known phenomenon in the treatment of substance dependence. Family and couples therapy is increasingly being used in treatment programs for these reasons. Family therapy is the treatment of choice for the substance-abusing adolescent.

Wikler[7] has developed a learning-theory model that drug dependence is contingent upon pharmacological and social reinforcement. The primary reinforcement for drug use is the powerfully pleasurable experience associated with use of the drug (the "flash" or "rush" or "hit"). The drug is positively reinforcing and this leads to repeating the behavior. The most highly effective reinforcers are the opiates, cocaine, and amphetamines. Moderate reinforcers are barbiturates and alcohol while drugs like mescaline or chlorpromazine are ineffective reinforcers. Wikler sees that the original reinforcement includes an escape *from* unpleasant states *to* pleasant states. Later when the drug relieves withdrawal symptoms, it takes on a new rewarding aspect—the avoidance of pain. Conditioning operates also in the association of primary reinforcement with the social milieu of the drug-dependent individual. Thus drug-seeking behaviors—"hustling, copping, fixing"—become self-reinforcing also. This explains why some drug-abusing and dependent individuals, when exposed anew to a social milieu similar to the original drug scene, will re-experience the original craving for the drug. Social reinforcement is important to the extent it fosters and continues the development of pharmacologic dependence.

Chein[8] also emphasizes that for many people being an addict has positive value. For the ghetto or suburban dweller living in a deprived and psychotoxic environment, drugs offer three things. They give that person a clear identity— "dope fiend"—which may well be looked up to in a small subculture and may be easy to exemplify. Being an addict gives the person a place in the subsociety where he/she is unequivocally accepted as a peer. The addict acquires a career in which he/she can be reasonably competent. This often contrasts sharply with the nondrug experience of the world. Finally the person avoids the pervasive feeling of helplessness and emptiness and replaces that with pleasure by taking drugs. Drug dependence then offers both the avoidance of pain and the promise of pleasure.

SUMMARY

Drug dependence has multiple causes. An individual born with varying lability to dependence. He/she develops a personality with some areas of weakness. The subculture further contributes to the development of dependence by attitudes and values that overtly or covertly support drug use. Once drug use has begun— most often by peers or physicians—continued use is reinforced by the positive presence of pleasure or by the absence of pain or both. A deviant identity is established around drug abuse, and further dependence is insured by a wish to avoid withdrawal symptoms, however mild. Clearly there would be no drug dependence if there were no mind-altering chemicals—equally clear is the fact that drugs per se become a threat only when an individual uses them as a response (or in response) to his/her inability to deal with social and personal problems. Unfortunately or not, we are a society who sees "a better life through chemistry," and drugs seem a simple solution to complex problems.

GENERAL DEPRESSANT DRUG SYNDROMES *(Includes Alcohol, Barbiturates, Benzodiazepams, and Other Sedative-Hypnotics)*

Because of the similarity of the syndromes of acute intoxication, overdose, and withdrawal among all CNS depressant drugs, we have decided to discuss the common syndromes, in order to acquaint you with general characteristics. We will make reference to important exceptions to the rule for various drugs.

CNS Depressant Intoxication

Acute intoxication is familiar to nearly everyone in some degree: The person is "drunk." More specifically, this refers to a generalized slowing of mental functioning, with poor comprehension and memory, decreased reaction time, poor judgment, and limited attention span. The person may be ataxic and slur his/her speech. Emotional changes are related to disinhibition and may include drowsiness, relaxation, relief from anxiety or lability of mood with aggressive and/or sexual behavior and irritability. The person may be belligerent and hard to deal with.

Chronic intoxication causes many of the same symptoms and signs, but may also result in general social decline with loss of family and job. There may be a variety of neurological effects, including vertigo, nystagmus, hypotonia and dysmetria. Chronic alcoholics are generally malnourished, which may lead to peripheral neuropathy and Wernicke-Korsakoff psychosis. Chronic alcoholics also have a variety of related illnesses which need not be described here.

Treatment of acute intoxication is generally observation and support. Physical exam, blood level of drug (if available) and blood glucose should be done in all patients. If intoxication is mild, and other results are normal, the person may be sent home with a friend or relative to "sleep it off."

If intoxication is moderate (i.e., stupor), or if there are complicating illnesses or no friends with whom the person can stay, then observation for several hours in the emergency room may be necessary. Always look for trauma, especially head trauma, in an intoxicated individual; he himself often is not aware of it. If in doubt, further workup, including neurological exams and skull x-rays, is indicated.

Always inquire about depression and suicidal thoughts. Is the intoxication the result of a suicide attempt? If there is any doubt about this, or if the intoxicated person admits to suicidal thoughts, observation and psychiatric consultation are indicated.

If the individual is agitated and/or belligerent, firm limit-setting and possibly seclusion and restraints may be necessary. Generally, most intoxicated persons can be "talked down" by a firm yet empathetic staff. If necessary, Haldol 2-5 mg IM is also helpful, especially in alcohol intoxication.

The management of chronic intoxication is similar, except that there are often a whole variety of medical complications. In addition, one must deal with the overriding concern of helping the individual get treatment for the drug problem. Additionally, it is likely that withdrawal will be a major problem that needs to be addressed. In general, it is best to attend first to acute toxic/overdose and urgent medical problems, second to withdrawal and other medical problems, and finally to drug dependency treatment. While it is senseless to talk to an intoxicated individual about his drug problem, that should always be the long-term priority.

Severe Intoxication/Overdose

While tolerance develops to a variety of effects of CNS depressants, there is often a thin line between intoxication and overdose, especially in the chronic user. Thus, accidental overdosage is common. Of course, intentional overdosage for suicidal and/or manipulative reasons is possible. Drugs are often mixed, especially alcohol and sedative-hypnotics, and the mixtures are more toxic than either drug alone.

The main danger in overdose is from the depressant effects, particularly on the brain-stem arousal and respiratory centers. Coma, progressing to apnea, shock, and cardiorespiratory collapse and death, may occur. Treatment is basically supportive, with attention paid to monitoring vital signs, airway maintenance, fluid and electrolyte management, and treatment of shock, if it occurs. Naloxone should be given to alleviate any CNS depression occurring from opiates. Gastric lavage should generally be done after the insertion of a cuffed endotracheal tube if the patient is comatose. There is no specific antidote, and hemodialysis is rarely done. If the individual survives the overdose and is a chronic user, then he/she is likely next to exhibit a withdrawal syndrome.

Withdrawal

The effects of abrupt withdrawal from CNS depressants are essentially the same for all depressants. However, they may occur with different intensity and over a different time-course, depending on the half-life of the drug. Additionally, there is a wide range of individual variability, depending on the drug, dosage, and duration of use. In general, the syndrome is a result of CNS stimulation due to the absence of CNS depression, to which the body has become accustomed. Thus, irritability, excitability, agitation, anxiety, insomnia, tremulousness and weakness all occur with regularity. Seizures may occur as well. These symptoms generally take place within the first 24-48 hours following the last ingestion of short-acting drugs such as alcohol and short-acting barbiturates, and constitute the *Minor Withdrawal Syndrome.* During this time, the individual generally is clear-headed and exhibits drug-seeking behavior.

If no treatment is instituted, and sometimes even if it is, the person may develop the *Major Withdrawal Syndrome (the DTs).* This generally begins 2 to 4 days following cessation or marked reduction of a short-acting drug, and may last up to 7 to 14 days. It consists of delirium with disorientation, short-term memory loss, agitation, hallucinations and delusions, hyperthermia and hypertension, and may result in death if not properly treated.

Long-acting drugs, such as the long-acting barbiturates and benzodiazepams, produce similar syndromes. However, because the blood levels of these drugs fall more slowly, the withdrawal syndromes tend to be less intense, occur later, and may be more prolonged. A patient may develop a major withdrawal syndrome with few or no symptoms of the minor syndrome. This should be considered in any patient who develops an unexplained toxic psychosis 2 to 10 days after hospitalization. There is a wide variability between individuals even if the duration and amount of drug use is the same. Additionally, many patients have been taking more than one drug. If these include both short, and long-acting drugs, a mixed syndrome will occur.

Treatment of the depressant withdrawal syndrome is controversial. Some authorities, such as Whitfield,[9] hold that detoxification can usually be done without drugs if an experienced, supportive staff provides emotional support for the patient. However, this generally occurs only in specialized settings designed for this purpose. His data, though, combined with the fact that many narcotic addicts can withdraw without symptoms, raise the question of how much of the syndrome is a product of the drug and how much is a result of an interaction between the individual and the setting. It may be as Cummings[10] states: "Degree of pain is directly proportional to the proximity of the sympathetic physician."

With those qualifications in mind, it is also true that common medical practice often or usually involves drugs in the treatment of withdrawal. With some addictions, such as barbiturates, it is *mandatory,* since untreated withdrawal can be extremely dangerous. With others, such as alcohol and the benzodiazepams, drug treatment for withdrawal is relative, depending on the individual physician, setting, patient, and degree of dependence. Withdrawal from short-acting barbiturates is the most dangerous for this class of drugs. It should always be monitored in a hospital. Abrupt withdrawal can lead to severe seizures and status epilepticus resistant to treatment. It can be fatal. Few physicians in general medical practice perform detoxification from barbiturates.

Withdrawal from benzodiazepams and long-acting barbiturates is also rarely seen. However, it may become more common with the high-use patterns of these drugs. Generally, treatment consists of general supportive care and the use of either the agent from which the individual is withdrawing or something like it. It is used in amounts sufficient to mitigate withdrawal symptoms when and if they occur, rather than treating for withdrawal before symptoms occur.

While many agents have been used to treat alcohol withdrawal, including paraldehyde, alcohol itself, and chloral hydrate, the benzodiazepams are the most commonly used now. Chlordiazepoxide is perhaps the best of them. Diazepam is said to produce a high preferred by alcoholics (they often become addicted). Generally, 100 mg of chlordiazepoxide is given orally (intramuscular injection is absorbed slowly and erratically) with the first signs of withdrawal, and then repeated every two to six hours as needed with a maximum of 500 mg in the first 24 hours. The dose is then halved the next day (to prevent excess accumulation) and withdrawal proceeds at 25 to 50 mg/day. Alcoholics often have other complicating illnesses.

SPECIFIC SYNDROMES *(Barbiturates and Similarly-Acting Sedatives or Hypnotics)*

All hypnotics and minor tranquilizers in Table 8-2 are cross-tolerant with barbiturates, produce a similar dependency syndrome, and have a similar life-threatening potential upon withdrawal. The depressants are the most frequent and the most serious drug dependency problem in North America other than alcohol. Thirty tons of barbiturates are produced annually in the United States. This provides enough barbiturates for a 30-day supply for every man, woman, and child annually. About 50 percent of the total annual production is misused or diverted into illegal channels. Barbiturates are responsible for 70 percent of drug deaths, whether accidental or suicidal.

Pharmacology. The model of depressant dependence is dependence on a derivative of barbituric acid. The primary effect of the barbiturates is depression of neural and muscular activity. All drugs in this class decrease dreaming sleep; upon cessation of drug use, patients describe an increase in unpleasant dreams, nightmares, insomnia, and feelings of having slept poorly. This is the ideal situation for insuring continued use and ultimate dependence. Tolerance does develop with depressant drugs but develops unevenly. As tolerance for the sedative effect develops, the patient comes closer to the lethal toxicity. Cross-tolerance develops with other depressants and with alcohol. These drugs are generally metabolized in the liver and excreted by the kidney.

Medical Use. Barbiturates have been commonly used in medical practice for sedation, as a hypnotic, and as an anticonvulsant. As we become increasingly

Table 8-2. Depressant Drugs.

Generic Name	Trade Name	Street Name	Usual Dosage	Dependency Dosage	Withdrawal Syndrome
Barbiturates					
Amobarbital	Amytal	Barbs, candy, peanuts, downers, sleepers, goof balls, blue devils	100–200 mg		
Pentobarbital	Nembutal	Yellow jackets, nembies	100 mg	400 mg/D 600 mg/D	Minor S/S Anxiety, tremor, weakness
Phenobarbital	Luminal	Phennies, dolls	32–100 mg	800 mg/D	Weakness, tremor, anxiety, convulsions (75%), DT picture (60%)
Secobarbital	Seconal	Reds, red devils, seggies, pinks	100 mg		
	Tuinal	Touies, double trouble, rainbows	50–200 mg		

			Dose	Max Dose	Withdrawal
Hypnotics					
Ethylchlorvynol	Placidyl		500–1,000 mg		
Glutethimide	Doriden	Goofers	250–500 mg	1,250 mg/D	Rare
Methyprylon	Noludar		200–400 mg		
Methaqualone	Quaalude	Ludes	50–300 mg	2,000 mg/D	90% show insomnia, tremor, muscle twitching, anxiety, weakness
Chloral Hydrate	Noctec	Mickey Finn	250–1,000 mg		
Minor Tranquilizers					
Meprobamate	Equanil		1,200 mg	2,400 mg/D	
	Miltown		1,600 mg	3,200 mg/D	90% have withdrawal, 50% severe with convulsions and DT-like picture
				6,400 mg/D	
Chlordiazepoxide	Librium		30–75 mg	80 mg/D	Some patients become intoxicated
Diazepam	Valium		15–70 mg	300 mg/D	Insomnia, anorexia, agitation, twitching, sweating, convulsions (late)
Doxepin	Sinequan		75–300 mg	60–120 mg/D	

aware of their ultimate failure as hypnotics and sedatives except on a very short-term basis, their primary indication is as anticonvulsants. Barbiturates remain useful in anesthesia and in the treatment of strychnine or cocaine overdosage.

The hypnotics described in Table 8-2 have little valid use except for "one-night stands."[11] Of the drugs available, glutethimide (Doriden) is the most dangerous because of the difficulty in the treatment of acute overdosage. Glutethimide rapidly becomes protein bound and is excreted with great difficulty by the comatose patient. Chloral hydrate in 0.5 gm or 1.0 gm doses or flurazepam (Dalmane) in 30 mg produces the least suppression of REM sleep and thus may be the best of the lot. The minor tranquilizers should be prescribed cautiously. Many physicians prescribe them in situations where psychopharmacological approaches are not indicated (see Chapter 7). All minor tranquilizers can produce a barbiturate-like dependency.

The complaint of "trouble sleeping" is never a disease. It is a common symptom of acute-stress situations and also of depression. A missed diagnosis of depressive insomnia results not only in the failure to provide appropriate treatment for depression, but may also provide the patient with the means to commit suicide. One fourth of deaths by suicide are due to barbiturates. This must be kept in mind by the clinician as he/she reaches for his/her prescription pad. No one has ever died from lack of sleep.

Street Use. "Downers" enjoy wide popularity by our sedation-seeking society. They are used for "kicks" because at low doses they release inhibitions. At higher doses they cloud consciousness and reduce awareness of a stressful reality. Downers are often used in combination with heroin or with psychostimulants, thus producing the "upper-downer" cycle.

Prescription use of depressants is widespread. About one fourth of all patients seen in a general medical clinic will be given a sedative and another sixth a minor tranquilizer. Ninety million prescriptions for minor tranquilizers were written in the U.S. in 1977. The proportion of these users who become dependent suffer essentially from preventable iatrogenic disease. In the past year, drug use statistics show the following:

Drug	Use by Women	Use by Men
Minor Tranquilizers	12.7%	7.5%
Hypnotic	9.5%	7.4%
Sedative	8.9%	4.1%

Clinical Syndromes. The most common clinical syndromes are:

1. *Acute intoxication.* This acute OBS (organic brain syndrome) is characterized by disorientation, intellectual impairment, motor uncoordination, disinhibition of affect and behavior, drowsiness to coma, shock, generalized depression, and death. Early medical intervention is imperative. Symptomatic support of all levels of function will result in recovery for most of

these patients. The patient with an acute overdose may wake up and proceed into barbiturate withdrawal as described below.

2. *Chronic intoxication.* This patient may have only a few signs or symptoms, such as slightly-slurred speech and motor uncoordination. The patient's friends or family often describe a recurring change in level of consciousness along with irritability and some emotional lability. The diagnosis and treatment of chronic intoxication merges with the depressant withdrawal syndrome.

3. *Depressant withdrawal syndrome.* The diagnosis based on history is simple. Unfortunately an accurate history is often not available because the patient 1) is reluctant to provide an accurate history because of fear of legal, moral, or familial consequences; 2) may be in early withdrawal and be disoriented, disorganized, or psychotic; or 3) is stuporous because of an acute overdosage which masks his chronic abuse. Withdrawal begins 12 to 16 hours after the last dose. Symptoms include restlessness, irritability, trembling, nausea and vomiting, and abdominal cramps. Later, muscle spasms, rigidity, hyperactivity leading to grand mal seizures or status epilepticus within 48 to 72 hours are noted.

The simplest diagnosis is made on the basis of a positive history. Consider depressant dependence in all cases of delirium. Obtain a blood or urine specimen and analyze for barbiturates and other depressant drugs. The possibility of depressant dependence is a medical emergency requiring immediate steps to evaluate this diagnosis. Immediate hospitalization is indicated. Fortunately there is a readily available and simple test that can be performed to rule out physiologically-significant dependence.[12] Since the depressants are cross-tolerant, all depressant dependence can be evaluated using pentobarbital. In this simple test the patient is given 200 mg of pentobarbital orally. Debilitated or elderly patients may be given 100 mg while severely-dependent patients may be given 300 mg. Sensorium is evaluated one hour after administration. Response to 200 mg pentobarbital is as follows:

Patient's Response	*Degree of Dependence*
Asleep but arousable	None

Awake but somnolent
    Nystagmus
    Trouble focusing eyes
    Slurred speech
    Ataxia
	Tolerant to 500-600 mg/day

Awake but not somnolent
    Lateral nystagmus only
    No ataxia
	Tolerant to 800 mg/day

No signs of intoxication	Tolerant to 1,000+ mg/day

Treatment. The test dose gives you the appropriate range for beginning detoxification in the hospital. The patient should be stabilized at this dose, using pentobarbital in divided doses for two days. On this amount the patient should show mild sedation and intoxication. If the patient is oversedated, the daily dosage should be reduced, while presence of abstinence signs and symptoms requires an increase in dosage.

Following stabilization, withdrawal proceeds *at no greater than 10 percent* of the original total dose per day. Thus, withdrawal proceeds over a 10-day period. The night-time dosage is the last dose to be given up. Seizures should not occur on this schedule, but if the patient does have a convulsion, rapid re-intoxication with 100-200 mg is necessary. Dilantin® has little effect on barbiturate withdrawal seizures. Other medications are not indicated. The staff must be aware of the seizure potential. These patients may secretly obtain drugs from friends or family while in the hospital.

Phenothiazines are contraindicated in the treatment of the psychotic features of this abstinence syndrome because of their potential for lowering the seizure threshold. Intercurrent medical problems may necessitate slower withdrawal.

Following acute detoxification, management is aimed at preventing further dependency on depressant drugs and alcohol. The patient should be informed that insomnia and irritability are common in the post-withdrawal period and may continue for months. This period is crucial, since the tendency to reestablish dependence during this time is high.

Maximal support by the clinician through this period is important. Referral for more extensive psychotherapeutic treatment is often indicated. Group therapy and family therapy offer much in terms of rehabilitation. Some patients will benefit from involvement with ex-addict therapeutic groups.

Clinical Course and Prognosis. The major effort of physicians should be directed at prevention, since most depressant-dependent patients begin their problem with a physician's prescription. The following three rules would markedly reduce the numbers of depressant-dependent individuals:

1. Consider why you are prescribing a depressant drug. Insomnia is a symptom rather than a medical problem. Insomnia may be the result of a social situation and as such will not respond to psychoactive medications. Often insomnia is a symptom of depression, anxiety, conflict, or stress, and requires specific rather than symptomatic treatment.
2. Never prescribe sedatives or hypnotics for more than three days; beyond that period they become physiologically antitherapeutic. Hence, *never give refillable prescriptions.*
3. Remember the tendency of all patients to combine depressants—alcohol and benzodiazepines most commonly—with disastrous synergistic effects. Assume that Murphy's law will apply—if a mistake can be made it will be made. With depressant drugs these single and synergistic effects are associated with accidents, accidental overdoses and suicidal overdoses.

PSYCHOSTIMULANT DEPENDENCE

The search for euphoria repeatedly leads people to dependence on "euphoria"-producing drugs. The history of psychostimulant dependence is remarkable in its demonstration of man's inability to learn from previous mistakes. A simple rule is that any agent which produces a sense of well-being either *directly* or *through relief of pain* has potential for abuse and dependence.

The psychostimulants in common use are the amphetamines and amphetamine-like drugs (see Table 8-3).

Pharmacology. Amphetamines are sympathomimetic amines similar to epinephrine. The peripheral effects include increased blood pressure, increased heart rate, increased peripheral vascular tone, pupilar dilatation, smooth muscle relaxation, and secretion of thick sparse saliva.

The central stimulating effects are especially intriguing. The members of this class produce arousal. This effect is demonstrable behaviorally and electroencephalographically. The central arousal effect is useful in the treatment of narcolepsy and in improvement of performance by offsetting fatigue and sleepiness. Psychostimulants improve motor performance only and this only in subjects who are sleep deprived. The subjective feeling of increased mental powers and euphoria is not substantiated by objective performance. Tolerance develops rapidly with continued use of psychostimulants.

Most amphetamine-type drugs are excreted in the urine and acidification of the urine speeds elimination.

Medical Use. Psychostimulants, introduced into clinical medicine in 1932, have been widely prescribed for a great variety of problems. Currently the only recognized uses of these drugs are for:

- Narcolepsy
- Hyperkinetic children

They are not recommended for treatment of depression or weight control.

In depression they may "activate" the patient to carry out suicidal ideation. A rebound depression is common when the stimulants are discontinued. There is little evidence that they are effective in weight control when one considers the risk/benefit ratio.

The use of psychostimulants to facilitate studying is widespread. Between 44 and 54 percent of medical students report use of amphetamines.[13] There is no evidence that objective performance is improved, and the false sense of self-confidence may impair judgment and performance on exams.

Amphetamines can be used in acute situations of fatigue where motor performance needs enhancement. Again the associated side effects may outweigh the benefits. Psychostimulants are used in a wide variety of sports. Available evidence indicates that it does not improve performance in the conditioned athlete.

Table 8-3. Psychostimulant Drugs.

Generic Name	Street Name	Trade Name	Therapeutic Dosage	Abusive Use
Amphetamine	Uppers, lid proppers, truck drivers, wake ups, diets, pep pills, splash, spliven, grease rhythm, jolly beans	Benzedrine	5–30 mgm/day	30–750 mgm/day
d-Amphetamine	Roses, cartwheels, bennies, whites, peaches, hearts	Dexedrine	5–30 mgm/day	15–500 mgm/day
Methamphetamine	Co-pilots, oranges, dexie	Methedrine	2.5–30 mgm/day	20–2500 mgm/day
Benzphetamine phenmetrazine	Meth, speed, crystal, bombido	Didrex, Preludin	50–75 mgm/day	100–1750 mgm/day
Phendimetrazine diethylpropen	Phennies	Plegine, Tepanil Tenuate	75 mgm/day	75–7500 mgm/day
Phentermine chlorphentermine		Fastin, Ionamin Pre-Sate	65 mgm/day	not yet reported
Clortermine methyphenidate		Voranil Ritalin	10–60 mgm/day	100–400 mgm/day
Fenfluramine pipradol		Pondimin Meratran	2.5–7 mgm/day	not yet reported
Pemoline ephedrine	Freddy	Cylert	20–150 mgm/day	75–700 mgm/day
Cocaine	Coke, snow		topical use	variable
Caffeine		No Doz® etc.	variable	variable

Abuse and Street Use. In 1970, fifty doses of amphetamines were produced for every man, woman, and child in the United States, many times more than required for medical use. The syndromes of misuse, abuse, and dependency often start in the doctor's office. Physicians must take the responsibility for systematically ignoring reports of abuse potential, which were recognized as early as 1938.

It is simpler to prescribe a drug than to confront the patient guilty of subtle misuse—"for weight control" or "because I'm tired all of the time" or "I need to cram for exams." One third of all patients who develop the abuse syndromes described below first received amphetamines from their physician. Population studies indicate that 1.6 percent of the people in the United States use prescription amphetamines "for diet purposes" at least six times a month—with an additional 0.8 percent using amphetamines with similar frequency for other reasons. Most physician-produced problems started with the prescription of amphetamines for depression or weight reduction purposes.

Psychostimulants are widely abused on the street scene, and "speed freaks" have become a subculture within this scene. Illegal manufacture and distribution serve this population. Five million dosage units are stolen each year and yet only 2 percent of psychostimulants seized in drug arrests are from legitimate domestic manufacturers.[14] Street users are aware that "speed kills," and speed freaks are the pariahs of the street scene. Because of the paranoia and potential for violence, speed freaks are avoided in most scenes. Speed kills in other ways. The physical deterioration of heavy users is apparent with weight loss, malnutrition, and hepatitis. The "crash" following a run is a profound depression with an attendant high risk for suicide. Multiple drug dependence is also common, since "downers" or heroin may be used to soften the "wired up" experience of "speed."

CHRONIC DEPENDENCE

Case History

The patient is a 30-year-old nurse. Because she had a weight problem, an amphetamine was prescribed. She was the only child of an absentee alcoholic father and a rejecting mother and was brought up by various relatives and a foster home. She went into nursing with mixed feelings. An early impulsive marriage ended unfortunately. It was followed by a pattern of involvement with older men "destined to terminate in suffering."

She began to rely increasingly on amphetamines to get her going and depressants to help her sleep (the upper-downer cycle). Her use of amphetamines increased and she began "stuffing down handfuls—eight or nine 10-milligram tablets at a time." Her daily intake reached 600 milligrams and during this phase she became increasingly active. She worked incessantly, often going 72 hours without sleep, and lost 60 pounds. Attempts to give up the drug made her depressed, and resuming it produced anxiety.

Finally, she entered psychotherapy. Withdrawal from amphetamines produced marked irritability and apprehension as well as hypersomnia and depression. She described amphetamines as making her more talkative, cheerful, and freer in the expression of anger. Subjectively, she experienced euphoria, optimism, energy, and gregariousness along with tachycardia, rambling talk, forgetfulness, and persistent tremor. She had urinary frequency, dryness of the mouth, and increased sexual desire with decreased sexual satisfaction. She had skin lesions produced by digging at her arms and face. She noted a major difference between the effects of barbiturates and amphetamines—both of which gave her a "jag." Barbiturates made her "confused, falling apart, and excited but threatened." Amphetamines left her "exhilarated, but more in control." Over a prolonged course of psychotherapy she took amphetamines sporadically until her personal problems diminished.

The following are characteristics of the psychostimulant-dependent individual. There is often a personal or family history of dependence on alcohol or other drugs. The patient begins use of the drug through medical channels but rapidly shows a tendency to increase the dose. There is an overpowering desire or need to take the drug and often to obtain it by any means. This leads the patient to obtain prescriptions from many physicians or by forging prescriptions, stealing the drug, etc. There is a clear psychological dependence on the drug and this culminates in effects which are deleterious to health or social functioning.

Treatment. The psychostimulant-dependent individual must be evaluated carefully. The underlying problem may be depression, anxiety neuroses, or family conflict. Immediate withdrawal from the drug is necessary. Evaluate the possibility of a mixed dependency, particularly on depressants. Keep in mind that the withdrawal "crash" can produce a profound depression and possible suicide. The patient should be aware that physiological effects of withdrawal in the form of sleep disturbance and psychological effects such as lassitude and irritability persist for weeks or months. Group therapy is quite useful, especially when other ex-users are involved.

Amphetamine Psychosis. "Amphetamine psychosis" is somewhat of a misnomer since it applies to the psychosis associated with any psychostimulant— including methylphenidate and phenmetrazine. The following case report is typical:

Case History

Dr. A. is a 30-year-old man hospitalized for a paranoid psychosis. He described using intravenous methylphenidate (Ritalin®), 100 to 200 mg daily. His use of methylphenidate had begun three or four years before admission, when a coach recommended it to him for use just before competitive athletics. He experimented with other drugs but did not use them regularly. At the time of his marriage, one year before admission, he began using methylphenidate more frequently. About nine months before admission, he began to use methylphenidate in "runs" of "shooting up" every 15 minutes for four to six hours.

Three months before admission, distortions of reality began. His wife, who was also taking the drug, began to suspect that people were following them. For several weeks the patient dismissed this idea; later, he began to wonder. He then identified "worms" coming out of the air conditioner. He came to believe he was infested with worms or bugs, which "explained" his frequent episodes of sleepiness and lethargy. He described peculiar sensations in his skin that he attributed to parasites. He considered himself to be the object of an extremely complex plot to help him get off drugs.

When admitted he was oriented, and his thought processes were normal except for the delusions and paranoia. For the first nine days in the hospital, he was lethargic. When discharged, he was much improved and entered outpatient psychotherapy. He and his wife soon returned to the use of intravenous methylphenidate, and his paranoid psychosis returned. After several months, he was again hospitalized briefly. His wife returned to her parents' home, and he then returned to outpatient psychotherapy alone. With discontinuation of methylphenidate, his paranoid psychosis ceased. The avoidance of methylphenidate was extremely difficult for him, and he frequently thought of "shooting up," knowing that "Ritalin® is my one dependable friend." There was no evidence of schizophrenia or other functional psychoses at that time.[15]

Paranoia is quite common in psychostimulant abuse and contributes to violent behavior. Delusions of infestation are also frequent. The patient may have either a withdrawal state of mild proportions characterized by lethargy and sleeping, or a profound rebound depression upon withdrawal. The latter may lead to a suicide attempt or renewal of the abuse pattern.[16]

The psychosis associated with psychostimulant abuse is characterized by suspiciousness, visual or auditory hallucinations, increased motor activity, decreased ability to concentrate, labile mood, obsessive thoughts, and compulsive behavior. The patient is not disoriented, and often has a thought disorder identical to that seen in schizophrenia. Early in the course the patient retains insight into his paranoid delusions. He knows he is paranoid and that it is due to amphetamines. The patient reports loss of appetite, weight loss, insomnia, and impairment of memory. He may be "wired up" (high) or "crashed" (depressed). Physical findings may include mydriasis, tremor of the hands, facial twitching, tics, or writhing (athetoid) movements of the upper extremities. Many patients will have self-inflicted skin lesions of the face, arms, or scalp in addition to needle tracks. Malnutrition and hepatitis are common.

Treatment. The major hindrance to proper treatment is a missed diagnosis. Patients with a psychostimulant psychosis are indistinguishable clinically from schizophrenic patients. It is worthwhile screening all schizophrenic patients for amphetamine dependence. In one urban study, it was revealed that up to 15 percent of schizophrenic patients were taking psychostimulants without that information being known to the clinician.[16] Treatment consists of hospitalization and withdrawal from the psychostimulant. In most cases the psychostimulant psychosis will clear in three to five days upon withdrawal. Use of antipsychotic medications may facilitate the recovery, as does acidification of the urine, which speeds excretion. Failure of the psychosis to clear in a short time may be related to continued use of drugs in the hospital or to the exacerbation of a basic schizophrenic process by the psychostimulants.

A major treatment problem involves the "rebound" depression following the cessation of psychostimulant use. The depression is related both to physiological changes in sleep patterns and to psychological factors. They are experienced subjectively as trouble sleeping, nightmares, restlessness, and irritability and depression while awake. The patient needs to be told explicitly that this is a withdrawal phenomenon. Many patients will return to psychostimulant use during this period because of their discomfort, or alternatively will turn to depressants to treat their sleep disturbance.

Once the psychosis remits, the major task is resocialization and rehabilitation. Depending upon the patient's motivation, various psychotherapeutic modalities can be tried. Blockade of the effects of amphetamines by other drugs is thus far experimental.

Medical Complications of Psychostimulant Dependence. Psychostimulant abuse has been associated with some specific complications. These include the foreign-body granulomata in the lungs, spleen, kidneys and retina—the result of shooting crushed tablets—hypertension and subsequent cerebrovascular accidents; direct cardiac toxicity with cardiogenic shock; and exfoliative dermatitis. "Overamping" (i.e., taking too much "crystal") can result in transitory episodes of aphasia or paralysis. Dyskinesias are also seen. Many of these complications may be related to blood vessel constriction and hypertension. A common complaint of the chronic user of psychostimulants is memory loss. There is some evidence that chronic heavy use does in fact lead to a chronic brain syndrome with associated impairment in memory. Occasionally a patient will suffer a more apparent cerebrovascular accident.

Clinical Course and Prognosis. The major effort of clinicians should be directed at prevention. The only legitimate indications for psychostimulants are narcolepsy and the hyperkinetic syndrome. Both of these diagnoses require consultation with experts—a neurologist, child psychiatrist and electroencephalographer at a minimum. Indiscriminate use of psychostimulants is inappropriate. Once begun, psychostimulant dependence tends to be cyclic and difficult to treat. The highly-motivated individual, medically dependent and on low or moderate doses, has a good prognosis. Experience with "speed freaks" has been uniformly poor.

COCAINE

Cocaine, an alkaloid from *Erythroxylon coca*, is often considered quite separately from other psychostimulants. It is in essence a central stimulator and peripheral anesthetic. It is classified under narcotic regulations as if it were an opiate, and, while it is highly reinforcing, it rarely produces an intense physiologic dependence. Its effects are to produce a striking "high" with garrulousness, restlessness and excitement. It increases the ability to perform work by decreasing the sense of fatigue. Sherlock Holmes used cocaine in this way, to Dr. Watson's eternal disapproval.

Cocaine use in the United States has increased dramatically over the past decades. The eighties may well be the "coke" generation.

Cocaine is readily absorbed from mucous membranes, and in this way has been used since Freud's early studies of it as an ENT anesthetic. "Snorting" or inhalation is a main route of street administration. Smoking the cocaine alkaloid with tobacco or marijuana—especially "free basing"— is reported to produce a more rapid euphoria although it has inherent risks for severe psychological dependency, toxic reaction, overdose, and "burns."

Clinical Syndromes: Psychosis. The subject notes decreased hunger and indifference to pain. In higher doses patients develop a psychosis identical to amphetamine psychoses. The hallucinations are reported to be more vivid with cocaine and more often effect multiple modalities, olfactory and tactile as well as auditory and visual. The stimulatory effect plus the vividness of the hallucinations often lead the cocaine psychotic to act antisocially.

Acute Intoxication. Acute overdoses are not rare. Severe toxic effects can be seen at doses as low as 20 mg, and lethal doses as low as 1.2 gm taken intravenously. The patient moves rapidly through excitement and psychosis. One notes hyperactive reflexes and the patient complains of a headache. The pulse becomes rapid and respiration shallow and irregular. Cocaine is a powerful pyrexic and the temperature rises rapidly, followed by delirium, convulsions, coma, death from respiratory depression and arrest. Early on the patient complains of nausea and abdominal pain and may report "bugs crawling on his skin." Early and rapid intervention is mandatory. Treatment consists of attempting to reduce absorption of the cocaine while beginning administration of intravenous short-acting barbiturates. Use of drugs such as amphetamines to counteract respiratory depression is contraindicated.

Dependence. Dependence on cocaine is fairly rare in this country because of its expense on the street market. There is some question as to whether true tolerance to cocaine develops or whether its rapid metabolism explains the apparent tolerance to larger doses. There is no physiologic dependence in that no clear abstinence syndrome develops at cessation of regular use. However, the primary reinforcement of the euphoria produced by cocaine is very effective, and dependency is rapidly developed and very difficult to give up. Cocaine is snuffed by some (and may cause septal perforation due to its vasoconstriction effects) and injected either alone or with heroin (speedball) by others. In either case its short duration of action and powerful euphoric effect make cocaine a drug that is very difficult to give up.

OPIATES (*Opium, Opium Alkaloids, Their Derivates, and Synthetic Analgesics with Morphine-like Effects*)

Introduction. More attention has been paid to "opiate" dependence in recent years than to any other drug dependency problem. This is related to the development of methadone as a potential treatment and to concern about the "dope-fiend" stereotype which is part of our cultural heritage. It is interesting to speculate whether 500,000 heroin addicts cause more harm to society than the estimated 10,000,000 alcoholics. Current estimates suggest there are 500,000 active addicts in the United States, a ten-fold increase from 1967. The drugs discussed here are indicated in Table 8-4. The large majority of these dependent individuals are using heroin.

Pharmacology. An opiate is any substance similar to morphine in creating an addiction or addiction liability, or any substance that can be converted into such a substance. Opium itself comes from the sap of paper somniferium. Heroin came onto the scene in 1898 as a "nonaddicting" substitute for morphine. Heroin differs from morphine in its analgesic affects; it is two to four times more potent than morphine and produces a higher degree of euphoria. Both heroin and

Table 8-4. Opiates.

Generic Name	Proprietary Name	Analgesic Potency	Therapeutic Dosage
Morphine	Morphine	1	32–60 mg/day
Heroin	None	4	None
Codeine	Codeine	0.1	120–240 mg/day
Oxycodone	Percodan*	1	20–60 mg/day
Dihydromorphinone	Dilaudid	4	4–8 mg/day
Oxymorphone	Numorphan	10	4 mg/day
Meperidine	Demerol	0.1	75–150 mg/day
Anileridine	Leritine	0.25	100–300 mg/day
Diphenoxylate	Lomotil**	—	—
Methadone	Dolophine	4	20–60 mg/day
Levorphanol	Levo-Dromoran	4	4–12 mg/day

*Also contains homatropine, APC.
**Also contains atropine.

morphine are compounds containing natural opium alkaloids. Synthetic opiates include percodan, methadone, demerol, etc.

Tolerance to the sedative, analgesic, euphoric, and respiratory depressant effects of these drugs develops rapidly, and dependence is established after two weeks of daily administration of 60 mg of morphine or its equivalent.

Opiate receptor sites in the central nervous system trigger a descending inhibitory apparatus. This alters nerve function such that a stimulus is felt but perception altered. This results in analgesia and a kind of tranquility. The opiates in therapeutic doses constrict the pupils, decrease respiratory rate and volume, decrease gastrointestinal tract motility and secretions, increase peripheral vasodilatation and histamine release resulting in flushing and itching, produce nausea, and reduce urinary output. Metabolized primarily by the liver, they are excreted by the kidneys, thus allowing for urine testing by a wide variety of techniques.

Medical Uses. The available generic drugs are used primarily for relief of pain. The usual total dose of morphine for 24 hours to relieve agonizing pain would be something like 60 mg. Morphine is also used to relieve shortness of breath due to pulmonary edema. Less potent opiates are used for cough suppression (Codeine) and diarrhea control (Paregoric and Lomotil). Relative strength is indicated on Table 8-4.

Street Use. Accurate statistics are not available. From 1955 to 1968 the number of reported opiate "addicts" in the United States was stable at 50,000. In the late 60's and early 70's this number ballooned to 500,000 and dropped to perhaps 450,000 by 1978. About 25 years ago, opiate dependence problems were seen in the white population with equal distribution in rural and urban areas. Now minority groups are vastly over-represented. Blacks constitute more than half of the known population, and Chicanos and Puerto Ricans represent large minorities. Opiate dependence is now a problem of urban ghettos and a problem of adolescence rather than youth. The age of the average New York City addict dropped from 25 in 1963 to 17 in 1971. Major cities and major ports of entry contain the most addicts.

Factors Leading to Dependence. The road to "H" is not all that mysterious. Opiate dependence develops in phases. The process often starts in a social situation where legitimate means to achieving culturally-accepted goals are not available. In this context—most often in a ghetto setting—the child or early adolescent turns to a peer group for a sense of identity and for security. This peer group often chooses delinquency as the most available method of achieving goals. Delinquent behavior precedes drug dependence.

Within the subculture, drug abuse is common and valued positively. The youth uses alcohol and marijuana in a social situation with much group support. The "evil pusher" plays no role in induction to the addict role. The step from marijuana to heroin is taken if the drug is available and the peer group supports it.

In Viet Nam, for instance, large numbers of GI's used heroin. Half of those who tried it became addicted—usually within five to 12 months. Dependence on heroin is a result of the rapid tolerance that develops. Once established, dependence is continued because of identification with the addict role.[17]

This identification is a positive one. For many users this is their first and only real identity. The addict subculture becomes a potent social force and provides a life quite separate from that of the "straight" world. "Hustling" and "copping" are valued experiences over and above their functional utility in maintaining a habit. Boredom with other drugs and the promise of a "junkie" identity seduce some people. Users who "chip" and "do" low-potency "dope" may increase the frequency of their use, develop tolerance, and become dependent even though "it can't happen to me." The opiate euphoria is in itself a powerful reinforcer, especially in the face of an otherwise psychotoxic environment.

Some opiate dependence is clearly iatrogenic. Medical addicts are of two major types.

The Chronic-Pain Patient. These patients' problems begin with an accident or surgery and ultimately develop into a chronic-pain syndrome. Pain medications, casually managed by the physician or nursing staff, lead to prolonged or excessive in-hospital use. Patients not only seek the pain relief and/or positive euphoria from their primary physician, but also often doctor hop. Codeine, Percodan, Dilaudid, and dihydrocodeine are the primary drugs used this way. The prevention of this addiction is exceedingly simple—careful attention to the prescription of pain medications in all situations. The treatment of such patients is much more difficult. Referral to a regional pain center may be the best approach in what are complicated situations.

The Physician (Nurse, Health Care Team Member) Addict. Easy access to drugs increases the potential for their abuse. Physician-addicts use drugs initially for relief from fatigue or pain. Prevention is much easier than cure. Physician-addicts have a strikingly solid record of rehabilitation in programs that monitor behavior and are not hesitant about restricting or removing licensure.

Clinical Syndromes: Acute Opiate Poisoning (Narcotism). Acute opiate poisoning is a medical emergency. This may be the result of a conscious overdose, an accident, the outcome of heroin roulette (never knowing the potency of the heroin one "shoots"), or the result of a "hotshot" (high-potency heroin given to an unknowing user).

The patient is brought to the emergency room *comatose* with:

1. Marked respiratory depression with hypoxia
2. Constricted pupils, or dilated pupils with no corneal reflex when hypoxia is severe
3. Needle tracks—seen in only 50 percent of cases
4. Pulmonary problems in 50 percent of cases

5. Pulse rate and rhythm regular except in profound central-nervous-system depression
6. Blood pressure normal or low
7. Hypothermia in severe cases

Medical treatment is as follows:

1. Assure adequate ventilation of the patient. This may often require intubation and the use of mechanically-asserted respiration. You may need to use muscle relaxants where hypoxia is evident yet the patient is still thrashing about.
2. If there is not a rapid improvement use naloxone (a morphine antagonist) intravenously, in doses of 0.4 to 0.8 mg, judiciously repeated over the course of 20 to 30 minutes. If the diagnosis is correct, you will see a dramatic change for the better, with improved respiration and level of consciousness. Failure to get any response places serious doubt on the diagnosis of opiate overdosage unless an additional complication is present.
3. If the patient has responded to the test dose of naloxone, you may give repeated doses if respiratory depression recurs. This recurrence is very frequently observed and may recur after long periods such as three to six hours. Naloxone, being an antagonist, will cause violent withdrawal symptoms in the dependent addict. Thus some caution is indicated in its use. Naloxone-precipitated withdrawal is very difficult to control.
4. As the patient becomes more stable, investigation should begin for pulmonary edema. A chest x-ray, arterial blood gases and an electrocardiogram should be done. Since the cause of the pulmonary edema is in the lung, phlebotomy, digitalization and diuresis are of little benefit. Intermittent positive-pressure breathing becomes the mainstay of treatment.
5. Large doses of steroids may be used because of their effect on the "allergic" component of the pulmonary edema and have been shown to improve oxygenation.
6. Multiple blood cultures should precede any antibiotic treatment in order to aid in the diagnosis of endocarditis and other infectious processes.
7. Withdrawal symptoms from other dependency-producing drugs such as barbiturates and alcohol should be considered at all times, since multiple drug dependence is common.
8. Immunization of these patients against tetanus is in order prior to their release to a rehabilitation program.

Chronic Intoxication. Repeated use of morphine or heroin leads to the development of tolerance. Morphine given in 15 mg doses four times daily over two weeks is enough to produce abstinence reactions when administration of the drug is stopped. The addict uses heroin to avoid the abstinence syndrome as in the following examples:

Time since last dose

12 hours	Yawning, running nose, tearing, gooseflesh
18 hours	Muscular aches, twitches, abdominal cramps, loss of appetite
24 hours	Agitation, insomnia, profuse sweating, vomiting, diarrhea, hypertension, elevated or lowered blood sugar
48 hours	Maximum intensity of all signs and symptoms
72 hours	Rapidly-decreasing intensity
7 days	Persistent insomnia, irritability, anxiety
6 months	Stable state

In the chronic state, ACTH production is depressed, and the male heroin addict may be impotent. Frequently female addicts stop menstruating.

The predominant feature of the street addict is "hustling." In order to pay for an increasingly expensive habit, most addicts turn to property crimes. They rarely are involved in violent crime, and the amount of property crime is probably exaggerated by both the addict and the police. Hustling often has a manic quality to it and provides the addict with a clear identity. The role of "addict" is a positive one often accorded status within the subculture. Hustling brings the addict into contact with straight society only when the "square" can be "used" as part of a "con." The addict has often been described as withdrawn from society and as being "passive." "Hustling" and "copping" are quite the opposite. The heavy user works an 18-hour day to maintain a habit. It may well be that some of the sociopathic behaviors described in the addict are a function more of situation than of personality.

If untreated the abstinence syndrome is fatal only in patients with significant intercurrent disease.

The abstinence syndrome of other opioids, including methadone, is similar to heroin with the exception of meperidine (Demerol). Myoclonic jerks and generalized seizures occur in meperidine withdrawal and are preceded by extreme restlessness, profuse sweating, and isolated muscle twitches.

Treatment. Long-term treatment of the opiate-dependent patient should be conducted by physicians trained in this treatment. Acute treatment of chronic opiate dependence requires admission to a drug-free environment where complete medical and psychiatric examinations with appropriate laboratory studies are carried out. Keep in mind:

1. The patient may both wish to withdraw and be reluctant to withdraw. The latter side of his ambivalence may lead him to "cop dope" while in the hospital or to bring his "stash" along.
2. Multiple drug abuse is common. A careful history regarding use and abuse of other drugs—especially barbiturates and other depressants—is man-

datory to avoid the mixed barbiturate-opiate withdrawal, which may terminate fatally if untreated.

Three choices of treatment are open:

1. *"Cold turkey:"* The regimen is simple: do not substitute or continue opiates. The abstinence syndrome may be softened by the use of phenothiazines or minor tranquilizers. Phenothiazines (chlorpromazine 25 to 75 mg every four to six hours) are preferable because of their sedating, antianxiety, and antiemetic qualities. Chloral hydrate may be given at bedtime. This may be the preferred treatment for pseudoheroin addicts where clear-cut physiological evidence of the abstinence syndrome is not apparent. The severity of "cold-turkey" withdrawal varies with the setting in which it takes place.
2. *Rapid reduction:* The patient is stabilized for two days on a dose and frequency of morphine sufficient to prevent the appearance of abstinence phenomena. This rarely requires more than 30 mg of morphine every six hours. Withdrawal of the drug then takes place over a period of five to ten days. This may be extended in cases of significant intercurrent disease. Meperidine-dependent individuals should be stabilized on meperidine and then withdrawn.
3. *Methadone substitution:* This is the preferred method, since it avoids parenteral drugs. Initially the patient is stabilized on a dose of oral methadone sufficient to suppress opiod withdrawal phenomena. Since methadone is relatively slow-acting, it is useful to start with 20 mg orally on admission, provided clear-cut signs (not symptoms) of abstinence phenomena are present. This dose may be repeated in 12 hours. Day 2 should be at the same level. Methadone is then withdrawn over a period of 3 to 7 days. Insomnia is treated with a sedative such as chloral hydrate, an antihistamine, or phenothiazine.

Abstinence phenomena persist for as long as six months. As with depressant dependence this is a crucial period, and maximal efforts at resocialization and rehabilitation are necessary. Long-term success has been claimed for several different kinds of treatment programs such as:

1. *Ex-addict programs.* Run by ex-addicts, these programs require a high degree of motivation. In return they offer a supportive setting for the ex-addict.
2. *Enforcement programs.* Physicians on licensure probation because of addiction respond well to this approach.
3. *Methadone maintenance programs.* Started by Dole and Nyswander in New York, these programs maintain addicts on levels of methadone (80 to 120 mg/day) or methadone substitutes which block euphoria. This substitute addiction allows for social rehabilitation of the addict and decreases the

economic loss to society. Methadone maintenance programs remain somewhat controversial. With selected addicts and adequate rehabilitation services, they have effectively returned addicts to social functioning. Unselected addicts in poorly-run programs with few rehabilitation services continue to use a wide variety of drugs and continue their criminal careers.

4. *Morphine antagonist programs.* These programs involve maintaining the addict on small doses of morphine antagonists such as cyclazocine. The antagonist makes the patient highly resistant to the euphoric as well as physiologic effects of morphine or heroin. According to conditioning theory, these drugs provide immunization against drug-seeking behavior by elimination of the reward properties of the heroin.

Clinical Course and Prognosis.   The likelihood for recovery from opiate dependence improves over time. Something like a two-percent annual recovery rate is reasonable, as is a two-percent annual death rate. A cohort of addicts thus will disappear over 25 years, half dying prematurely, half becoming abstinent. The realization that traditional treatment programs (such as the Public Health Hospital at Lexington) had practically no impact on long-term outcome led to the development of newer programs. It seems clear at this point that ex-addict therapeutic communities, parole programs, and methadone maintenance programs each improve the long-term outcome while appealing to different subcategories of opiate-dependent individuals.

Medical Complications of Opiate Dependence.   Heroin is now a leading cause of death of teenagers in New York City. The mortality and morbidity of opiate dependence is impressive. The two-percent annual death rate stems both from violent deaths (homicide, suicide, accidents and OD's) and medical complications. Septic problems plague the heroin-dependent individual. Ranging from local infections at the injection site through "cotton" fever to raging septicemia, it includes endocarditis, mycotic aneurysms, septic pulmonary and cerebral emboli, hepatitis, tetanus, malaria and tuberculosis. The invading organisms may be highly unusual. In addition heroin has been associated with transverse myelopathy, paraplegia and encephalopathy. Opiate dependence may give biologic false positives in serologic tests.

Significant numbers of addicted mothers give birth to addicted infants. Signs of withdrawal in the newborn include irritability, hyperactivity, tremulousness, vomiting, diarrhea, fever and protracted high-pitch cry. Treatment can be in the form of tincture of opium one to two drops per pound of body weight as needed to suppress withdrawal, with reduction in dosage over the next ten days.

As methadone maintenance programs expand, more and more parents leave their methadone-laced orange juice in the refrigerator. The minimum lethal dose is 75 mg in adults and 10 mg in children. Daily maintenance in addicts is often in the 80-to-100 mg range, so one dose may be lethal to unsuspecting friends or family. In children and adults respiratory depression is the major problem.

Therapy is nalorphine 0.1 mg/kg intravenously repeated in one half to one third of the original dose two or three times at ten-minute intervals. Initial improvement is transitory and fractional doses of nalorphine may be required for longer periods. Analeptics are contraindicated and continuous attention to adequate ventilation and fluid and electrolyte balance is mandatory. Respiratory depression can persist for 48 hours.

CANNABIS ABUSE OR DEPENDENCE

Marijuana (grass, pot, gage, griefs, hay, hash, hemp, jive, locoweed, manicure, Mary Jane, Mezz, mor a grifa, mutah, rope, weed, Texas tea, Acapulco gold, etc.) is smoked (as a joint, reefer, roach, stick) in a holder, roach clip or pipe, or ingested in food. By 1976, 21 percent of all American adults had tried marijuana and eight percent were current users. The use of marijuana in high-school students increased throughout the 70's but now appears to have leveled off.

Dependence on marijuana remains a controversial issue. As research into its cognitive, behavioral and developmental effects proceeds, a complex picture develops. Clinically, dependence on marijuana most closely resembles dependence on alcohol or sedative-hypnotics. The concern and controversy over marijuana are more related to sociopolitical and moral-legal issues than to pharmacologic or psychiatric issues.

Pharmacology. Marijuana is derived from the plant Cannabis sativa. The resin, flowers, and leaves contain tetrahydrocannabinol (THC)—the active agent of marijuana. The potency of marijuana varies with its origin. Marijuana grown in the United States contains 0.2 percent of THC. In Mexico it has a THC content of one percent, while Jamaican and South Asian marijuana may have two to four percent THC. Hashish is composed of only the drug-rich resinous secretions of the flowers and is 5 to 12 percent THC. The effects of THC are dose dependent; the method of use, prior experience, set, and setting will significantly alter effects.

Tolerance does develop to the effects of THC, but requires high-frequency (more than once daily) use of "strong" marijuana over a prolonged period (two to ten years). As tolerance develops, intake is increased to reach the original level of "high." Almost no American users can be described as meeting the criteria of heavy usage of strong preparations for two years or more. Most of the American experience involves short- or long-term use of preparations containing low THC.

THC has mixed depressant and hallucinogenic properties. It is not a narcotic. The usual social "joint" will contain 2 to 10 mg of THC. The physical effects of this dosage are reddening of the conjunctiva, increased heart rate, dryness of the mouth, and irritation of the throat. It does not have a regular effect on appetite.

The psychological effects of low dosage include euphoria (high) with a feeling of detachment and relaxation. Sensations are more intense. Time is drawn out, and distance perceptions are distorted. There is a tendency toward distractibility, suggestibility, sociability, and hilarity. An individual at this level of "high" is not noticeably different from his normal state. At higher doses short-term memory impairment occurs as with alcohol. The ability to drive a car is significantly impaired. At higher doses psychedelic or psychotomimetic phenomena begin to appear.

Medical Use. Marijuana or THC currently has no legal medical use in the United States other than for research. THC has a variety of interesting properties being investigated for medical potential. Of particular interest is its potential use in glaucoma and as an antiemetic for those patients on cancer chemotherapy. This latter use shows particular promise.

Street Use. In some parts of the country users outnumber nonusers. The majority of men and women who have used marijuana appear to be reasonably conventional. The "pot head," stereotype and "antiestablishment" youth with an "amotivational syndrome" (lazy, slovenly-dressed hippie) is as inaccurate a picture of the marijuana user as is that of the skid row bum for the alcohol user.

Marijuana is used primarily in a social setting. It is not "pushed" by a pusher but rather offered by a friend. The "stepping-stone" theory that most heroin addicts used marijuana previously is accurate but does not go far enough. One can make an even better case for tobacco or alcohol as the drug of escalation. Probably the association of marijuana and heroin use is more related to their image as "underworld" drugs than to anything else. The "drug store" in the street scene sells both drugs. The situation is in some ways comparable to the liquor store selling colas, beer, and whiskey. There is a subtle inducement to "move up" to the "hard stuff."

Clinical Description of the Syndromes. Adverse reactions to marijuana are not common. In part this is related to the low THC content of marijuana used in this country. The majority of unpleasant reactions to marijuana are anxiety reactions or panic and occur in the novice. These panic states are related to the interaction of drug setting and set effects. The illicit nature of marijuana creates anxiety and fears of police and discovery by family. The anxiety leads to marked mood changes when mild distortions of self-image and time perception take place. Panic states and acute paranoia then appear. These reactions are transient and disappear quickly with gentle friendly reassurance. Flashbacks have been reported but apparently seldom need treatment.

Psychosis has been reported following long-term use. This has been seen mainly in Eastern countries where high-potency preparations are available. Early reports of psychosis or brain damage have not been replicated in the United States. Cannabis use among schizophrenic and borderline patients seems clearly to increase the risk of exacerbation of symptoms.

An acute delirium characterized by disorientation, confusion and memory impairment associated with heavy use has been described but is also rarely seen in this country.

Studies of long-term heavy users in Jamaica and Greece failed to reveal any evidence of deterioration of physical, mental, or social functioning which could be attributed solely to heavy cannabis use. The current research into the possibility of brain damage or potential for genetic damage is controversial, with neither effect proved nor disproved. Continued attempts to document subtle long-term behavioral or endocrine effects have also yielded little that is conclusive.

There are no known cases of death directly attributable to marijuana. That cannot be said of any other drug discussed in this chapter.

There are risks inherent in marijuana's use. The use of any psychoactive drug to provide a solution to a social or intrapsychic problem cannot be justified. Achieving sociability or intimacy or happiness with marijuana may prevent achieving the same state without continued use of drugs. Regular use of any drug to achieve important personal goals is likely to be self-defeating.

Medical Complications. By itself THC has not been shown to cause significant disease or death. The smoking of marijuana can cause decreased pulmonary function and long-term use can cause permanent lung damage resembling that found in other smokers. Cannabis use does induce tachycardia and may have a negative inotropic effect on the heart and thus should not be used with patients suffering from heart disease. Chronic use does cause a decrease in sperm production although the effect of this is unknown.

Clinical Course and Prognosis. Panic reactions clear up with little or no trouble. Psychotic reactions have a good prognosis. Developmental arrest is infrequent but can be serious.

Decriminalization continues to be a controversial sociopolitical issue. In effect decriminalization has been practiced in the courts for many years now. The direct costs of effective law "enforcement" and the indirect costs of criminalization of large numbers of youth are recognized as outweighing our prohibitive concern. Regulation seems inevitable. Prevention seems logical in the sense that all people need an education about drugs. Proper appreciation of effects of all drugs is most likely to produce wise use and less abuse of all drugs.

PHENCYCLIDINE TOXICITY

Phencyclidine (PCP, peace pill, angel dust, hog, "crystal," inside-outer) is a drug with complex effects and increasingly wide abuse. The complexity of its effects is revealed by the fact that emergency room physicians correctly identified only 8 of 61 patients as under PCP intoxication. The wide abuse is evident from recent studies indicating that 15 percent of high-school-age students have used PCP.[18] PCP has been discussed previously in Chapter 3.

Phencyclidine was developed originally as a surgical anesthetic, but removed from human use in 1965 because of emergent reactions (in anesthetic recovery).

In 1967 it became available for veterinary use, and ultimately all legitimate manufacture was stopped in 1978.

Abuse of PCP began in the 60's, and it was often used to "cut" other hallucinogens. It is often sold as "THC," mescaline, or "strong" gold marijuana.

One of the reasons for its current popularity is the ease with which it can be made at low cost in a "basement" lab.

Pharmacology. Phencyclidine has central-nervous-system depressant, convulsant, psychotomimetic, and sympathomimetic qualities. It can induce a "dissociative" state characterized by an "eyes open" coma similar to the dissociative anesthetic ketalor. PCP is available as a white powder or crystal—often sold as "crystal"—but it is also sold in tablet or capsule form. It is usually smoked in a "joint" but may be sniffed, ingested orally, injected intravenously, used in eye drops or rectally. The typical dose in a single "joint" is 1-3 mgs. PCP is a very lipid soluble and excretion is primarily through the kidneys and is enhanced markedly by the presence of acid urine. Effects generally begin within 5 minutes if smoked or 30 minutes if ingested and last 5 hours to a week or more depending on the dose. In the typical situation, 48 hours are required until the person feels normal. Chronic users may exhibit symptoms for extended periods after discontinuing use.

Phenomenology. In normal volunteers PCP produces a state nearly indistinguishable from schizophrenia and characterized by body image changes, loss of ego boundaries, depersonalization, insensitivity to pain and a related great physical strength.

Clinical Syndromes. Acute Overdose—Individuals with PCP overdose will become delirious, then progress through stupor, coma, convulsions and possibly death, depending on the dosage. There may be alteration of coma and hyperactivity. The coma is of the "eyes open" type with intact or hyperactive muscle tone in contrast to sedative OD in which the muscles are flaccid. Pupils are miotic or normal; often there is nystagmus. There is usually tachycardia with systolic and diastolic hypertension which may reach dangerous levels. Irregular respiratory patterns are seen. Rhabdomyolysis with myoglobinuria may be present.

Treatment is largely supportive. No drug has been found to be specifically helpful in PCP overdose. If the patient is comatose, gastric lavage should be done after intubation. Blood and urine samples should be sent for analysis. PCP is often adulterated with anticholinergic substances, so the use of phenothiazines, which are also anticholinergic, is generally not helpful and may exacerbate symptoms. Physostigmine may be helpful in these cases, but should not be used routinely and must be used with caution. Acidification of the urine with ascorbic acid 2 gms every 6 hours) may speed excretion. Specific therapies aimed at specific problems (i.e., intubation and ventilation for hypoxemia, diazoxide for hypertensive crisis or Dilantin for seizures) should be employed where indicated. Often, if the patient recovers from acute OD, he will progress to toxic psychosis.

Acute Confusional State. This may be the presenting state, or it may follow acute overdosage. It is characterized by disorientation, confusion, agitation, hallucinations, drooling, sweating, and delusions. A "blank stare" is often seen. Depending on dose and route of administration, it will typically last one to eight hours, but may persist for a week or more.

Treatment. The patient should be placed in an environment which minimizes sensory stimulation. Restraints may be necessary. Vital signs should be monitored. Although no drug has been shown to be very effective, diazepam 10 to 20 mg orally may help calm the patient and may be repeated in doses of 10 to 15 mg if not used over a prolonged period of time.

Schizophreniform Psychosis. A psychosis much like paranoid or catatonic schizophrenia has been reported to persist following the above acute reactions. This may occur following one or several exposures. Clinically it is not distinguishable from schizophrenia, but it may be treatment resistant and persist for weeks. Treatment is similar to any functional psychosis, and phenothiazines are not contraindicated.[18]

Typical "Trip." The typical experience of a person taking the usual dose of 1-5 mg will be sedation and mild euphoria. Hallucinations and other perceptual distortions similar to LSD are common. Flashbacks are more common than with LSD.

Cohen[19] suggests that the amnesia induced during an acute episode may explain why users with a "bad trip" will continue to use PCP.

HALLUCINOGEN ABUSE

The psychedelic or psychotomimetic era is of relatively recent origin. Although hallucinogens have been readily available throughout history, their use until recently took place most often in a religious or mystical setting and was limited to a few people. Hoffman described the mind-altering effects of LSD-25 in 1938. Huxley wrote persuasively of the effects of hallucinogens in *The Doors of Perception* in 1954. The major impetus for hallucinogen use came in the late 1950's and early 1960's with the deification of Timothy Leary by a growing subculture.

Pharmacology. LSD-25 is the model drug, but the class includes both naturally-occurring and synthetic chemicals (see Table 8-5). These substances have similar characteristics. Although they may be habituating, they do not create physical dependence. Tolerance develops rapidly and disappears rapidly. They are extremely potent in that minute quantities produce major effects, yet they are safe in terms of direct drug morbidity and mortality. Their mode of action is unknown.

Table 8-5. Hallucinogens.

Chemical Class	Common Name	Natural Source
Lysergic Acid Derivatives		
d-lysergic acid diethylamid	LSD, Acid	
	Oloiuqui	Rivea Corymbosa
	Morning Glory Seeds	Ipomea Tricolor
Phenylethylamines		
	Mescaline	Lophophora Williamsii (Peyotl)
2–5 dimethoxy-4 ethylamphetamine	Doet	
2–5 dimethoxy-4 methyl amphetamine	DOM (STP)	
Myristicin		Nutmeg
Indolealkylamines		
	Psilocybin	Psilocybe Mexicana Heim
	Bufotenin	
Dimethyltryptamine	DMT	
Diethyltryptamine	DET	
Indolic Derivatives		
	Harmine	Peganum Harmdla
	Ibogaine	Tabernauttie Iboga
Piperidyl Benzilate Esters		
Phencyclidine	PDP (Sernyl)	
Cyclohexamine		
Tetrahydracannabinol	THC	Cannabis Sativa

Medical Use. The hallucinogens have been used in Europe in the course of psychotherapy. Research performed in the U.S. in the early 1970's on hallucinogen use in dying patients and in alcoholism never demonstrated conclusive positive results. Hallucinogens currently are not used clinically in the United States.

Street Use. Hallucinogens enjoyed a burst of popularity in the 1960's and early 1970's. Recent estimates indicate that they enjoy a small but continuing popularity. Motivation for use of psychedelics varies. Originally they were used to produce a religious-mystical state. Later they were used for their therapeutic or insight-providing potential. Widest use came when they were espoused as "mind or consciousness expanders" and as a means of "tripping." Route of administration was almost invariably oral.

Clinical Syndromes. The effects of the hallucinogens have specific dose-related impacts producing alteration in mood in association with a psychotic-like state of relatively brief duration.

The onset and length of the "trip" varies with the drug and the dosage. Characteristic of the hallucinogen psychoses is the vividness of the visual experience and the perceptual distortions—often useful as an aid in diagnosis. For most individuals the experience is impressive but neither profound nor malignant. Prolonged psychoses are possible, and acute panic reactions are common and potentially dangerous. Repeated use of hallucinogens almost never occurs in patients with a prior stable background.

The major risks in hallucinogen abuse stem from their use to facilitate "closeness" or reduce "personal problems." A second risk is accidental or suicidal death during the acute intoxication. The third problem is that of subsequent "flashbacks" occurring up to 18 months after the last dose. These brief recurrences of a state similar to the original episode are anxiety producing, because the subject is aware he has not taken the drug and fears for his sanity. The use of low dosages of phenothiazines is helpful for patients experiencing troublesome flashbacks.

Clinical Course and Prognosis. The acute "trip" is short-lived. Most persons will recover spontaneously in 24 to 36 hours. During this period they may need protection from doing harm to themselves or others. Referral to a local self-help peer group is often preferable to hospitalization. Since the subject can never know exactly what drug he has taken, use of phenothiazines is contraindicated in the acute situation. Diazepam or Benadryl can be used to calm or sedate the acutely-agitated patient experiencing a "bad trip."

Most persons who take hallucinogens soon become disenchanted with them. Less than one percent of one-time users will go on to a repeated chronic use and become "acid heads."

The early findings of chromosome changes associated with hallucinogen use have not proven to be clinically relevant. However, these early findings served to dissuade many youths from using hallucinogens.

OTHER DRUGS OF DEPENDENCE AND ABUSE

Any agent that 1) produces a sense of well-being, however transitory, and/or 2) reduces pain and/or 3) produces an alteration in the state of consciousness has potential for abuse and dependence. Thus there are instances where people have become dependent on steroids because of their tendency to produce a mild sense of euphoria. A wide variety of pain-reducing agents have potential for dependence, in addition to analgesics already discussed under opiate dependence. Attention should be paid to a problem thus far poorly recognized in this country— abuse or dependence on aspirin, phenacetin and propoxyphene (Darvon).

Aspirin

Few people consider aspirin a drug and thus ignore its potential for medical mischief. In the U.S. some 44 million tablets of aspirin are ingested each 24 hours. The problems associated with this high level of use/abuse are many. Everyone should be aware of aspirin's corrosive effect on the gastrointestinal tract, with associated increase in blood-loss leading to or aggravating peptic-ulcer disease or gastritis. In addition, aspirin is a potentially lethal drug in an acute overdose. The fatal adult dose can be as low as 60 "adult" aspirin. Chronic salicylism is associated with dizziness, tinnitus, headache, decreased hearing and increasing mental confusion. At higher levels aspirin can produce a toxic encephalopathy with incoherent speech, hallucinations, distortion, hypoglycemia, convulsions and ultimately coma and death.

Phenacetin

Phenacetin is even more dangerous than aspirin when used abusively. "APC" is widely available in over-the-counter products and is being compounded in many prescription drugs as well. It is most commonly abused by persons who are primarily anxious and/or depressed or by other persons with chronic pain. Abuse is currently defined as ingestion of 1 gm per day for one year or more, although smaller doses over longer periods also qualify. Phenacetin abuse can lead to hemolytic anemia, interstitial nephritis and urinary-tract cancer.

Propoxyphene

Darvon's potential for abuse is also poorly recognized. Although rarely a drug of preference, it is often abused as a substitute for opiates by heroin addicts. It is used by amphetamine abusers to counteract the effects of injecting large doses of amphetamines. It's worth noting that in some areas Darvon is used to produce "highs" among high school students. Its ready availability for this purpose makes its potential for abuse high. We know, for example, that over 80 percent of people familiar with Darvon will use it to treat themselves without consulting their physician. Overprescription of Darvon by physicians is a major factor in its abuse. It can cause death rapidly when taken in a suicide attempt.

Finally there is a wide variety of substances which are usually sniffed, inhaled or ingested to produce an altered state of consciousness. A list of the more common deliriants follows:

Gasoline	
Commercial Solvents	In glue, lighter or cleaning fluids, toluene, xylene, benzene, naphthol, hexane, acetone, trichlorethylene, carbon tetrachloride.
Aerosols	Propellants in many household and commercial aerosol sprays such as insecticides, deodorants, glass chillers and hair sprays.
Anesthetics	Chloroform, ether, nitrous oxide amylnitrite.
Miscellaneous "hallucinogens"	Wheat and aspirin, rosewood seeds, niacin, clinitest tablets, dog ricket tablets, antiparkinson drugs, mandrax, romilar, many atropine-like drugs, insulin.

There is an endless supply of these products available from the average grocery or hardware store. For the most part they are volatile hydrocarbon solvents. The effects parallel the effects of alcohol or barbiturates. At low doses they are disinhibiting, while at higher doses they produce delirium, progressive sedation, and culminate in coma and death. There is a multitude of medical and psychological complications attendant upon deliriant abuse, including acute kidney, bone marrow, and liver toxicity, as well as temporary and permanent alteration in psychologic and neurophysiologic function. The mortality associated with use of deliriants can be the result of respiratory arrest due to central-nervous-system depression, cardiac arrest, or simple suffocation by the too-common plastic bag.

SELF-MEDICATION BY PHYSICIANS

Clinicians often use denial, the unconscious mechanism which allows one to resist recognition of an aspect of reality. When this is combined with a sense of omnipotence most clinicians share, they may use dependency-producing drugs with the conviction that "dependence can't happen to me!"

Clinicians may rationalize both initial use and continued use on one of several grounds. "I give so much to my patients, I deserve a little relief from pain." "I need it to keep me going." "The patients need me, so I can't stop taking it now." The reasons given by clinicians for their original use of dependency-producing drugs are "overwork," "chronic pain," and "fatigue." Little do these clinicians realize that the "overwork" and attendant "fatigue" are often the result of the clinician's neurotic "need to be needed."[20]

Many clinicians are unaware that tension or depression is a frequent antecedent to drug dependence. Tension or depression may accompany success in clinical practice, because success can lead to overwork and fatigue which drugs may seem to relieve at first (a touch of Demerol, a couple of drinks, or some Ritalin). About one or two percent of physicians will become dependent on drugs in their careers. Abuse of mood-altering drugs is the most common sign of psychiatric illness in physicians.

Ready access to drugs is an important contributing factor. The clinician has a ready supply. Access to "samples" makes the temptation to seek relief from discomfort or fatigue by use of self-prescribed medication hard to resist. Further increasing the likelihood of self-medication is the clinician's reluctance to ask colleagues for treatment of minor problems. A useful aphorism in this regard is "a doctor who treats himself/herself (or his/her own family) has a fool for a doctor and an idiot for a patient."

Prevention is much more important than treatment. Clinicians should know that self-medication is a prelude to dependency. A sensitivity to depression in oneself may allow one to seek professional help. Once a dependency problem develops, physicians have a good prognosis in programs which require compulsory supervision, with one's licensure hanging in the balance. Some 92 percent of drug-dependent California physicians in such a program become abstinent.

Drug dependency strikes one's family and colleagues with some regularity. The earlier this is recognized and confronted, the better the outcome.

Drug Dependence—Alcohol

Alcohol is the most widely used and abused drug in the U.S. today, if nicotine and caffeine are not included. Current estimates indicate that there are approximately 10 million alcoholics. It is used by over 70 percent of the population and, of those who drink, about 18 percent are heavy drinkers. It is one of the most common problems encountered in the practice of medicine, accounting for 10 percent of all health care costs in the United States. Yet it continues to be underdiagnosed in all but the more advanced stages.

Recognition and the Role of the Physician

Attitudes regarding alcohol use and abuse are important. Many of us have positive attitudes toward drinking and drinkers in general (and many or most of us drink), yet we as a society and as professionals still morally condemn those with drinking problems. Alcoholism is often seen as a sign of moral weakness. How we view our own use is obviously important. Alcohol and drug abuse is prevalent among physicians. It is estimated that one in ten physicians who drink has a problem with alcohol. How many of us fail to see problem drinking in our patients because then we would have to confront our own possible vulnerability?

Ignorance is another important factor, although not as important as attitudes. Common myths held about alcoholism are that "a typical alcoholic is a skid row bum" (only three to five percent are), "alcoholics don't respond to treatment" (up to 60 to 80 percent of alcoholics may be helped by treatment), and "there's nothing I can do for them until they stop drinking" (you can do a lot, although you can't make them stop drinking). Ignorance is related to negative attitudes, in that the myths justify the attitudes.

Diagnosis (also see previous section). It is more complicated with alcohol since it is a legal, social drug. In practice an alcoholic is often defined as someone who drinks more than the doctor! The best overall definition of alcoholism is probably "use of alcohol in such a way as to interfere with function, socially, occupationally, interpersonally, and/or physiologically." Several diagnostic systems have been proposed. Diagnosis in the early stages of problem drinking (often before any evidence of physiologic damage) is more difficult yet much more helpful. It is important to ask about alcohol use with *all* of your patients. Questions such as "How do you use alcohol?" as part of the *regular* history are more productive than "How much do you drink?" If you suspect a problem, asking directly whether the patient thinks he/she has a problem is helpful and often productive. The Michigan Alcoholism Screening Test[21] is an adjunct to collecting data and facilitating discussion.

Pharmacology. Alcohol is primarily a CNS depressant, most similar to barbiturates and other sedative-hypnotics. It exerts its effects first on the cerebral cortex, thus affecting those functions requiring the highest integration, such as abstract thinking, and those functions based on prior experience and training. The "stimulant" aspect of alcohol comes from its disinhibiting effect. That is, depressing cortical function reduces self-restraint, so the intoxicated individual feels better about doing and feeling things he/she normally wouldn't. Thus, while alcohol physiologically depresses sexual function in humans, people often feel more sexually enhanced while intoxicated. The same is true of most motor functions such as driving.

The effects of alcohol are, in general, directly related to the blood level. However, more marked effects are noticed when the blood level is rising than when it is falling. It is rapidly absorbed from the stomach and small intestine. Oxidation occurs in the liver and is almost complete, so that little is excreted unchanged. This occurs at a constant rate dependent on body and liver weight; in the average person this is about 10 ml per hour (two-thirds to one ounce of whiskey). Intoxication in most people is obvious with blood levels of approximately 100 to 150 mg percent, but the "legal" level varies from state to state. Levels of 400 to 500 mg percent are often lethal.* The CNS depressant effects of alcohol and other sedative-hypnotics are synergistic, a fact of which patients taking sedative-hypnotics should be made aware.

Tolerance. Tolerance to both the behavioral and physiologic effects of alcohol can be developed. As with other CNS depressants, there is increased metabolism of the drug, but much of the tolerance occurs because the individual learns how to act while intoxicated. Cross-tolerance occurs with other CNS depressants, such as sedative-hypnotics and general anesthetics.

ALCOHOLISM

There is no unitary syndrome of alcoholism; alcoholism is a broad term used to describe a range of behaviors, difficulties, and syndromes. In our opinion, no attempt to date to classify the various "subtypes" of alcoholism has proved clinically useful. DSM-III is too new to make comment on. There are, however, important commonalities in classification we think are useful.

The most important of these is that drinking progresses along a continuum from abstinence, through social drinking, to problem drinking and alcoholism. It is common to distinguish between a predepressant, or prodromal phase, and a problem, dependent, or addicted phase. Thus, alcoholism begins with learning to drink, often beginning in the teenage years. Social drinking is characterized by a

---

*Four ounces of whiskey taken on an empty stomach normally produces a blood level of about 65 to 90 mg percent alcohol.

"take it or leave it" kind of feeling about alcohol: It doesn't matter to a person whether he drinks or not. Social drinkers seldom, if ever, become significantly intoxicated. During this first phase, the pre-alcoholic will notice *relief from distress* or emotional pain associated with alcohol. Progression to heavy drinking and seeking out this relief follows. It then becomes the primary mode of dealing with emotional distress. This constitutes the earliest stage of alcoholism. Drinking becomes more common and begins to occupy an increasingly central role in the affected individual's life. For example, the availability of alcohol at a party becomes more important than the people there. The individual becomes pre-occupied with drinking, and may begin to look forward to the next drink, such as after work or at noon luncheon. Tolerance may develop, necessitating increased amounts and/or frequency of drinks, and drinking episodes lead to more severe intoxication more frequently.

As the illness progresses, the first indication of problems usually occurs in the interpersonal relationships of the early alcoholic, that is, with the spouse and family. This occurs because of the preoccuption with alcohol (it becomes more important than the spouse) and also because the early alcoholic, often, but not always, becomes a different person while intoxicated. This often means abusive or self-destructive behavior which is disinhibited by the alcohol. At this point, "blackouts" may begin to occur. Blackouts are episodes of amnesia not associated with gross intoxication. The individual simply doesn't remember events that occurred while he was intoxicated.

During this state of problem drinking or early alcoholism, the drinking episodes are well-rationalized ("everyone does it," "just having a little fun with the boys/girls"), and its destructive effects are denied. Denial, in fact, is characteristic of alcoholics and occurs both in the drinker and spouse. Denial is an unconscious mechanism and, as such, the individual is actually not aware of or selectively ignores aspects of reality. Thus, the drinker will not be aware of gradual isolation from spouse, or failing work performance, or will rationalize these events, using alternative explanations. The spouse and family may ignore repeated incidents, and not confront the alcoholic with their perceptions of difficult behavior. The family, employer or colleagues and friends often unwittingly help the alcoholic stay alcoholic. When this occurs, it is termed "enabling the alcoholic." The most important aspect of enabling is that it protects the alcoholic from the natural consequences of his actions, thus facilitating the denial inherent to the illness. An example of this is the husband who "overlooks" his wife's obvious intoxication when he gets home, or explains it away by saying, "She's bored, sitting home all day. What are a couple of drinks?"

As the illness progresses, alcohol becomes increasingly central in the person's life, and drinking may become almost continuous. Isolation from the family continues and worsens and may result in expulsion from the family. Blackouts become more common. The alcoholic may be arrested for drunk driving and/or become involved in accidents. Job performance fails and job loss is common. Health effects begin to show up as weight loss, malnutrition, peptic-ulcer disease, liver disease, and so forth.

In this more advanced stage it often becomes increasingly difficult for the individual to maintain denial. Following one or more of these major sequelae from drinking, the person will seek help, frequently from Alcoholics Anonymous. Many make some recovery, some totally recover. A few (3-5 percent) will continue on the downhill course and elect a skid row type of existence. It is also in this stage that doctors will be more likely to make the diagnosis, although even here many will not. It is also here, in the stage of chronic alcoholism, that many of the physiologic sequelae become manifest. The description of the numerous physical illnesses associated with chronic alcoholism is well-covered in most internal-medicine texts and will not be dealt with here.

Thus, an important commonality underlying this concept of alcoholism is that it is a progressive, chronic, relapsing illness. In this way it is analogous to diabetes mellitus or rheumatoid arthritis. Another important point is that the person destined to become an alcoholic starts by social drinking and that there are indications of problems early in the illness. One does not have to wait until it reaches end-stage proportions to make the diagnosis.

Management. The single most important aspect of management is recognition. One cannot treat something that is unrecognized. As with most illnesses, early recognition offers greater chances for successful treatment. Thus, it is important to have an idea of your own attitudes towards drinking and alcoholism and to examine your own drinking behavior. Will your attitudes impede your recognition and treatment of problem drinking in others? Secondly, it is important to keep the characteristics of the illness in mind, and to look aggressively for signs of problem drinking in *all* your patients. Use of standard questions and questionnaires (such as MAST) are helpful.

Once you have identified drinking as a possible problem, it is important to discuss your concern with your patient, and the spouse if necessary. This should be done after a complete history and physical examination and when laboratory results are back so that you can present the evidence of problem drinking to the patient. It is important to do this in a factual and nonjudgmental way. Expect defensiveness, denial, and hostility since these are part of the disease. Try to minimize your response to these provocations.

Remember that it isn't up to you to make the patient quit drinking, but rather it is your responsibility to advise of your diagnosis, recommendations, and concern. Don't be discouraged by an initially-unfavorable response; often it takes several such confrontations to erode the denial, but you may plant seeds that will bear fruit in the future.

Don't be an enabler yourself, minimizing or ignoring signs of problems. Don't prescribe sedative-hypnotics to someone with a drinking problem unless it is for withdrawal. Many alcoholics seek these out, and most often their use only complicates the problem.

Timing is important in that alcoholics are more likely to be willing to confront their problem during a crisis. One such time, often missed by doctors, is after an accident or illness associated with drinking. The "reflective lull" following a binge is another good one.

Once the diagnosis is established and accepted by the patient, at least to some degree, what do you do next? First, does the patient need detoxification? If so, see the section on depressant-drug syndromes in Chapter 7. Also, there may be a facility in your community that specializes in detoxification/withdrawal.

As for long-term management, the first thing to do is decide how involved you want to be. If you find you "can't stand" alcoholics and can't get over that even after reflection, then referral may be the best choice. If you want to be involved, you can do so to the extent you choose. Again, recognition is the single most important aspect of management.

At any rate, get to know your community resources for the treatment of alcoholism. You may want to visit them to establish a liaison and to get a better idea of which patients would do well there. Go to an AA meeting—most AA groups are more than happy to have you visit.

Once you've done the above, we hope you'll begin to be actively involved in the treatment of those patients with drinking problems. The long-term treatment generally consists of group and individual psychotherapy, and education about alcoholism. The family is becoming more and more involved in treatment. AA and Al-Anon (an AA-like organization for families of alcoholics) are still a mainstay of treatment. A comprehensive discussion of the long-term management of alcholics is beyond the scope of this book.

Disulfiram (Antabuse). You should consider prescribing disulfiram to all your alcoholic patients. Disulfiram is a drug that interferes with alcohol metabolism. When a person taking disulfiram drinks even a small amount of alcohol (7 ml) there is an accumulation of acetaldehyde in the blood which causes a very unpleasant syndrome consisting of flushing, headache, nausea and vomiting, sweating, hypotension, anxiety and weakness. In severe reactions, it can be dangerous and even fatal, but death rarely occurs. The usual dose of disulfiram is 250 mg daily.

All patients taking disulfiram should be warned about the effects, and given a wallet card stating they are on Antabuse. The drug causes few if any problems by itself. It is useful primarily in helping an alcoholic to get over an impulse to take that first drink. Relative contraindications include psychosis or dementia, severe depression, suicidal impulses, or severe cardiovascular disease.

Psychotic Syndromes Associated with Alcoholism

There are several syndromes of psychotic proportions associated with alcohol use. These include pathological intoxication, alcoholic hallucinosis, and alcoholic paranoia (see Chapter 2). These are rarely used terms that describe a variety of disorders which manifest psychotic symptomatology, such as auditory hallucinations or paranoid delusions, and seem to be associated with alcohol use. They can occur while the individual is intoxicated, or may become more manifest following withdrawal, and they may persist for months after the last use of the drug. They are generally treated with neuroleptics such as Haldol. Such individuals should be referred to a psychiatrist.

Alcoholism and Depression

The exact relationship between alcoholism and the affective disorders remains controversial. Some authorities see alcoholism as a manifestation of an underlying or "masked" depression, or as a syndrome to be included in a "depressive spectrum." That there is some genetic link between the two disorders has been suggested but not conclusively demonstrated. It may also be that depression is a phenomenon secondary to alcoholism. At any rate, we believe the best course of action is to achieve abstinence for several weeks or months before attempting a trial of antidepressants, in the absence of clear indications such as severe or suicidal depression.

REFERENCES

1. Becker HS: Becoming a marijuana user. *AJS* 59:235-42, 1953
2. Mendelson J, Mello N: Biologic concomitants of alcoholism. *NEJM* 301:912-921, 1979
3. Pihl RO, Spiers P: Individual characteristics in the ideology of drug abuse progress. *In Experimental Personality Research*, Vol. 8, New York, Academic Press, Inc., pp. 93-195, 1978
4. Frederick C: Current trends in suicidal behavior in the U.S. *Am J Psychother* 32:172-200, 1978
5. Blum RH: *Society and Drugs.* San Francisco, Jossey-Bass, 1970
6. Rockwell, D: Alcohol and marijuana-social-problem perspective. *Brit J Addict* 68:209-14, 1973
7. Wikler A: Dynamics of drug dependence, implications of a conditioning theory for research and treatment. *Arch Gen Psychiatry* 28:611-17, 1973
8. Chien I, Gerard D, Lee R, et al: *The Road to H: Narcotics, Delinquency, and Social Policy*, New York, Basic Books, 1964
9. Whitfield C, Thompson G, Lamb A, et al: Detoxification of 1,024 alcoholic patients without psychoactive drugs. *JAMA* 239:1409-10, 1978
10. Cummings NA: Turning bread into stones, our modern anti-miracle. *Am Psychol* 34(12):1119-1129, 1979
11. _____. *Sleeping Pills, Insomnia, and Medical Practice.* Institute of Medicine Study, National Academy of Sciences, Washington, D.C., 1979
12. Wikler A: Diagnosis and treatment of drug dependence of the barbiturate type. *Am J Psychiatry* 125:758-65, 1968
13. Watkins, C: Use of amphetamines by medical students. *South Med J* 63:923-29, 1970

14. Ellinwood EW, Sudilovsky, A: Evolving behavior in the clinical and experimental amphetamine (model) psychosis. *Am J Psychiat* 130:1088-93, 1973

15. Spensley J, Rockwell D: Psychosis during methylphenidate abuse. *NEJM* 286:880-81, 1972

16. Rockwell D, Ostwald P: Amphetamine use and abuse in psychiatric patients. *Arch Gen Psychiatry* 18:612-16, 1968

17. Lindesmith A: *Addiction and Opiates.* Chicago, Aldine, 1968

18. Lerner S, Burns RS: Phencyclidine use among youth. *In* Peterson R, Stillman R: NIDA Monograph 21, Washington, D.C., U.S. Government Printing Office, 1978

19. Cohen S: PCP (Angel Dust) new trends and treatment. *Drug Abuse and Alcoholism Newsletter* 7:1-3, 1978

20. Vaillant G, Sobowale N, McArthur C: Some psychological vulnerabilities of physicians. *NEJM* 287:372-75, 1972

21. Selzer ML: The Michigan Alcoholism Screening Test (MAST). *Am J Psychiatry* 127:1655-59, 1971

9

Practical Guide to Management of Common Sexual Problems

HOBART SEWELL, M.D.

Dramatic changes in attitudes about sexuality and sexual behavior have occurred in the past few years. More patients are coming to health care clinics with questions and problems regarding human sexuality. Patients continue to expect health professionals to be authorities on sexual issues. One survey indicates that between 15-25 percent of patients seen in the general practice of medicine have significant sexual problems. Sexual dissatisfactions are present in at least 50 percent of marriages. Increasingly, patients are requesting professional advice. This is due, in part, to the greater liberalization of the subject plus recent advances in the field. Yet, with all the information and changes, myths, misconceptions, conflicts and malfunctions continue to plague our society and our patients. Sexual maladies are and will always be a part of the human condition.

Most sexual problems can be diagnosed and treated by primary care professionals. This is especially true if an adequate sexual history is obtained and if the disorder is properly diagnosed. In probably no other area can primary prevention be more effective than in the area of sexuality. Estimates are that 75-90 percent of sexual problems can be resolved in the office by the informed, concerned health care professional.

ASSESSMENT OF SEXUAL PROBLEMS

Sexual History

A sexual history should be routinely included in the assessment of all psychiatric and medical patients. General principles to be taken into consideration when obtaining the history are:

1. Ask specific detailed questions—the most important principle.
2. Never assume a patient's sexual information is totally accurate or complete.
3. Be supportive and nonjudgmental.
4. Try to use language appropriate to the patient without compromising information gathering.
5. Maintain a professional attitude with a sensitive, positive regard—a patient should feel, even be told, that if the discussion becomes uncomfortable, it can be stopped at any time.
6. There is never an uninvolved partner in sexual dysfunction in a relationship lasting more than two years; therefore some assessment of the relationship is important.
7. Sexual problems can be devastating to people's lives.
8. Offer education and information throughout history taking, as well as realistic positive reassurance that something can be done about the dilemma.

The patient should be encouraged to present his concerns (present illness) in detail, and this can be followed by more specific questions to better outline the origins, course, and differential diagnosis of the problem.

As a part of every complete non-crisis history and physical examination, open-ended nonintrusive questions should be asked. They could be included as part of genitourinary systems review, or on a history form reviewed by a nurse practitioner, paramedic, nurse, or doctor.

Examples of open-ended nonintrusive questions are:

1. Have there been any problems with your sexual relationship?
2. Has there been any change in your sexual relating?
3. Has anything been affecting your sexual interest and activity?

If there is a positive response on the part of the patient, the health professional will want to pursue the history-taking to determine the specific nature of the sexual difficulty. The most effective question is, "Tell me what happens in a typical encounter." Many patients reply, "What do you mean?" One then says, "How often do you have sex? Who initiates it? How is that communicated? How long is foreplay? What happens in foreplay? How long does intercourse last? Do both have orgasm? What happens after orgasm?" It would be important to know if there was a time when sexual relating was satisfying to the patient and partner. If so, what things happened to bring about the change? This is important for differential diagnosis as well as prognosis. Questions related to specific sexual disorders for men and women will further delineate the problem:

I. *Male dysfunctions*
  1. Erectile dysfunction (impotence):
    A. What percent of time do you experience erectile failure?
    B. Are there times when you do not have erectile difficulties?
    C. Do you have problems with erections during masturbation?
    D. Do you have the same difficulty with other partners?
    E. Do you have early morning erections?
  2. Premature ejaculation:
    A. How many strokes before ejaculation occurs?
    B. What affects the length (frequency, partner, alcohol, drugs, etc.)?
    C. Is the same problem present with masturbation?
    D. Has this always been the pattern?
  3. Retarded ejaculation:
    A. What percent of the time do you have ejaculations?
    B. Has this always been the pattern?
    C. Do you ejaculate with masturbation? Oral stimulation? Partner stimulation? Anal penetration?
    D. Do you experience the same problem with other partners?

II. *Female dysfunctions*
  1. Preorgasmic (never experienced an orgasm):
    A. Degree of arousal and stimulation:
      (1) As you are being touched and stimulated, do you become excited? How?
      (2) How much lubrication or wetness do you have?
      (3) Does your partner stimulate you in the right way?
    B. Attention to erotic stimulation:
      (1) While your partner (or self) is stimulating you, what are you thinking about?
      (2) Tell me about the last time you tried to reach orgasm. How did you feel?
    C. Partner interaction:
      (1) What does your partner think about your being nonorgasmic? What does he do and say? Do you talk about it?
  2. Secondary nonorgasmic:
    A. Ask the following questions:
      (1) When was the last time you had an orgasm?
      (2) What percent of time do you have successful orgasmic experiences during love-making?
      (3) Do you experience nonorgasm with all partners?
      (4) What do you think keeps you from having orgasms?

   B. Explore psychological causes for inhibition:
      (1) Attitude of partner.
      (2) Performance anxiety.
      (3) Degree of anxiety.
      (4) Depression.
      (5) Fatigue.
      (6) Stress.
   C. Explore physiological causes for inhibition:
      (1) Alcohol intake.
      (2) Drugs.
      (3) Medical complications (diabetic, etc.).
      (4) Pain.
      (5) Surgical complications (hysterectomy, etc.).
3. Vaginismus (involuntary vaginal spasm leading to dyspareunia):
   A. Explore the possibility of:
      (1) Rigid restrictive, strict moral background, religious or otherwise.
      (2) Rape, molestation, incest or other traumatic incidences.
      (3) Ignorance and misinformation about sex.
      (4) Severe guilt from sexual conflicts.

III. *Sexuality, intimacy, life events*
   1. Relationship between sex and other areas of functioning:
      A. What other problems are present? Which are the most pressing?
      B. What is the relationship between them and sexual dysfunction?
      C. How well do you relate with your partner in general?
      D. Can you talk about sexual problems?
      E. Do you love your partner?
      F. What happens if your problems (including sexual) are not resolved?
      G. What attempts have you made to correct the problems? How helpful have they been?

Assessment and Differential Diagnosis

The examiner must be familiar with the physiology and nuances of human sexuality. Much of the pioneering work in these areas has resulted from the investigations of Masters and Johnson,* and it is summarized below:

Female
   Excitement (the early stage of sexual arousal):
      Lubrication—10-20 seconds.
      Inner ⅔ of vagina lengthens and distends.
      Uterus pulls up and away from the vagina.

---

*Author's summary. Refer to 1) Masters WH, Johnson VE: *Human Sexual Inadequacy*. Boston, Little, Brown and Co., 1970, and 2) Masters WH, Johnson VE: *Human Sexual Response*. Boston, Little, Brown and Co., 1966.

Clitoral shaft swells (length increases 2-3 times; diameter increases also).

Labia minora increases in size 2-3 times.

Labia majora retract from midline.

75 percent of individuals experience sex flush (maculopapular rash) (epigastrium, chest, neck, face and forehead).

Nipple erection (myotonia) and breasts increase in size (25 percent).

Plateau (high stage of sexual excitement):

Orgasmic platform—outer ⅓ of vagina contracts to produce grasping effect.

Clitoris retracted under hood.

Sex skin reaction—labia minora increase in size (3 times) and turn bright red.

Uterus—fully elevated in the false pelvis.

Bartholin's glands secrete 1-3 drops.

Sex flush spreads over the breasts and lower abdomen, etc.

Breasts increase in size.

Areolae engorgement (cause nipples to appear less erect).

50 percent reduction in total length of clitoris just before orgasm.

Orgasm (total body response) (loss of voluntary control):

Orgasmic platform—strong rhythmic contractions (3-5 in mild orgasm to 8-15 in more intense ones—.8 seconds apart).

Uterus undergoes contractions similar to labor.

Seminal pooling of vaginal secretions.

Sphincter contractions.

Blood pressure increases systolic 30-80/diastolic 20-40.

Labia majora flattens, labia minora protrude.

Urinary meatus dilates.

Resolution (5-10 minutes):

Perspiration response—(back, thighs, and chest wall; occasionally forehead and upper lip).

Outer ⅓ vagina returns quickly to normal.

Inner ⅔ vagina returns more slowly to normal (5-8 minutes).

Clitoris returns to normal position out from under the hood in 5-10 seconds, and returns to normal size in 5-10 minutes.

Sex flush disappears in 5-10 seconds.

Breasts return slowly to normal size in 5-10 minutes (areolar swelling disappears in 5-10 seconds).

No refractory period.

Male

Excitement:

Erection—arteries dilate/vein valves close (reflex).

Nipple erection 60 percent.

Urethra lengthens and dilates (2 times).

Urination difficult or impossible.

Urethra meatus dilates.

Plateau:

   Cowper's gland secretion.

   Scrotum thickens and increases in size 50 percent; testicles increase in
      size 50 percent.

   Testicles fully elevated and rotate anteriorly.

   Ejaculatory inevitability (2-4 seconds).

   Corona of glans becomes more swollen.

Plateau and Orgasm:

   Carpopedal spasm (hyperextension of arch of the foot and claw-like con-
      tractions of the toes).

   Spastic contractions of the arms, legs, back, lower abdomen.

   Involuntary opening of the mouth in a gasping reaction to hyperventilation.

   Widespread vasocongestion—generalized myotonia.

   Facial muscles contract involuntarily.

   Involuntary, rapid pelvic thrusting immediately prior to orgasm.

Orgasm:

   Urethra and penis rhythmical contractions.

   Hyperventilation (greater than 40/minute) (3 times normal).

   Heart rate—100-180 (2 times normal).

   Blood Pressure—increases systolic 40-110/diastolic 20-50.

   Stage 1: Contractions of the accessory organs of reproduction—the vas
      deferens, the seminal vesicles, the ejaculatory duct, and the prostate—
      work to collect sperm and seminal fluid, which are compressed into the
      entrance to the prostatic urethra. The urethral bulb becomes greatly
      distended, this signals the inevitability of orgasm.

   State 2: Ejaculation of the seminal fluid is caused by regularly recurring
      contractions of the urethra and the muscles at the base of the penis and
      around the anus (2-4 seconds). Eight-tenths second intervals between
      the first 3-4 major responses. The urethra continues to contract slightly
      and irregularly for several seconds after the initial expulsive response.

Resolution

   Penis decreases to 50 percent larger than unstimulated state.

   Testes descend.

   Refractory period (15-20 minutes).

   Perspiration reaction immediately after ejaculation (soles of feet, palms
      of hands—occasionally on torso, head, face and neck) (⅓ of men).

Sexual problems have multiple etiologies. For this reason, it is important to
obtain a complete psychiatric and medical assessment and place special focus on
life events and the interaction between the patients and their partners. Many
patients will require a physical examination and indicated laboratory tests (e.g.,
CBC, Chem Panel, hormone levels). A drug history is essential as adverse effects
may interfere with sexual performance.

Common Sexual Myths. Many sexual concerns result from mistaken information or biases about human sexuality. In recent years, more scientific information has become available, and a more liberal view on normal sexual behavior has been accepted. Yet sexual myths remain common, and some of them include:

1. Anatomical differences, e.g., size of penis, vagina, breasts.
2. Masturbation being perverted, causing mental illness, etc.
3. Oral and anal sex as being perversions.
4. Simultaneous orgasm is necessary for satisfaction.
5. Sex during menstruation is harmful and taboo.
6. Deep penetration is harmful because semen may get into the abdomen.
7. Menopause or hysterectomy signals an end to sexual responsiveness.
8. Circumcised males have more trouble controlling ejaculation than uncircumcised males.
9. When Bartholin glands are gone, lubrication disappears.
10. Clitoral size, swelling and contact are necessary for orgasm.
11. Sex during pregnancy will precipitate labor or damage the baby.
12. Not having a vaginal orgasm (in today's world not being multiorgasmic) means you are less of a woman.
13. "If I can't satisfy my wife, I'm not much of a man."
14. "My husband must be homosexual, because he doesn't make love to me anymore."
15. Vaginal surgery alters female responsiveness.
16. "My son must be homosexual, because he doesn't have a steady girlfriend."

At times these myths can be corrected by simple reeducation and permission giving for change in sexual relating. At other times, they may persist.

Underlying Psychological Disorders. Individuals with major psychiatric disturbances frequently have sexual disorders. These include the personality states where the individual may be shy, distrusting, or inhibited; the neurotic, who fears intimacy; the depressed or manic, with marked changes in sexual interests; and the psychotic, with bizarre sexual ideation. Treatment should be directed towards the underlying psychiatric disturbance with psychotherapy and psycho-active medication.

Biologic-Medical Disorders. Most all major medical (metabolic, cardiovascular, degenerative, genitourinary, gynecologic, etc.) and surgical (genitourinary, cardiovascular) disorders will interfere with sexual performance. The general debilitation may also produce malaise, pain, and depression, with reduction in sexual interest.

Drug use and abuse also affect sexual functioning. CNS depressants (alcohol, etc.) tend to reduce interest while CNS stimulants (amphetamines, cocaine, etc.) may increase interest. Prescribed medication (e.g., antihypertensives, neuroleptics, anticholinergics) may impair sexual physiology. Patients may also be embarrassed about discussing sexual concerns and may prefer to focus on somatic complaints. Often the concerns presented are vague and deal indirectly with sexual issues. In these cases, it is helpful to directly question the patient and obtain a sexual history.

Treatment approach includes evaluating and correcting, if possible, the underlying state. With persistent disorders (coronary artery disease, paraplegia), it is important to discuss techniques, restrictions on frequency, and realistic expectations by both partners.

Sexual Aversion. A fear of sexuality may be present in both men and women. Frigidity was the common term given to women with this disorder. In men, aversion typically is diagnosed by withdrawal and disinterest in sexual relating. At times it may be associated with homosexuality and with an aversion toward heterosexuality. At other times it may be with individuals with special physical or psychological characteristics. Causes are multiple and include biologic factors, prior sexual experience, highly inhibited life styles, and myths. In individual relationships, general dissatisfaction and especially repressed anger may be responsible.

Treatment approaches include individual or couples' therapy and behavior modification. It is important to look for the presence and source of repressed anger in both men and women.

Relationship Dysfunction. Sexual problems are commonly symptoms of a troubled relationship. Often there are many dissatisfactions which are noteworthy, yet the couple or the patient focuses more exclusively on sexual concerns. Loss of sexual interest is a frequent complaint, and outside relationships may be present.

In such cases it is important to focus the questioning on the interaction. Couples' therapy is the treatment of choice. Focusing merely on the sexual disorder will have limited beneficial effects or result in treatment failure.

Sexual Dysfunction. Cases do present where the specific sexual dysfunction (impotence, premature ejaculation, anorgasmia, etc.) is primary and where the disturbance in the relationship has followed. Sex therapy is the treatment of choice. Results are normally favorable, especially if motivation for treatment is present and if both partners are agreeable to accepting change.

OFFICE MANAGEMENT OF COMMON SEXUAL PROBLEMS

Most sexual problems can be readily diagnosed and treated by the primary care professional. The more complicated or refractory cases can be referred to the psychiatrist or sex therapist.

Male Sexual Dysfunctions

Secondary Impotence. This is a common problem and, in contrast to primary impotence, there is a better prognosis if impotence has not been lifelong.

General instructions to the patient (and partner) include the following:

a. No sexual intercourse for two weeks.
b. Get the partner involved in non-demanding stroking and sensate touching of the man who should focus exclusively on his own sexuality.
c. The partner should be supportive and cooperative of the masturbation.
d. Initially a sustained and repeat penile erection is the goal. Later intercourse is attempted.
e. Sexual fantasy is encouraged unless it distracts from maintaining a penile erection.

Premature Ejaculation. Ejaculatory control is present when a man can experience high levels of excitement that characterize the plateau stage of the sexual response cycle without ejaculating reflexly. Premature ejaculation exists, in contrast, when ejaculation is beyond the man's control and occurs prematurely and by reflex. This reflex can occur independent of sexual conflict and can be conditioned from voluntary early release with masturbation or from early anxiety-laden sexual experiences.

Sensory feedback is the essential element in learning this control. The hypothesis underlying the treatment of premature ejaculation is based on the assumption that the ejaculatory reflex occurs automatically, so that these patients function much the same as victims of spinal cord injury or individuals who have been deprived of sensory feedback for physical reasons. Some men with premature ejaculation do not clearly perceive the sensations premonitory to orgasm, which deprives them of the regulatory power of the higher nervous system, and therefore, treatment is analogous to biofeedback techniques which bring automatic functions under voluntary control.

Therapy is highly effective and allows for greater voluntary control over ejaculation and lengthening of intercourse.

The Squeeze Technique. The frenular squeeze technique for treatment of premature ejaculation was developed and utilized by Masters and Johnson. Briefly, the therapy consists of two parts—the first, application of the "squeeze" by the female, but with the couple abstaining from any sexual intercourse, and the second—a combination of the frenular "squeeze" and sexual intercourse.

This technique is designed to be applied at least a half dozen times during each session of touching, at the discretion of the female or upon signal from the male, and not simply when ejaculatory inevitability is reached. Each application of the squeeze as shown below (Figure 9-1) consists of a firm pressure applied for 10-20 seconds. A constant pressure is important, and the patient and his partner should be reminded that a firm pressure can be applied without pain or injury.

1. *For the First Week.* (One daily practice session which includes at least six applications of the "squeeze.") No sexual intercourse allowed.

    Naked, and in the position of the female sitting below the male, the female is instructed to explore the male sensually, caressing with hands, mouth or

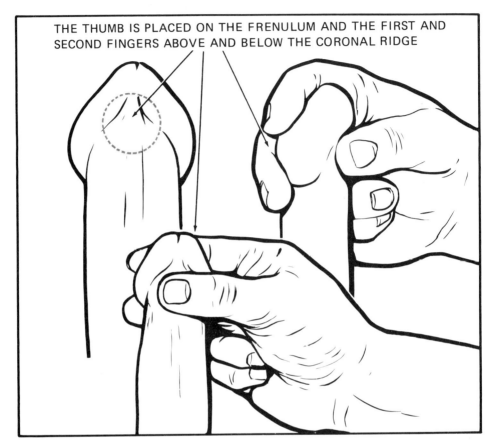

THE THUMB IS PLACED ON THE FRENULUM AND THE FIRST AND SECOND FINGERS ABOVE AND BELOW THE CORONAL RIDGE

Figure 9-1. The Squeeze Technique.

by any other means short of intercourse that is pleasurable to both. If the man's penis becomes erect while his partner is caressing it, she can at any time that feels right to her, apply the "squeeze" to his penis. The male, too, can give verbal feedback about sensations he is having, and tell his partner when to apply the "squeeze." He communicates this when the sensation of coming first appears. Above all, the couple should not wait for ejaculatory inevitability to start. As both partners feel more comfortable with the technique and as the male feels able to take a more active role, partner pleasuring should be included.

The "squeeze" should be applied at least six times in each pleasuring session, but with practice will need to be applied fewer and fewer times during each half hour practice.

2. *For the Second Week.* (One daily practice session which includes at least six applications of the "squeeze.") Sexual intercourse is allowed.

The instructions for body pleasuring are the same, except that after the first application of the "squeeze," the penis is then inserted into the vagina.

Occasionally, KY jelly may be needed to facilitate this but should be used sparingly.

After initial insertion, both male and female remain quiet without any pelvic thrusting movement. This allows the male to experience a "quiet" vagina. As the male feels high levels of excitement approaching, he signals for the female to apply the "squeeze." This she does by lifting up, removing the penis from the vagina and applying the frenular "squeeze." When the sense of urgency to ejaculate has passed, she again inserts the penis into the vagina, and the procedure is repeated.

Again, at least six applications of the "squeeze" should be included during the first sessions. As the male is better able to control, fewer and fewer applications of the "squeeze" will be needed during the practice time.

The patient should be told some amount of erection will be lost but will return with renewed stimulation.

Stop-Start Technique. When, during thrusting, ejaculatory inevitability approaches, the male is instructed to cease all thrusting movement and press the pubic bone against the partner's pubic bone, thus pushing the penis all the way into the vagina. Then both partners stop moving. When the urgency to ejaculate subsides, movements may again be resumed. This procedure will need to be practiced several times in a row over a two-to-three week period until the male no longer feels the urgency to ejaculate prematurely. In the treatment, the male must focus his attention on the sensations of impending orgasm while he is making love to his partner.

1. The couple engages in limited foreplay, only to the degree that this brings the male to erection. The male is to lie on his back while the female stimulates his penis manually or orally. The patient must focus his attention exclusively on the erotic sensations from his penis where he is being stimulated. Concurrently, he is not to focus on his partner, or be distracted in other ways. When he feels premonitory orgasmic sensation, he instructs his partner to stop stimulating him. After a few seconds, he will notice the sensation has disappeared, but before his erection is lost, stimulation is resumed to be stopped just prior to orgasm.

   The patient is to repeat this procedure a second and third time, and on the fourth time is to ejaculate. At no time is the patient to try to exert conscious control over orgasm, beyond signaling his partner to stop stimulation.

2. After the patient is able to concentrate on his sensations and able to recognize the intense sensation that occurs just prior to orgasm, he is instructed to repeat the exercise this time with the penis lubricated with a non-drying, nonirritating massage lotion. After three to six of these extra-vaginal practice sessions with ejaculation occurring on the fourth erection in each session, the partners then move to include intercourse. The initial attempt should be conducted in the female superior position. Now, the stop-start

procedure is employed and thrusting movements should stop when the preorgasmic level of sensation is reached by the male. At this point, the penis remains motionless in the vagina until after the sensation disappears at which time thrusting is again resumed. Coital orgasm may occur after the fourth session.

3. After intercourse in the female superior position has been successful, the couple is instructed to attempt intercourse lying on their sides. The stop-start exercises are again employed and emphasis is placed on the "focusing of attention" on the sensations during lovemaking.

4. The last part of this therapy involves the male in the male superior position. The stop-start techniques are again used at this level. It cannot be emphasized too strongly that the "focus of attention" is essential therapeutically in the treatment of premature ejaculation by this method. Ejaculatory control in the female superior and side-to-side position is generally obtained in three to four weeks. However, the time required in the male superior position varies.

Eight-Step Desensitization Program. This eight-step program is indicated for premature ejaculating men who do not have a steady partner. The patient should complete successfully each step before moving to the next. This method is also often highly successful. It also has the advantage of allowing the patient to pace himself, observe progress, and build confidence by mastering the previous steps.

During each of the eight steps, the male must concentrate on the sensations he is experiencing in his penis. He should stop when these sensations become too intense, but before ejaculation is inevitable, and to resume "pleasuring" after the intense feelings subside. Awareness of his breathing patterns is helpful, as the focusing on deep breathing allows for continued relaxation and sustaining the erection without ejaculating.

Steps one and two are done by the male alone, either with or without the partner present.

1. Stimulation of the penis via self-masturbation. Do not use lotions or oils— "dry."

2. Stimulation of the penis via self-masturbation using oil or lotion to mimic vaginal secretions—"wet."

3. "Dry" stimulation of the penis via *partner* masturbation.

4. "Wet" stimulation of the penis via *partner* masturbation.

5. Sexual intercourse with the female in the "female superior" or female-on-top position. Neither the male nor the female are to do any thrusting or moving. It is an opportunity to experience intervaginal containment and a "quiet" vagina.

6. Sexual intercourse in the female superior position with the woman controlling all thrusting movements.

7. The partners experience intercourse with the male *only* initiating thrusting movements, first in the female superior position and then in the male superior position.

8. Both partners thrust together during intercourse, each initiating movements as desired.

Female Sexual Dysfunctions

Preorgasmic Women. Studies have indicated that often women have little knowledge of their anatomy and physiology. A pelvic exam with their mate present, and a general review of the anatomy and physiology of the sexual response are essential first steps in treatment. It is important for women to realize that they must assume a responsibility for their greater enjoyment of sex. As part of this, the woman must have an understanding of her own arousal and be able to communicate this with her partner. Factual information is supportive and helpful: Kaplan estimates that 75 percent of women achieve orgasm and for most of these, there is the need for clitoral stimulation to assist with sexual arousal and to achieve orgasm.

Steps in Treating Preorgasmic Women. Lo Piccolo and Lobitz have developed a program of direct masturbation which they find helpful in treating preorgasmic women. This approach can be used by a physician or physician's assistant to help preorgastic women to become orgastic. Each step should be accomplished and gone over before proceeding to the next.

Initially for desensitization purposes:

- Ask patients what percentage of people masturbate.
- Explain that masturbation produces physiologically the most intense orgasm for both men and women.
- Deal with patient's attitude towards masturbation.
- Self-disclosure about masturbation may be helpful.
- Get cooperation from partner to support masturbation.
- Male partner should tell the mate about his masturbation.

Specific assigned techniques (each step should be mastered before proceeding).

Step 1. The woman should experience self-awareness by herself, i.e., examine her nude body—appreciate beauty of her sex organs; suggest doing this after bathing. Ask her to take a trip through her body assessing what she likes and doesn't like. Assure the patient that everyone likes or dislikes parts of his/her body. Kegel exercises can increase the tone and vascularity of pelvic musculature. Instruct the woman to tense and relax her pubococcygeal muscles three times a day at least ten times.

Step 2. Next, the woman explores her genitals tactually and visually without expectation or intent of arousal. Some women may feel some apprehension, but encourage them that this will disappear after awhile.

Step 3. Require visual and tactual exploration of the genitals to locate sensitive areas that produce pleasure and arousal. Explain exploration of all areas, i.e., clitoral shaft and hood, major and minor labia, vaginal opening, whole perineum and suggest the use of a mirror.

Step 4. Next, discuss techniques and variations of masturbation (be as graphic as possible). Some use videotapes effectively at this point. Focus her concentration on pleasurable manual stimulation, i.e., a "love-in" for herself. The use of a lubricant may enhance pleasure and prevent friction. The patient may reach orgasm.

Step 5. Suggest increasing the duration and intensity of masturbation (30 to 45 minutes). Also, recommend developing erotic fantasies, romantic stories, or whatever else turns the patient on.

Step 6. If orgasm hasn't been achieved, ask the patient to purchase a vibrator. Using the vibrator, lubricant jelly, and erotic fantasies, suggest stimulation as long as it remains comfortable and erotic (up to 45 minutes).

Step 7. Once orgasm is achieved, have the woman masturbate with her partner present. He learns the techniques effective for her genital stimulation. Co-involvement and desensitization occur.

Step 8. Have the partner do for her what she has been doing for herself (manually or with a vibrator).

Step 9. Finally, have the couple engage in intercourse with her partner and/or herself concurrently stimulating the woman by the proven successful method. Position suggested: female on top, lateral or rear entry in order to allow easy access to the clitoris.

Vaginismus. Vaginismus is the involuntary spasm of the vagina, partially or totally. It is always associated with some degree of dyspareunia, if intercourse is possible at all. With these patients it is very important to rule out organic causes, document the course, and seek possible relationship with interpersonal and life events.

Often, the patient will have underlying psychological problems and referral for therapy is indicated. The treatment should begin with a thorough pelvic examination with partner present, going over anatomy and physiology of sexual response. Knowledge reduces anxiety.

If there are any associated organic causes of coital discomfort and pain, obviously this must be completely corrected first. Hegar dilators are gradually introduced. Partners are instructed in doing this at home and intravaginal containment of larger and larger objects is accomplished. Much support and gradual nonpressured accomplishment is encouraged. The clinician must take time to explain each thing he does and do as much as he can to put the patient at ease, asking questions in order to dissipate anxiety, correct prevailing myths, and defuse any painful sensations as they arise. Deep breathing and relaxation exercises are useful adjuncts.

SEX AND AGING

Sex activity need not be reduced in frequency or satisfaction with advancing age. Myths about declining interest are false. Yet, adjustment needs to be made for failing health or loss of a spouse.

Some natural changes occur in the sexual response cycle with aging. Also, as a woman ages, the vaginal walls may become atrophic with drying and reduced elasticity. Fatigue may occur more rapidly, and the man may have more difficulty maintaining an erection. The response cycle changes with aging, as indicated below:

Male

Excitement: Increased time for erection.

Erection is not hard.

Plateau: Reduced desire to ejaculate and thus more ejaculatory control; therefore intercourse lasts longer.

Therefore, it is important to the man to be allowed to ejaculate at his demand level.

Pre-ejaculatory secretion is less.

Orgasm: Inevitability stage shortened (to 2-4 seconds from 1-2).

Shorter or may not occur at all.

One-stage ejaculation is common (hormone deprivation).

Semen expulsion less forceful.

Resolution: Loss of complete erection in seconds (shorter resolution, longer refractory period).

Female

Excitement: Lubrication slower (5 minutes).

Less lubrication.

Smaller clitoris (still functional).

Plateau: Less elevation of uterus.

Less increase in size of vaginal canal.

No sex skin reaction.

No changes in labia majora.

Orgasm: Shorter phase, 4 or 5 contractions.

1 or 2 uterine contractions.

Painful spastic uterine contraction (hormones low).

Resolution: Faster.

Treatment is often educative with encouragement of an active sexual adjustment. Vaginal hormonal creams and lubricants may be helpful.

Health care professionals need routinely to give accurate information about the effects of aging processes on sexual response to older patients. Many couples needlessly stop all intimacy because of complications and myths around penis-in-vagina sex.

SUMMARY

The health care professional's role in dealing with the sex-related concerns of his patients is an important part of total health care. It is possible in a busy office practice to deal with many of these issues. A brief history model for common sexual problems and a screening model for their management and treatment are presented. People do suffer from sexual infirmities. For some, this means their lives and relationships are devastated. These sexual difficulties can also undermine health. We have an obligation to help them when we can.

SUGGESTED READING

Normal Sexual Response
   Brecher R, Brecher F: *An Analysis of Human Sexual Response.* Signet, 1966
Abnormal Sexual Response
   Belliveau R, Richter L: *Understanding Human Sexual Inadequacy.* Bantam, 1970
Sex Therapy
   Kaplan HS: *The New Sex Therapy.* New York, Brunner Mazel, Inc., 1974
Overview
   Kalodny R, Masters W, Johnson V: *Textbook of Sexual Medicine.* Little, Brown & Co., 1980
Men
   Zilbergeld B: *Male Sexuality, A Guide to Sexual Fulfillment.* Bantam, 1978
Women
   Barback L: *For Yourself.* New York, Doubleday & Co., 1975
   Dodson B: *Liberating Masturbation.* San Francisco, Goddess Books, 1977
   LoPiccolo J and Lobitz W: The role of masturbation in the treatment of primary orgasmic dysfunction. *Arch Sex Behav* 2:163-165, 1972
General
   Comfort A: *The Joy of Sex.* New York, Crown, 1972
Couples
   Bach G: *The Intimate Enemy.* New York, W. Morrow, 1968

10

Geriatric Psychiatry

GABE J. MALETTA, Ph.D., M.D.

Geriatric psychiatry is the study of psychopathology during a time in life which can be considered the end stage of a long, ongoing continuum. Therefore, by definition, it is the study of a unique kind of pathology, at once similar, yet different, from the psychopathology seen during earlier times in the life cycle. Old age can be considered as another phase of development in the life span of the individual; developmental in the sense that, like its predecessors, it is a dynamic, non-static time. Each phase of the human life span has its own unique traumata, specific to that age group; and the aged are no different. However, this particular group carries with them the accumulation of exposures to the multiple problems

191

and sufferings of an entire lifetime, and that makes their psychic burden a particularly heavy one.

One must add to this concept the relationship between the aged individual and his significant environment. Social pressures and inadequate resources certainly contribute to dysfunctional features associated with old age. Also, elderly people are frequently seen as separate from the mainstream of society, rather than in terms of being in continuity with it. Unfortunately, this tends to create a negative stereotype of an aged individual, and in many ways makes it easy for society to adopt a posture of unconcern and even active neglect.

Therefore, the concerns of psychiatry, particularly in the geriatric population, must always consider the individual in terms of the much larger social milieu in which he exists, not only when attempting to understand causes of psychopathology, but also when considering appropriate treatment.

It has only recently become generally acceptable that aged patients actually have treatable mental illness. Previously, most pathologic behavior in the elderly was thought due to "old age," or "senility," or "hardening of the arteries." This attitude prevailed even when dealing with those patients who presented with symptoms of a predominantly paranoid or depressive nature, with no signs at all of any sensorium deficiency.

Besides dementing illnesses, aged patients frequently exhibit typical or atypical psychiatric disorders, including psychosis, anxiety and depression. Further, psychotropic medications are clearly useful in the treatment of these disorders. However, it is also known that age does influence the action of a medication and may impair the predictability of drug effects, since pharmacological principles concerning drug effects depend on evaluation of the drug, projected against the physiologic system changes that occur with aging, as well as in terms of existing disease and other drugs already being taken. (For an in-depth review of this area, refer to Maletta, 1979.)

Deleterious side effects of psychotropic medications are more common in older patients for a variety of reasons, including polypharmacy, drug interactions, unique receptor sensitivity, inappropriate dosage, and diet, to name a few.

The definition of an aged, or "old" patient should be clarified. Sixty-five years is used by convention as the lower limit when considering an aged patient. It is well-known that more than 10 percent of the population of the U.S. (or 22 million people) presently are over the age of 65, and the proportional number continues to grow year by year. It is estimated that 20 percent of the population (or 56 million people) will be over 65 by 2035. However, it should be kept in mind that not all patients over 65 should be considered "old." Indeed, from age 65 to age 90 is a span of 25 years, which makes lumping everyone over 65 in the category of "old" as illogical as calling everyone from age 1 to 25, "young." Those patients less than 75 years have recently been called "young-old," while those over that age are considered as "old-old," in an attempt to further quantify and individualize patients.

This chapter will discuss behavior, both normal and abnormal, in the aged patient, and then present information on the differential diagnosis of the unusual behaviors. Finally, treatment will be discussed, both practical and psychopharmacologic.

BEHAVIOR IN THE ELDERLY PATIENT

Normal Psychologic Changes

Before discussing the common psychiatric problems encountered in the aging population, it would be of benefit first to briefly outline the normal psychologic changes seen in the elderly individual.

Fundamentally speaking, today's generally accepted psychosocial theories suggest the basic psychologic needs do not really change as one ages, but instead should be viewed as a function of both developmental stage and life style.

Basically, the needs reflect a necessity for continuing adaptation throughout the life span. There is a steady decline with time in the functional capacities of most organ systems, with a decreased efficiency to maintain a constant internal environment, i.e. homeostatis, following stress.

Therefore, several adaptive tasks become necessary as one ages. One is the perception that aging is in fact occurring, with the concomitant acceptance of a realistic definition of limitations. That realization calls for a frank and honest redefining of one's physical and social "life space," and perhaps substituting alternative sources of need satisfaction (for example, switching from handball to the less strenuous game of tennis). Another important adaptive task is the need to critically reassess criteria for self-evaluation and perhaps even reintegrating one's values and life goals.

In that context, four major *areas* must be considered: the internal resources of the individual; one's cognitive abilities; the concept of "self;" and the inevitable progression with aging from independence to dependence.

Internal Resources of the Individual. These obviously vary among individuals, and an attempt to quantitatively separate the relative contributions of heredity versus environment in this particularly subjective area would prove fruitless. Nevertheless, one might consider many unique factors, including:

- Philosophy of life
- Attitude towards others
- Ability to cope effectively with stresses
- Appreciation of esthetics, i.e., one's relationship to nature and beauty
- Spiritual and religious beliefs

Cognitive Abilities. Many investigators believe that learning ability does not necessarily decline with aging. However, what does seem to change is the rate, or speed, at which one can learn new material. Therefore, learning may be facilitated if the older individual is allowed to set his own comfortable pace.

There is an interesting concept which compares "crystallized" and "fluid" intelligence with aging. Crystallized (or static) intelligence, which is thought to be based on past experiences, seems to undergo a slight, but not significant decline with old age. On the other hand, fluid (or dynamic) intelligence, which is thought to be biologically mediated, gradually declines with aging, beginning from young adulthood.

Self-concept. This is also known as self-esteem, or a "sense of self." In psychiatric terms, in order to have a positive sense of self, one needs a healthy and intact ego, a so-called "ego-integrity." In the aged individual, this comes from basically accepting one's life as having been inevitable, appropriate and meaningful. Inescapable physiologic and anatomic changes concomitant with aging must be accepted, e.g., graying hair, wrinkled skin, loss of physical stamina and endurance, etc. Further, there must be a gradual acceptance of the inevitability of loss, e.g., loss of spouse and/or significant others, loss of work role.

If ego-integrity is absent, a sense of despair may result as one ages, especially after retirement, when feelings of self-worth may be minimized. There may be fear of death, and the individual's life cycle is not accepted as having been adequate enough. The despair is further amplified because one may feel that time is now too short to begin anything new, and no clear-cut alternative avenues toward trying to achieve ego-integrity are seen.

Independence to Dependence. This situation might be viewed as a gradual down-turning spiral, with a continuum which progresses from independence through interdependence, and finally to dependence. The place that the older individual occupies on this continuum is influenced by many factors, including one's physical, emotional, social and economic situation.

Common Psychiatric Problems

The most common psychiatric conditions seen in older patients can be classified into three broad categories:

- The so-called "functional" brain disorders, including psychogenic thought disorders, and the affective disorders, primarily depressive reactions.
- Drugs of abuse, including alcohol. This is an important area in aging which deserves a comprehensive discussion, and will not be covered in detail in this chapter. See Schucket (1977) for more information.
- The so-called "organic" brain disorders, of which delirium and dementia are the two classic sub-categories.

FUNCTIONAL DISORDERS IN THE ELDERLY PATIENT

Schizophrenic Syndromes

Psychotic thought disorders are now considered to be common problems in the aged population. However, some confusion exists, not only concerning diagnosis, but also in terms of time of onset. It is generally accepted that most older schizophrenics developed the problem in their early years and carried it with them into old age, with few having the initial onset of illness late in life. Usually the onset is seen in the late teens or young adult period, so that a 65-year-old may have a 40 or 50-year-history of illness, the so-called chronic, long-standing schizophrenic.

Also, thought disorders can present in the elderly as other than a straight-forward functional illness, usually in a patient who has had schizophrenic-type symptoms for many years with no signs of progressive intellectual decline ("dementia"). It may also be seen as part of a schizophrenic-like symptom complex in some elderly patients who have a dementing type illness.

These two ends of a spectrum, both considered by some as "psychosis" in the elderly, underline the confusion seen when an attempt is made to quantify the operational definition of psychosis in the aged population.

To add to the diagnostic fuzziness, there are other groups of elderly patients who could be considered psychotic or schizophrenic (unfortunately the two words are frequently, and inappropriately, used synonymously). As already mentioned, one group is those elderly patients with a seemingly first-time, acute onset of a schizophreniform illness and no evidence of dementia. Another is a group of patients with a long-standing dementia who may have no observable thought disorder or hallucinations, but do have enough disorientation and general intellectual impairment to cause considerable distress to themselves or those around them.

As in early life, schizophrenias in the elderly are characterized by disturbances in thinking, mood and behavior. Loss of reality testing, such as hallucinations or illusions also may be present.

Late-occurring Paranoid States

Although paranoid thinking may be part of the symptom complex seen in schizophrenia, it is listed here separately because late-occurring paranoid states in an elderly patient frequently represent a first-time phenomenon of mental illness. Symptoms of this psychotic illness, which is characterized by delusions and/or hallucinations of a grandiose or persecutory type, may not occur until age 60 or later.

It is thought by some that this late onset of paranoid symptoms may represent an unconscious "face-saving" device by the elderly patient against the gradual loss of self-mastery and control that is being experienced, and the fear and helplessness implicit with it.

Affective Disorders

Depression. If there is a common psychologic disturbance in the elderly, it is depression. Depression can be viewed as a syndrome interrelating somatic, psychic and behavioral symptoms and signs.

Some common somatic manifestations include: anorexia, insomnia, fatigue, reduced sex drive, headache, and constipation.

Common psychic symptoms include: sadness, irritability, anhedonia (inability to experience pleasure), guilt feelings, difficulty in concentration, pessimism, loss of interest, somatic concerns or delusions and suicidal thoughts.

Behavioral signs are exemplified by: poor grooming, withdrawal, crying, motor retardation (or agitation), self-reproach and suicide attempts.

Depression in senescence is commonly over-looked, because it does not always follow the same pattern or have the same symptoms and signs as in the younger age group. The onset is likely to be more gradual and is likely to be primarily somatic in its manifestation, thereby being easily confused with the physical illnesses which are so common in the older patient. The usual affective symptoms and signs of depression such as sadness, crying spells, guilt and self-deprecation may be absent, and instead an atypical clinical picture may be seen. Depressed elderly patients may demonstrate a considerable impairment of memory, concentration and comprehension, along with psychomotor retardation and loss of initiative. These may be so prominent as to easily confuse a depression with a dementing illness in an elderly patient.

It is essential that this differential diagnosis be made, because frequently an elderly patient who is depressed receives a diagnosis of dementia and is treated accordingly by staff. This unfortunately may result in the elderly patient beginning to conform to the situational ambience of his environment, with demented activity and behavior eventually following.

Late onset depressives, in comparison with early onset patients, seem to have been better adjusted emotionally, socially and psychosexually. The majority of severe first depressive attacks appear after the age of 60, in both men and women. It appears that the onset may follow the occurrence of some traumatic event, which also differs from younger depressed patients, where specific precipitants are usually not evident.

These precipitating events can be classified as the occurrence, in a depression-prone individual, of multiple losses, either experienced or feared. These losses include: health, bereavement over death of spouse, relatives and friends, loss of the work role because of retirement, loss of financial security, moving away of children, loss of status, loss of familiar physical surroundings, and an underlying fear of the inexorably approaching end of life.

Mania. Although manias are far less frequent in late life than are depressions, they do occur. Frequently, these episodes are part of a bipolar disorder, which may have been overlooked in the elderly patient. It usually follows a depressive reaction, and the manic symptoms, e.g., pressured speech, flight of ideas, etc., may be mistaken for aggressiveness or overactivity and the diagnosis overlooked. Hostile and/or paranoid behaviors may also be present in these elderly patients, which may further complicate the diagnosis of mania.

Neuroses

Although many authors suggest that most neuroses seem to improve with aging, their incidence is pronounced in the elderly. Neuroses, defined as "emotional maladaptions arising from unresolved unconscious conflicts," are much more prevalent in the aged than are psychoses. However, since they manifest neither gross personality disorganization nor gross distortion of external reality, much less attention is paid to them than to the more visible psychoses. As is the case with younger patients, neuroses in the elderly are classified according to their predominating symptoms.

Anxiety Neuroses. Anxiety is defined as an apprehension that stems from the anticipation of danger, the source of which is largely unknown. A neurosis of this type is characterized by increased muscle tension, gastrointestinal and urinary system disturbances, headaches, irritability, disturbances in regular heart rhythm, excessive perspiration, and even a vague sense of impending doom.

Since all too often, real-life situations which are anxiety provoking occur quite frequently in the older patient, it is no wonder that anxiety states are common.

Compulsive Neuroses. These kinds of disorders which occur in the elderly are similar to those which occur earlier in life. Orderliness, perfectionism, attention to minute details, self-doubt and feelings of inadequacy are some common signs of the compulsive person. Repeated acts of a penitential nature occasionally appear in elderly patients, and may be an attempt at protection against particular guilt-arousing fantasies.

Hysterical Neuroses. Such neuroses, especially the conversion type, i.e., loss of function of a particular body part, are uncommon in the elderly. However, what is frequently seen in older patients is a preoccupation and possible exaggeration of the severity of minor physical symptoms and complaints.

Chronic Fatigue. This type of neurosis is also known as neuroasthenia, and is characterized by complaints of chronic weakness, fatigue and exhaustion. It is obviously difficult to highlight this particular problem in older patients because of their propensity to tire quickly and recover more slowly than younger individuals. One theory for the increase in emotional fatigability in the aged is that as gratifying experiences decrease with advanced age, so does an individual's interest, and therefore, he is apt to tire more quickly.

It should be stressed that a diet of satisfying accomplishments is more in order for an older patient with this problem than the often heard suggestion to "take a long vacation and get away from it all." "Rests" of this type may actually exacerbate the lethargy and emotional fatigue.

Hypochondriasis

Although technically this phenomenon is classified as a neurosis, its prevalence is high enough in the elderly population to consider it separately. Hypochondriasis, or the inordinate preoccupation with one's bodily functions, is an especially common disorder in the aged.

The symptoms seem to be focused mostly on various aspects of the gastrointestinal system, although no system is excluded from involvement. It is suggested by some that this preoccupation among the elderly with feeding, digestion and evacuation is involved psychodynamically with the unconscious expression of dependency needs, i.e., the desire to be taken care of, as when one was an infant.

Sleep Disturbances

It is generally thought that older individuals need as much sleep as they did in their earlier years. However, periods of sleep my be shorter and less sound, i.e., less stage 4 sleep, in this age group, and complaints about lack of sleep are common. It is better to categorize these complaints as sleep disturbances, rather than sleeplessness. These disturbances may be due to more frequent nocturia than when younger, with a subsequent inability to fall back to sleep quickly. Also, many uninvolved, inactive older persons take several naps during a typical day, thereby obviating the ability, or the need, to achieve an uninterrupted full night's sleep.

Special Problems

Stress. Aged persons are susceptible to many stresses and strains that significantly influence not only physical and mental parameters, but also the capacity for social self-maintenance and self-sufficiency.

These stresses include physiologic stress related to decreased functional capacity, as well as acute and chronic illness; and psychologic stresses involved with feelings of dependence, isolation, loneliness, and intra and interpersonal and intrafamily conflicts. Also, socioeconomic stresses occur, primarily related to losses related to retirement, widowhood, loss of family and friends, and loss of occupational status and adequate economic support. Many of the stress factors common to the elderly patient are listed below:

Physiological:
   Multiple chronic diseases
   Insidious degenerative processes
   Increased risk of injury
   Impaired general/cerebral metabolism
   Impaired neuromuscular/musculoskeletal/integrative systems
   Homeostatic imbalances

Nutritional deficiencies
Sensory deprivation secondary to receptor impairment
Gastrointestinal/genitourinary disorders
Economic:
Compulsory retirement
Reduced income
Substandard housing
Increased expenses for medical care/food/rent
Inadequate retirement benefits/insurance/social security
Psychological:
Cognitive/emotional disorders
Situational reactions
Psychiatric crises
Dementias
Neurotic episodes
Sociocultural:
Diminished social role
Loss of authority
Dependence on others
Deflated ego
Communication breakdown
Societal rejection
Denial of aging
Mortality anticipation
Social desolation
Withdrawal/isolation

The summated detrimental effects of this multitude of stresses over a long period of time are crucial regarding the outcome of illness in the elderly, and in fact may be as important as the specific effects of a particular mental or physical disorder.

Relationship Between Functional Disorder and Physical Illness. The intertwining of physical illness and mental status must be strongly emphasized. Physical health may be more relevant to psychiatric impairment than any other factor studied, both in hospitalized and community-resident elderly patients. There is a general decrease in physical capacity with time as one ages, usually heralded by a lessening of strength, vigor and coordination. There is also an increase in the likelihood of developing a chronic disabling disease, e.g., cardiovascular, renal, or pulmonary, as well as osteo or rheumatoid arthritis. Older individuals are increasingly more vulnerable to serious illnesses related to infection, malnutrition, accidents and drug and alcohol abuse. All of these may be associated with evidence of mental and/or emotional problems.

A decrease in sensory acuity occurs with aging. Visual defects or blindness occur in 4 percent of individuals in their 60s, and in 15 percent of those in their 80s. Hearing defects occur in 5 percent of those in their 60s, and in 25 percent of those in their 80s. Functional changes are known to occur at the level of sensory receptors, with an increase in the threshold level of stimulation necessary for activation. Also, functional changes occur in the afferent pathway (the input pathway to the brain) with aging, as evidenced by a decrease in nerve conduction velocity.

Changes in the nervous system at the sensory receptor and the afferent pathway account for only about four percent of the decrease in function noted in the aging nervous system. Most of the functional changes occur within the brain itself, with possible alterations occurring in resting membrane potential thresholds, neuroglial regulation, synaptic receptor number and sensitivity, change in excitation/inhibition ratios, or focal changes in blood brain barrier.

As far as the aged individual is concerned, changes become evident in all sensory modalities, including vision, audition, olfaction, taste, touch, vibration and pain. In terms of vision, there is a decrease in visual acuity, as well as a decrease in the ability to discriminate among colors, leading to problems with proper depth perception. Specific auditory problems of the aged, e.g., presbycusis, are manifested by a decreased acuity for high frequency sounds, as well as a decrease in the ability to discriminate among sounds.

Decreases in visual and particularly auditory sensation with aging are significant, since these changes tend to amplify the feelings of loneliness and isolation, which may already be prevalent in many elderly people due to psychologic factors. In fact, this situation of isolation, coupled with a borderline sensorium, and under conditions of severe stress, may frequently lead to an abrupt onset situation of delirium in an elderly individual, known colloquially as "sundowning." The name is derived from the frequent observation in hospitals that many elderly patients whose mental functioning is borderline during the day, frequently decompensate totally at night (after "sundown"), when their already compromised sensory input is even more severely curtailed.

CASE HISTORY—*SUNDOWNING*

Mrs. G. was a 75-year-old woman who was admitted to the hospital because of a fractured arm secondary to a fall. She lived with her 78-year-old husband and their daughter, who was married and had two teenage sons. They had lived in this environment very happily for the past 10 years and all family members were quite satisfied with the arrangement. Over the last one to two years, the patient became gradually more forgetful, and occasional periods where she seemed to be confused were occurring with greater frequency. Because of the mutual understanding among family members, the patient's gradual intellectual decline was not considered a problem. Also, her hearing and vision had gradually been deteriorating over the past five years, but without incident.

The fracture was set under a mild sedative, and late the first night in the hospital, after earlier appearing quite nervous, the patient was found standing naked in another patient's room, attempting to squat and urinate, and shouting incoherently.

The intern was called, and the patient was correctly diagnosed as having been "sundowning." She was given 10 mg Haldol IM and placed in her bed with soft restraints and was consistently reassured with appropriate reality orientation. Her care plan was revised to insure appropriate changes in her hospital environment, which stressed optimum sensory awareness and familiarity so as to prevent a reoccurrence. The rest of her hospital stay was without incident.

Inadequate nutrition is a significant problem in the elderly. Problems in this area are due to a variety of reasons, including lack of understanding of good nutrition, lack of money, and sometimes an inability to get out and shop. Also, feelings of loneliness, apathy and depression contribute to the lack of interest in eating and the unwillingness to try to achieve a good diet.

Suicide. Suicide occurs with fairly high frequency among the elderly, predominantly among white men. In fact, the highest rates for suicide in the entire population are for white male divorced individuals over 65. This high rate is thought to be directly related to ill health and depressive reactions, with the correlation depending, in part, on the fear of chronic disability and dependence that characterizes many of the elderly.

Suicide among the elderly is a serious problem, which in many cases is not really appreciated, either by professionals or the lay public. The seriousness of this danger is underscored by the fact that successful suicide attempts are more common than unsuccessful ones in old age. Also, the methods most frequently used for suicide, especially among aged men, i.e., shooting, hanging and drowning indicate the severity of the suicide intent.

There is some indication that suicides in the older age group in recent years may be decreasing, for reasons which are not at all clear, but this phenomenon still represents a serious problem in the elderly population.

DIFFERENTIAL DIAGNOSIS OF DEMENTIA

When evaluating a symptom complex in an elderly patient, it is extremely important to consider the possible multivaried etiology of what is being observed. The possibility that the unusual behavior being witnessed is due to a physical problem rather than to a mental one, or that drug toxicity is involved, or that there is a combined physical and emotional problem, becomes a real issue in this patient population.

In a small number of patients, what may look superficially like a thought disorder may in fact be symptomatic of an acute, temporary and reversible dysfunction in sensorium (a "delirium"), or a progressive, chronic, marked decline in intellectual function, usually irreversible (a "dementia"), brought on by any number of physical causes, and which can easily be misinterpreted by the casual observer.

It's important to point out that the general impression of the lay public that "senility" (dementia) is a natural consequence of aging is without real foundation. This idea has come to be part of our folklore; but in reality, only one in ten people 65 years of age, who are not institutionalized, have the diagnosis of dementia. For a population cohort of 80 years of age, 15-20 percent have a dementing illness. It could be argued that if one lived long enough, there would be a continuing increase in the percentage of individuals with dementia; however, these statistics suggest that a very small number of elderly people are afflicted with a progressive, chronic and marked decline in intellectual function (including perception, attention, memory, orientation, cognition and affect).

The concept of "final common pathway" should be discussed here. The nervous system has a limited range of reactions with which it can demonstrate abnormal functioning. Problems can arise in thinking, perception, attention, concentration, memory, orientation and emotional stability. Although the etiologies of the inappropriate behavior in an elderly patient may be very different, e.g., delirium vs one of the dementias vs. depression or other functional problem, the clinical signs of abnormality may be exactly the same, i.e., the final common pathway. This is analogous in some ways to the clinical sign of fever. The quantitative observation and measurement of a fever is the same, regardless of whether the etiology is due to a sunstroke or subacute bacterial endocarditis, i.e., a fever is the "final common pathway" for some very diverse etiologies. It is the same for the observation of abnormal or inappropriate behavior in an elderly patient.

As differential diagnostic ability improves, the separation of delirium from dementia from functional etiologies (especially depression) in an aged patient with a history of unusual behavior takes on greater and greater significance, when thinking in terms of treatment (Freeman, 1976; Katzman and Karasa, 1975). Elderly patients who exhibit unusual behavior frequently are quickly diagnosed as demented and therefore considered untreatable, when a careful look may reveal a treatable delirium or depression. This is not a frequent occurrence, but that in no way diminishes its importance. The significance of early differentiation between a treatable and a nontreatable cause of unusual behavior is obvious.

Further, the aged patient may be less a help than a hindrance in terms of his ability as a good, or even adequate, historian. There are frequently problems encountered in communicating, whether it be because of understanding, or some difficulty in coherent speaking. Perception, attention, memory and even orientation are all areas in which the aged patient may have a deficit. Many others, for a variety of reasons, are frankly unreliable in their reporting.

Frequently, lack of interest as well as the presence of sensory deficits may significantly and adversely affect the response of the patient.

Another point to consider is the fact that seldom does one see an aged patient who brings with him, to the first meeting, a copy of a comprehensive past medical history and physical examination.

Finally, even standardized psychological tests as well as clinical laboratory values are difficult to interpret when used with the aged patient, since the standard values for "normal" are almost always derived from a pool of healthy, young adults. It's not really clear at the present time as to the need and significance for therapy of "normal" aged psychologic and lab values. This entire area begs for further study and thought, and obviously the whole concept of appropriate differential diagnosis of mental aberration in an aged patient is a crucial one for later therapeutic success.

Delirium

This clinical state, also known as "acute brain syndrome," is defined as an acute onset of a fluctuating disorder of consciousness, perception and attention, with frequent loss of reality testing. A key component of this disorder is that it is due to no permanent damage of neural tissue, and is therefore a reversible state.

The major causes of delirium*† (sometimes referred to by neurologists as "secondary brain dysfunction" to differentiate it from the dementias, or "primary brain dysfunctions") are listed below.

Drug toxicity (prescribed; street; over-the-counter)
    Psychotropics, bromide, and antiparkinsonians, incl. Levodopa
    Digitalis, diuretics, antihypertensives, steroids, disulfiram
Acute alcohol abuse
Central nervous system
    Trauma causing subarachnoid or epidural hemorrhage
    Transient ischemic attack (TIA)
    Emboli leading to minor stroke (CVA)
    CNS lupus vasculitis
Cardiovascular
    "Silent" myocardial infarction in the elderly
    Onset of arrhythmia
    Congestive cardiac failure
Metabolic and endocrine
    Diabetes mellitus
    Hypoglycemia (also nonketotic hyperglycemia)
    Hyperglucocorticoidism (Cushings)
    Myxedema (also hyperthyroidism)

---

*Defined as a fluctuating disorder of consciousness, perception, attention, memory, orientation and judgment, with frequent lability of affect and loss of reality testing.

† Differential diagnosis must include depression ("pseudo-dementia" of aging); psychoneurosis; psychosis; and aphasia.

Hepatic failure
Renal failure (uremia)
Acute porphyria
Anemia (dietary or GI bleed)
CNS or systemic infections (with or without fever)
Fecal impaction in the elderly
Urinary bladder distention in the elderly
Dehydration and electrolyte imbalance
"Silent" pneumonia in the elderly

Dementia

Dementia is a clinical state comprised of gradual deterioration of intellectual function due to chronic, progressive degeneration of the brain. This global deterioration of function includes perception, attention, memory, judgment and emotional stability, and may follow a pattern of simple and gradual deterioration, or may involve rapid, complicated deterioration.

Many causes of dementia, e.g., space-occupying lesions, myxedema, normal pressure hydrocephalus and the nutritional deficiencies, can be arrested and may even be somewhat reversible if detected early enough. Unfortunately, Alzheimer's disease, which accounts for anywhere from 25 to 50 percent of the dementias, is due to progressive cerebral atrophy of unknown etiology. The final outcome, i.e., loss of total intellectual faculties, is the same, the only difference among patients is the length of time from detection to total disability (may range from several months to several years). The major causes of dementia* are listed below.

Alzheimer's disease†
Multi-infarct dementia
Space-occupying lesions
   Chronic subdurals
   Chronic abscess
   Frontal meningioma or a metastatic lesion
Myxedema (hypothyroidism) or other chronic endocrine causes
Pernicious anemia (Vitamin B_{12} deficiency)
Chronic arsenic or lead intoxication
Nutritional dementias
   Folate deficiency
   Niacin deficiency (pellagra)
   Pyridoxine deficiency
   Thiamine deficiency (Korsakoff's)

---

*Defined as a gradual deterioration of intellectual function due to chronic, progressive degeneration of the brain.

† Alzheimer's disease (of unknown etiology) of the elderly is a progressive cerebral atrophy, formerly known as "senile dementia," which may make up about 25 to 50 percent of the dementias reported. Pick's disease may be a variant of the same disorder.

Alcoholic dementia
Chronic normal pressure hydrocephalus
Dementia pugilistica
Neurosyphilis
Other infectious agents (viral; tuberculous; cryptococcal)
Specific neurologic syndromes (including Wilson's, Parkinson's, Huntington's, cerebellar degeneration and multiple sclerosis)

The study of Alzheimer's-type dementia from an epidemiologic focus may eventually prove the most worthwhile regarding a specific causative agent.

There are four major hypotheses presently considered as important by epidemiologists:

Genetic Hypothesis. This hypothesis states that the age of onset and the type of dementia are related to the family history of disease and causes of mortality. Among key questions, the following are of interest:

1. What association, if any, exists between a family history of dementia, Down's syndrome, cardiovascular disease, hematologic and other malignancies, and the diagnostic classification of subjects in the study?
2. With regard to the primary or secondary causes of death of parents and siblings of the demented patients and controls, is there a greater tendency for relatives of patients with dementia of the Alzheimer's type to die of infections or other illnesses indicating deficiencies of the immune system?

Immune Function Hypothesis. According to this hypothesis, either genetically preprogrammed or environmentally induced changes in the immune system directly preceding (five years) the onset of the dementia may be viewed as triggers for Alzheimer-type dementias. To examine this hypothesis, it would be worthwhile to obtain a good history of infectious and autoimmune diseases during the five years immediately preceding onset of the dementing condition. It is likely that the validity of this data would be greater than a history of disease in childhood and early adulthood.

It would also be of interest to examine the occurrence of events that could lead to either environmental (toxins, drugs, etc.) or psychological (death of spouse, etc.) stress during the five years preceding onset of the dementing condition. The hypothesis here is that these events may lead to a suppression of the immune response, which in turn may accelerate, slow or conceal virus infections. In Parkinson's disease, for example, patients often reach plateaus only to progress rapidly to a new stage of the disease with the death of a spouse.

Accelerated Aging Hypothesis. The basis for this hypothesis is the notion that older persons are more vulnerable to intellectual fallaway due to the cumulative loss of brain cells in certain brain areas and therefore, the loss of essential redundancy.

Many diverse factors, acting together, which compromise brain tissue during the life of the individual, would be viewed as predisposing the individual to a dementing condition. These factors include: alcohol and drug abuse, head trauma, brain infections, carbon monoxide poisoning and other environmental insults, poor nutrition, and uncontrolled epilepsy. The general hypothesis is that the more of these factors exist, and the more prominent each of these factors is, the earlier the age of onset of the dementing condition. It would also be important, of course, to investigate which individual factors were selective for particular categories of dementias (Alzheimer's, arteriosclerotic, etc).

Slow Virus Hypothesis. This hypothesis is likely to be the most difficult to investigate, because of the difficulty of obtaining valid data on early medical history. This approach involves the identification of events occurring at particular times during the individual's life, which may be related to the initial slow virus infection. Certainly, a history of childhood and adult infections, vaccinations and innoculations, as well as some time-related lifestyle variables (urban/rural, occupations, nutrition, etc.) would be worth inspecting. This type of hypothesis has been studied in multiple sclerosis extensively without much success at present.

Depression

Depression in geriatric patients is frequently overlooked, or misdiagnosed, largely because it does not follow the same clinical pattern as depression in younger patients (Wang & Busse, 1971).

Depression of later life is not so clearly manifested by a depressive "mood," such as sad, guilty and/or hopeless feelings, self-deprecatory thoughts, and crying spells, as it is in younger patients. Instead, psychomotor retardation, impairment of attention, somatic complaints, loss of libido and drive are much more common symptoms and signs in the older depressed patient.

It is extremely important to differentiate the diagnosis of depression from one of dementia in an aged patient, because depression is a reversible, usually easily treatable problem. Treatment, whether it be with ECT, TCAs, MAOIs, supportive psychotherapy, or combination thereof, can frequently and markedly improve the quality of life of the individual. For specific treatment of depression in the elderly, the reader is referred elsewhere (Davis, 1978).

Differentiation of Delirium, Dementia and Depression

Geriatric patients are frequently seen exhibiting signs of mental fallaway, including disordered intellectual function, emotional lability, memory dysfunction and disorientation. Because of the concept of final common pathway in nervous system dysfunction, as discussed earlier, the etiology of dysfunction in a particular patient may be a delirium, dementia, depression, or commonly, a mixed dementia-depression syndrome.

The physician is then faced with the substantial task of establishing a diagnosis based on symptoms common to these very disparate disorders.

It is extremely important to decide upon the correct diagnosis since treatment is, of course, based on proper diagnosis.

Also, prognosis may be quite different, depending on whether the patient has a clearly reversible and treatable delirium, a treatable depression mimicking an organic disorder, or an irreversible, nontreatable dementia. Therefore, proper initial diagnosis of the patient is imperative.

Probably the most important evidence for differentiating depression from delirium-dementia comes from assessing the patient's intellectual functions. The depressed patient, although his responses may be slow and difficult to elicit, can perform intellectual functions properly. A simple, standard bedside test for measuring sensorium is given here as an example.

1. 3 X items ('red,' 'table,' '23 Broadway') in five minutes
2. Where are you?
3. What kind of place is this?
4. Date (±3 days acceptable)
5. Day of week
6. Time (±1 hour acceptable)
7. Present President
8. Past Presidents in reverse
9. Largest city in U.S.?
10. Serial sevens (1x error acceptable) or serial threes
11. Spell "world" and "around" forward and backward
12. Days of week forward and backward

Correlate answers with observation of perception, attention, lability of affect and presence of thought disorder.

A much more sophisticated screening battery for eliciting diffuse cortical dysfunction (delirium or dementia) has been developed by Jenkyn, *et al.* (1977). It involves not only testing of intellectual function, but also some examinations of neurological functions which can be performed quickly at the bedside, and which have been found statistically to correlate well with diffuse cortical dysfunction. The Jenkyn screening battery follows.

1. Nuchacephalic reflex
2. Glabella blink
3. Suck
4. Upgaze
5. Downgaze
6. Visual tracking
7. Lateral gaze impersistence
8. Paratonia of both arms

9. Paratonia of both legs
10. Limb placement
11. Test of sensorium, esp:
    a. Accurate spelling of "world" in reverse
    b. Accurate order of Presidents in reverse
    c. Accurate recall of 3 items over time

Another approach used to differentiate delirium/dementia from depression (also sometimes referred to as "pseudodementia") is to attempt to rate, by clinical examination, various features which seem to differentiate these entities. (Table 10-1.) This approach to the problem is admittedly very generalized and qualitative; but if taken as a small sample of representative data in the context of many other tests of differentiation, these data could prove worthwhile.

Probably the best way to determine the specific etiology in a patient with mental fallaway is to utilize the binary logic flow chart system, beginning from the time the patient is first seen and ending at appropriate diagnosis and treatment. (Figure 10-1.)

Table 10-1. Rating Scale of Clinical Features Differentiating Depression from Dementia.

	Depression ("Pseudodementia")						Dementia
		1	2	3	4	5	
Duration of symptoms	short						long
Cognitive loss recognized by patient	very aware						unaware
Feelings of distress	frequently expressed						none apparent
Attention and concentration	preserved						defective
Typical answers	"don't know"						"near miss"
Evidence of disabilities	highlighted by patient						concealed by patient
Performance effort	low						high
Performance variability	marked						minimal
Affective change	pervasive						labile and shallow
Congruency of behavior with manifested cognitive impairment	incompatible						compatible

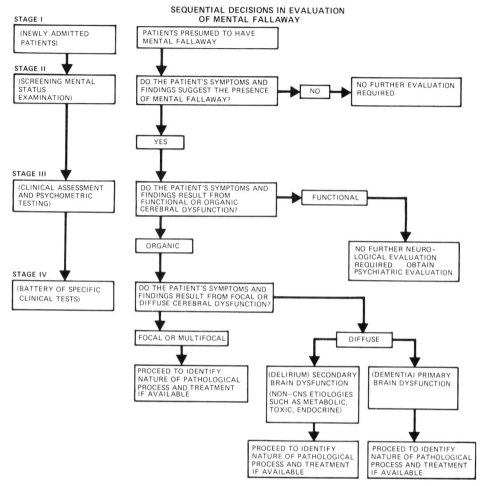

Figure 10-1. Sequential Decisions in Evaluation of Mental Fallaway.

Stage I describes those newly admitted patients presumed to have mental fallaway.

The decision at stage II as to whether or not the patient's findings suggest the presence of mental fallaway is based on a screening mental evaluation. The screening examination seeks historical findings consistent with intellectual and memory decline from the patient and from relatives, friends and/or letters of referral from health professionals. Historical findings suggestive of premorbid intelligence are sought, e.g., educational background. A mental status examination is performed to determine orientation, language abilities, attention, recent memory, general fund of knowledge, constructional abilities, and ability to handle calculations appropriate for educational background.

The decision at stage III as to whether the patient's apparent dementia results from organic or functional causes is made by a combination of traditional clinical assessment and a battery of psychometric tests. Functional causes are assessed by a traditional psychiatric interview. Based on a thorough examination, a clinical rating scale differentiating depression from dementia is employed (Table 10-1). In addition, the Hamilton Depression Scale and if possible, the Zung Self-Rating Depression Scale could be employed to assess and quantitate the degree of depression.

If functional causes for apparent dementia are excluded, then a full battery of neuropsychometrics is generally administered for the purpose of confirmation and quantification of the organic intellectual dysfunction. This battery should be administered by a qualified neuropsychologist and consists of at least the following tests:

Mental Status Interview
  • Orientation
  • Memory
  • Conversational and Expository Speech
Bender Visual Motor Gestalt Test
Apraxia Test
WAIS Vocabulary Subtest
WAIS Information Subtest
WAIS Digit Span Subtest
WAIS Block Design Subtest
WAIS Digit Symbol Subtest
Visual Discrimination Test
Spatial Orientation Memory Test
Luria Reading Test
Luria Object Naming Test
Partington's Pathways
Face-Hand Test
Wechsler Memory Scale Paired Associates Subtest
Oculomotor Scanning Test
Finger Tapping Test
Hamilton Rating Scale for Depression
Zung Self-Rating Scale for Depression
Wechsler Memory Scale—Logical Memory Subtest

The above battery routinely takes 1½ to 2 hours to administer. The tests are interpreted according to standard conventions and based on normative data, and an overall impairment index can be computed as well as inferred verbal and performance IQs.

The decision at Stage IV as to specific type of neurological dysfunction and specific diagnosis will be based on a battery of screening tests. The division of patients at Stage IV into focal or multifocal versus diffuse categories can usually be made by clinical neurological examination. Certain laboratory investigations, e.g., CT scan and EEG, may also be of benefit in some instances in making this determination.

The subdivision of the diffuse category into primary dementias (primary brain dysfunction) on the one hand, and secondary dementias (delirium caused by metabolic, toxic, endocrine encephalopathies, or of other non-CNS etiology) on the other hand, has much clinical importance. The latter in general has a more favorable prognosis and is reversible if the primary abnormality can be corrected. A clinical characteristic of this kind of encephalopathy is that a fluctuating level of consciousness is often seen.

The primary dementias consist of primary brain dysfunctions and only occasionally are reversible. As mentioned earlier, many of these may lend themselves to stabilization. Establishment of an accurate diagnosis is required to identify those primary dementias with treatable etiologies and for making a prognosis. Wells (1978) suggests a comprehensive diagnostic battery of tests. The following is a revised and updated version of this battery of laboratory studies for patients with organic intellectual decline:

Blood tests:
    Complete blood count
    Serological test for syphilis
    SMA-12
    Electrolytes
    T_3 and T_4
    Vitamin B_{12} and folate levels
    Serum bromide, barbiturate analyses, and other drug assay if appropriate
Urinalysis
Chest x-ray
Computerized axial tomography (CT scan) of the head
EEG
CSF analyses

CSF analyses consist of total protein, cells, glucose, VDRL, India ink, and cultures for bacteria and fungi. Further neurological evaluation may be performed, e.g., cerebral angiography, scinticisternography, nuclear brain scans, skull x-rays, serum ammonia, cryptococcal antigen, brain biopsy, as the clinical situation warrants.

Treatment. The treatment of diffuse mental fallaway is based on the established diagnosis. In selected cases treatment with thyroid hormone, vitamins, chelating agents, and antibiotics may be indicated. Also, surgical procedures, such as removal of subdural hematomas and tumors, and shunting for normal pressure hydrocephalus may be indicated.

Anticoagulants may be indicated in patients with a history or predisposition to thromboembolic disease.

CNS stimulants may bring about an increase in activity and some improvement in intellectual functioning, but studies showing drug efficacy are equivocal. These agents (amphetamines and methylphenidate) may cause increased confusion and paranoid ideation.

In addition, treatment of medical problems such as pulmonary, renal, or hepatic insufficiency is important. Some believe that a sudden decrease in mental functioning in the aged can be traced to general medical abnormalities in 50 percent, and to a primary change in neurologic function in about 33 percent.

Finally, some general care procedures are employed:

- Assign the same nurse every day
- Keep immediate surroundings as quiet as possible
- Put a clock and a calendar near the patient's bed
- Label articles with hospital's name, e.g. sheets, towels, etc.
- Frequently remind the patient where he is
- Post a list of the patient's daily routine
- Make sure windows are safe and secure
- Make night rounds every half hour
- Keep a night light near the patient's bed
- Assign the same nurses for each shift
- Be sure nurses and aides introduce themselves
- Try to minimize changes in routine
- Maximize sensory input with glasses and hearing aides
- Be on the alert for subclinical infections and pain since these may cause decompensation of marginal coping abilities
- If sedation is needed, use of mild or low-dose antianxiety agents on a short-term basis is indicated. If stronger medication is needed, use of high-potency low-dose, low anticholinergic, antipsychotic medications should be used, carefully biotitrated as to dose to each individual aged patient.

TREATMENT OF THE GERIATRIC PATIENT

This section on psychiatric treatment is divided into two parts, one on psychotherapy and one on psychopharmacology. It is, of course, an artificial separation of these two key components in optimum treatment of any psychiatric patient, young or old. In real life, one cannot separate treatment of a patient into neat compartments, but must instead carefully choose the most appropriate combination of psychotherapeutic and drug modes (ranging from all to none of one of the treatment modes, to any combination of the two).

Only in remembering that aged patients must be treated as individual human beings, with multivaried personalities and life experiences, can the most appropriate and effective unique treatment plan be devised for each patient. This "biotitration" of course compounds the difficulties involved with treatment of mental illness, but makes it all the more interesting for those practitioners involved.

Psychotherapy

As mentioned earlier, the geriatric population has a multitude of specific stresses with which to contend. The physiologic, psychologic and socioeconomic stresses are unique to the geriatric patient and the cumulative effects thereof over the course of a lifetime must be considered. However, allowing for reduced vigor and perhaps speed of learning, psychotherapy can probably be conducted along lines similar to those used at younger age levels. There may be a need to be more active and direct, since length of time available for therapy may be shortened among the geriatric population.

Also, working closely with the family of the geriatric patient can be very important, since families frequently are an integral part of the patient's personal care and well-being. It is essential that, when feasible, open lines of communication be maintained between family and therapist in order to foster high levels of understanding, and therefore optimum treatment of the patient. Too often, caring family members of an aged patient who are eager to help and could be elicited as co-partners in therapy, are kept in the dark by a reticent and noncommunicative therapist.

The type of psychotherapy utilized depends on the physical state of the patient, his suitability for therapy and his present capacity for establishing a workable relationship with the therapist. Also, are the presenting symptoms in the older patient new; or are they a continuation of a long-standing personality structure?

Psychotherapy can be conveniently described as a spectrum, with "supportive" psychotherapy at one end, to pure "insight" psychotherapy at the other, with the center of the spectrum somewhat fuzzy. Generally speaking, supportive therapy is directed at symptom relief and overt change in behavior, with no emphasis on modification of the patient's personality or resolution of intrapsychic conflict. The goals of insight-directed psychotherapy involve attempting to help the patient to achieve greater self-awareness and even some degree of underlying personality change. Also, there is an attempt to achieve some degree of overall psychological maturity, with increased independence and tolerance of stress. The type of therapy chosen for a geriatric patient of course depends on the individual makeup, needs and abilities, as discussed earlier.

Some general guidelines concerning treatment of geriatric patients can be listed.

1. Understand and try to minimize the insecurity and anxiety of the patient. This must be done with considerable tact in order not to shatter an older patient's pride. Somehow, the patient must be made to feel his dependency needs are being gratified, without having him feel he is leaning on someone else for support. A key point here is that by taking over functions for the aged, care-givers effectively, if inadvertently, rob them of self-mastery, independence and control. Unfortunately, takeover sometimes becomes necessary as a protective device from deficiencies in judgment. When possible, plans should be made with patients, not for them.

2. The aged patient should be allowed to adequately express himself. Impatience by the therapist, even when problems are repeated over and over again, is difficult to handle. Attention and empathy (not sympathy) are essential. Respect, not pity, is necessary for the patient to maintain his self-esteem and dignity.

3. An optimistic attitude is helpful when dealing with an aged patient. Patients should leave the psychotherapeutic session gratified, and feeling that something was accomplished. Admittedly, this is not always an easy thing to accomplish.

4. Aged patients should be directed into programs and activities which help enhance their physical and mental attractiveness. To be wanted increases one's self-esteem, and consequently, one's value to others. They also should be assisted into accepting a curtailment and redirection of activities when necessary, with the redirection into something gratifying and meaningful. In order to accomplish this, the therapist should be aware of the facilities in the community, the church and social agencies which have been established for the elderly. The geriatric patient should be helped to maximize his physical, mental and social capabilities. Remotivation techniques directly challenge the particular aged patient who desires to withdraw from life, or to die. One of the best ways of remotivation is to encourage the aged patient to become involved in helping relationships, and to take an active interest in the lives of others.

DEATH AND DYING

When discussing psychotherapy in the aged population, a word should be said about death and dying. According to Kubler-Ross (1969), psychiatrically it is important to appreciate that "in terms of the unconscious, we cannot conceive of our own death and that in addition, we cannot differentiate between the wish and the deed." Although people today have the same kind of thoughts and fantasies about death that occurred in their ancestors, today's society seems to be a death-denying one. There is the suggestion of an illusion that since man has mastered so many things, death will be mastered as well.

Some generalizations can be made, based mostly on Kubler-Ross' and others pioneering work (Hackett, 1962; Wake, 1959).

1. Almost all patients know when they are terminally ill, whether or not they've been told. Patients usually state that they would like to be told if their illness is serious, but not without hope.

2. Most, but not all patients seem to pass through five stages (denial, anger, bargaining, depression and acceptance) between their awareness of serious illness and their death. The physician, particularly one who is himself comfortable in facing the dying patient, can assist the patient in passing through one, some or all of these stages by appropriate verbal and nonverbal

support. The patient is particularly heartened when he realizes the physician will stay with him until the end.

Psychopharmacology

One can categorize general patterns of disturbed behavior seen, although not exclusively, in the aged population which suggest the use of psychotropic medication. They have been reviewed elsewhere (Stotsky, 1972) and are revised as follows:

1. Boisterous, aggressive, belligerent, verbally hostile and even assaultive.
2. Anxious, restless, agitated, motorically hyperactive (including pacing and hand-wringing), aneretic, sometimes even self-mutilating.
3. Elated, rapid-talking, hyperactive, with pressured speech, insomnia and disorganized thinking.
4. Depressed, aneretic, insomniac (particularly in the early morning), morbid, nihilistic and guilty thinking, preoccupied with death, retarded in thought, speech and movement, often exhibiting paranoid thinking.
5. Uncooperative, withdrawn, quietly negativistic, sullen, at times mute and even stuporous.
6. Delusions involving ideas of jealousy, persecution, influence, grandiosity, or erotic experiences.
7. Hallucinations, primarily auditory or tactile (formication).
8. Regressed behavior, including carelessness about personal appearance and a disregarding of lifetime moral standards, silly affect with grimacing common, deficit in perception, attention span, memory (both recent and remote) and orientation, poor insight and judgment.

A prolonged incidence of the above behavior, with no evidence of an organic etiology, as well as the failure of environmental manipulation, suggests intervention with psychotropic medications.

Psychotropic medications are defined here in the traditional manner, i.e., any medication which is capable of modifying mental activity, and is given with the intent to exert an effect on mental activity. Mental activity is a function of the brain by which an individual is aware of his surroundings and his distribution in time and space, and also by which he is able to attend, to remember, to reason and to decide, as well as to experience feelings, emotions, and desires.*

---

*Another definition of "mind," usually attributed to Ambrose Bierce, is less stuffy, more real, and supplies ample food for one's own thoughts. "MIND, . . . A mysterious form of matter secreted by the brain. Its chief activity consists in the endeavor to ascertain its own nature, the futility of the attempt being due to the fact that it has nothing but itself to know itself with."

The subgroups subsumed under the rubric of psychotropic medications are:

- Antipsychotics
- Antidepressants
- Antianxiety agents
- Sedatives and hypnotics
- Stimulants
- Cognitive-acting drugs
- Lithium carbonate
- A miscellaneous group usually associated with the aged, e.g. vasodilators, vitamins, hormones, possibly endorphins and encephalins.

It is not the intent of the chapter to go into detail concerning the specific therapeutic activity and side effects in the aged population of each of these psychotropic drugs. Rather, general concepts concerning use of psychotropic medications in the elderly patient will be discussed. Specific information on subgroups of psychotropics can be found elsewhere (Maletta, 1979).

It is well-known that aging in different organ systems occurs at varying rates, and that among individuals, the rates of functional decline of the same organ also differ. Further, disease processes that randomly occur in a cohort of same-aged individuals must be considered. This adds to the disparity in functional capabilities of organ systems. Therefore, each aged patient fits no general category and must be considered as a unique individual.

Given the sensitivity of aged individuals to drug dose and side effects and also keeping in mind the multitude of other medications frequently taken, the necessity of individualizing drug choice, dose, mode of administration, as well as time of day and length of treatment becomes paramount. This is the concept of biotitration of medication in the aged patient.

General guidelines should be established for choice and administration of all psychotropic medications, especially when used in the aged population. For example, the concept of a "standard dose" is a poor one with older patients. A good rule of thumb is "start low and go slow." One should be conservative in approaching drug treatment in an elderly patient, but not so conservative that one practices therapeutic nihilism and the patient winds up receiving no treatment at all. Some guidelines for administration of psychotropic medications include:

1. Medical history, including social history (alcohol, drugs, smoking, coffee, cola, chocolate, etc); allergies or adverse interactions; good medication history, recent and past (including nasal decongestants, eye drops, birth control pills, vitamins, dietary habits, etc).
2. Medications should be given initially at a high enough effective dosage (must be biotitrated for each patient), then decreased as soon as feasible to the minimum effective dosage necessary to provide the desired clinical result (exception: aged or debilitated patients—with them, begin low and

build up gradually). Consider initiation of therapy on an IM basis, to circumvent problems and GI absorption. This is not advisable for elderly patients because of the potential for postural hypotension.

3. Particular medication chosen should be the most effective against the particular target symptoms exhibited, and also because of its particular side effect profile, especially in elderly patients.

4. Medications should be administered for a sufficient period of time before deciding on efficacy (4-6 weeks, within practicality restraints). If possible, steps should be taken to ensure the medication has a serum level. Remember that serum levels may vary as much as 100-fold in different patients given the same dose of medication.

5. Be aware of FDA upper limits of dosage where given (not a constraint to individual clinical considerations, but is important to know legally).

6. Antiextrapyramidal agents (AEA) should not be routinely used on a prophylactic basis. When they are used, it should be no longer than three months continuously without discontinuation and observation. Avoid using AEAs in aged patients already on an antipsychotic and/or an antidepressant because of the potentiation of anticholinergic side effects.

7. The most optimum medication regimen is a single daily dose, if half-life permits, preferably at bedtime. A possible exception is an elderly patient who may be unable to tolerate the side effects of a single daily dose.

8. PRN antipsychotics should be thought about only on an initial treatment basis, and then switched to ongoing as soon as possible.

9. Medications should be discontinued once a year or sooner, to ascertain their continuing need and also in the case of antipsychotics, to observe possible onset of symptoms of tardive dyskinesia which are masked by the medication. Weekend "drug vacations" are probably not very effective regarding decreasing side effects.

10. Indiscriminate polypharmacy should be avoided. However, the concept of polypharmacy may be a useful one in many cases, e.g. an antipsychotic plus an antidepressant; dilantin and phenobarbital; a tricyclic plus a MAOI (provided their possible adverse interaction is understood); occasionally two antipsychotics might even be justified if a high dose of one which is effective causes toxic symptomology; a tricyclic plus lithium.

11. Avoid chronic use of minor tranquilizers or sleep medications, especially in elderly patients.

12. Avoid chronic use of IM medications.

13. If patient has been on an MAOI, wait at least two weeks before beginning an antidepressant tricyclic.

14. If new symptoms are seen after a medication is started, it's very important to decide whether they're due to the disease or the medication (or both). It is therefore a good idea to attempt to observe the patient in depth in order to get an adequate idea of his disease symptomology *before* beginning a psychotropic.

Particularly with antipsychotic medications, where mechanism and efficacy are generally considered to be similar among the various drug families, one should choose a drug in terms of its particular side effect profile for an individual aged patient. The drug should be best suited to the existing physiological ambience of the patient, both in terms of existing diseases, and other drugs already in the system. This minimizes the possibility of drug/drug and drug/system interactions, both of which are real and potential dangers in the elderly patient population on medications. It should be reiterated here, because of its importance, that one of the most common effects of drug-drug interactions in elderly patients is a toxic delirium, which is not infrequently mistaken for a dementing illness or even a psychosis.

CASE HISTORY—*TOXIC DELIRIUM*

Mr. R. was an 82-year-old man who was brought into the ER by his family because he was "acting crazy and senile." The behavior had started abruptly two days earlier following a visit to the patient's eye doctor for a routine examination.

The patient had a long previous psychiatric history, with a diagnosis of "chronic undifferentiated schizophrenia," and was presently being treated with Thorazine 600 mg/day and Cogentin 2 mg b.i.d. He was also placed on Elavil 150 mg/day about one month prior to being seen because of "depression" following the recent death of his wife of 60 years. Patient was also taking an over-the-counter sedative to help him sleep. It was discovered that the ophthalmologist had dilated the pupils of the patient during the exam in order to get a better look at his retinas.

On mental status exam, patient was found to be disoriented to time and place. His attention, concentration and perception as measured by digit span were found to be grossly deficient, and he remembered none of three items after five minutes. He was having visual hallucinations throughout the exam.

Patient was admitted to hospital, where his work-up for organic causes, including CT scan, was unremarkable. His medications were gradually stopped, and he was placed under close observation. Within seven days, his sensorium was perfectly clear and his MSE was completely within normal limits.

Other general areas to consider when discussing psychotropic drugs in elderly patients are:

1. Appropriate size and clarity of instructions on medication container labels.
2. Ease of opening of medication containers (surprisingly, "childproof" bottles can be a frequent barrier to the acquisition of needed medication by an aged patient with feeble hand and finger strength, or a declining adeptness at hand-eye coordination).
3. Medication ingestion and optimum dietary habits. Diet is a problem somewhat unique to the elderly patient. At best, it is erratic in terms of quantity and quality; and at worst, the diet may be nutritionally disastrous.

These habits impinge directly on the patient in terms of optimum medication ingestion, absorption and activity.

4. Optimum maintenance therapy. There is substantial evidence in the field of psychotropics, especially the antipsychotics, that fewer patients kept on medication had a relapse of symptoms when compared with comparable patients on no medication, or on a placebo. However, there is less substantial evidence that this is necessarily true for older patients (Davis, *et al.*, 1973).

Again, one must use clinical, individual judgment when deciding whether to maintain a particular aged patient on psychotropics, and if so, at what dose and for how long. Certainly, much stronger indications for maintenance treatment in an older patient would be needed than for a relatively younger one because of problems with side effects, both short- and long-term. Some indications to consider might be a) a history of relapse in the past following discontinuation of drugs, and b) if doses used in the past were very high when compared with other patients with the same diagnosis. A major point to remember is that under no conditions should all elderly patients be routinely placed on maintenance psychotropic medications for years at a time without a regular, periodic review.

5. Problems with side effects after long-term usage. This is particularly important with long-term usage of antipsychotics, because of the increasingly prevalent discovery of symptoms of tardive dyskinesia, not only in elderly patients, but patients in general who take these psychotropic medications. Those who prescribe and dispense these medications should maintain a constant vigil for early signs (such as resting tongue fasciculations) of this sometimes irreversible motor dysfunction, especially in the elderly population (Tarsy and Baldessarini, 1976).

REFERENCES

Asnes D: Psychopharmacology in the aged. Use of major psychotropic medications in the treatment of the elderly: case examples. *J Geriat Psychiatry* 7:189-202, 1974

Busse E and Pfeiffer E (eds): *Mental Illness in Later Life.* Washington, D.C., Psychiatric Association, 1979

Dewald P: *Psychotherapy—A Dynamic Approach.* New York, Basic Books, 1969

Jenkyn L, Walsh D, Culver C and Reeves A: Clinical signs in diffuse cerebral dysfunction, *J Neurol Neurosurg and Psychiatry* 40: 956-966, 1977

Kubler-Ross E: *On Death and Dying.* New York, Macmillan, 1969

Maletta G: Effects of psychotropic drugs in the elderly patient. *In*: Maletta G and Pirozzolo F (eds): *The Aging Nervous System.* New York, Praeger Press, 1979

Maletta G (ed): *Survey Report on the Aging Nervous System.* Washington, D.C., DHEW 74-296, 1975

Schuckit M: Geriatric alcoholism and drug abuse. *Gerontologist,* 17: 168-174, 1977

Verwoerdt A: *Clinical Geropsychiatry.* Baltimore, Williams & Wilkins, 1976

Wang H and Busse E: Dementia in Old Age. *In*: Wells, C (ed). *Dementia.* Philadelphia, F.A. Davis, 1971, pp. 151-162

Wells C: Chronic brain disease: An overview. *Am J Psychiatry* 135: 1-12, 1978

Wells, C: *Diagnostic Evaluation and Treatment in Dementia. In*: Wells, C (ed). *Dementia* Philadelphia, F.A. Davis, 1977

Wells C: Organic psychoses. *Psych Ann* 8:58, 1978

SUGGESTED READING

Ban TA: The treatment of depressed geriatric patients. *Am J Psychother* 32: 93-104. 1978

Brown BS: How do mental health and aging affect each other? *Geriatrics* 31: 40-44, 1976

Citrin R and Dixon D: Reality orientation. A milieu therapy used in an institution for the aged. *Gerontologist* 17: 39-43, 1977

Davis J, Fann W, El-Yousef M and Janowsky D: Clinical Problems in Treating the Aged with Psychotropic Drugs. *In*: Eisdorfer C and Fann W (eds): *Psychopharmacology and Aging,* New York, Plenum, pp. 111-125, 1973

Davis J and Garver D: Psychobiology of Affective Disorders. *Current Concepts,* Upjohn Co., 1978

Eisdorfer C: Evaluation of the quality of psychiatric care for the aged. *Am J Psychiatry* 134: 315-317, 1977

Fleiss J, Gurland B and Roche P: Distinctions between organic brain syndrome and functional psychiatric disorders. *Int J Aging Hum Dev* 7:323-330, 1976

Freeman FR: Evaluation of patients with progressive intellectual deterioration. *Arch Neurol* 33: 658-659, 1976

Gagleano L, Gianturco D and Ramm D: Treatment goals in geropsychiatry. *J Am Geriatr Soc* 23: 460-464, 1975

Gaitz C (ed): *Aging and the Brain.* New York, Plenum Press, 1972

Garetz F: Common psychiatric syndromes of the aged. *Minnesota Med* 57: 618-620. 1974

Goldstein S and Birnbom F: Hypochondriasis and the elderly. *J Am Geriatr Soc* 24: 150-154, 1976

Hackett T and Weisman A: The treatment of the dying. *Current Psychiatr Ther* 121-126, 1962

Katzman R and Karasu T: Differential diagnosis of dementia. In: Fields W (ed). *Neurological and Sensory Disorders in the Elderly.* New York, Stratton, 1975, pp. 103-134

Kay DW: Schizophrenia and schizophrenia-like states in the elderly. *Br J Psychiatry* 9: 19-24, 1975

Kral VA: Somatic therapies in older depressed patients. *J Gerontol* 31: 311-313, 1976

Raskind M, Alvarez C, Pietrzyk M, Westerlund K and Herlin S: Helping the elderly psychiatric patient in crisis. *Geriatrics* 31: 51-56, 1976

Sachar EJ: The concept and phenomenology of depression, with special reference to the aged. *Geriatric Psychiatry* 7: 55-69, 1974

Sathananthan G, Ferris S and Gershon S: Psychopharmacology of aging: Current trends. *Curr Dev Psychopharmacol* 4: 249-264, 1977

Simon A, Lowenthal M and Epstein L: *Crisis and Intervention.* San Francisco, Jossey-Bass, 1970

Snyder B and Harris S: Treatable aspects of the dementia syndrome. *J Am Geriatr Soc* 24:179-184, 1976

Sparacino J: An attributional approach to psychotherapy with the aged. *J Am Geriatr Soc* 26: 414-417, 1978

Stotsky B: Haloperidol in the treatment of geriatric patients. *In*: DiMascio A and Shader R (eds): *Butyrophenones in Psychiatry,* New York, Raven, pp. 71-86, 1972

Tarsy D and Baldessarini R: The tardive dyskinesia syndrome. *In*: Klawans H (ed): *Clinical Neuropharmacology,* Raven, pp. 29-61, 1976

Timiras P (ed): *Developmental Physiology and Aging.* New York, Macmillan, 1972

Turner R and Sternberg M: Psychosocial factors in elderly patients admitted to a psychiatric hospital. *Age and Aging* 7: 171-177, 1978

Van Praag HM: Psychotropic drugs in the aged. *Compr Psychiatry* 18: 429-442, 1977

Wahl C: The fear of death. In: Feifel H (ed): *The Meaning of Death,* New York, McGraw-Hill, 1959, pp. 16-29

III
TREATMENT CONCERNS

11

Guidelines for Administering Psychotropic Agents

PATRICK T. DONLON, M.D.

About 20 percent of all prescriptions written by physicians are for psychotropic agents. These agents make an important contribution to modern medicine, because psychopathological disorders are both disabling and distressing. In general, they are well tolerated and highly effective. Clinical indications and adverse effects were covered in the previous chapters: neuroleptics (3, 12), tricyclic antidepressants and lithium (5), monoamine oxidase inhibitors (6), and antianxiety agents (7). Following are 10 basic, yet practical and clinically oriented guidelines for the proper administration of psychotropic agents. These are followed by a discussion on the strategies for administering the four common classes of psychotropic drugs.

1. *There must be a strong indication.* The indications for the administration of psychotropic agents must be sound for two reasons: First, the likelihood of a positive response correlates highly with the recommended diagnostic indications listed on the package insert; and second, the potential merit of the agent must greatly outweigh the risk of adverse effects.

Often patients will request psychotropics for trivial symptoms, such as anxiety or insomnia. In such cases the origin of the complaint must be carefully assessed. In general, medication is never indicated for minor symptoms where other treatment recommendations (techniques to reduce stress, relaxation therapies, etc.) are in order. Also, if the symptoms are secondary to a medical or other psychiatric (e.g., depression) disorder, the focus of treatment should be directed there. If an antianxiety or sedative-hypnotic agent is to be prescribed, it should normally only be for a brief trial as anxiety and insomnia are typically episodic and dependence may become a concern with maintenance therapy.

Lithium, neuroleptics, and antidepressants are often indicated on a maintenance basis. But justification must be documented, and the patient should be given trials off the medication periodically to document continued need. Because long-term adverse effects are now being documented with neuroleptics (e.g., tardive dyskinesia/TD) and lithium (e.g., renal lesions), the risk and merits of ongoing treatment should be discussed in detail with the patient, and possibly an informed consent form signed.

2. *Many factors influence response.* The curative effects of drugs are often exaggerated, when in fact, the outcome of drug therapy is the cumulative effect of numerous determinants. Some of these factors are described below.

Among the most important factors are the pharmacologic actions, the effects of kinetics (absorption, metabolism, excretion, etc.) on bio-availability, and dosage schedules. These are discussed briefly later in this chapter where the individual agents are reviewed.

Diagnosis, natural history, and a doctor-patient relationship are important. A diagnosis is helpful in identifying the correct treatment, plus providing general guidelines for the prognosis and natural history. As it may be difficult to predict the natural history early in the course of an illness, it is helpful to discontinue psychotropic drug treatment from time to time to establish the need for further maintenance treatment. A patient may have a spontaneous remission or exacerbation of symptoms unrelated to drug treatment. Rapid remissions are not only the rule with anxiety and panic states, but also occur with depression, mania, schizophrenia, and organically impaired mental states. With a positive doctor-patient relationship, the patient often responds better to treatment and develops fewer adverse effects.

Another factor which affects treatment response is the patient's willingness to take the drugs as prescribed. There are many reasons why a patient may not follow the physician's instructions: misunderstanding of directions; denial of illness; concern with the interactional effects of other medications or alcohol; possible interference with socialization or recreation; inconvenient dosage scheduling; feelings of helplessness; discouragement of family, friends or other "authority figures;" past negative experience with the same or similar agent; and perhaps most importantly, concern with adverse effects. Regardless of the reason, the end result may be the same, namely, inadequate clinical response. The physician should routinely inquire about compliance, and if the agent is being taken irregularly, document why.

Various illnesses and life events can influence treatment. The patient may have mental symptoms from a medical illness or adverse effects from prescribed or illicit drugs. Thus, a complete medical history is a prerequisite to psychotropic drug treatment, and patients who fail to respond to drug treatment may require further assessment. In addition, the relationship between stressful life events and treatment response is strongly suggested by the terms "reactive," "functional," or "situational" psychiatric disorders. The relationship with life events may be more common with the milder in contrast to major psychiatric states. Nonetheless, all psychiatric illnesses can be influenced by a wide variety of concurrent or upcoming life events which can markedly influence subjective distress and thus affect response to treatment.

Nonspecific factors (characteristic of patient-doctor-agent-treatment setting, etc.) can greatly influence drug treatment. These factors also seem to be more influential in mild (vs. severe) psychiatric disorders. However, an enthusiastic attitude by the patient and doctor toward psychotropic drug treatment increases compliance and probably will result in a more favorable outcome. These nonspecific factors are important historically in medicine and also help to explain why healers in general achieve favorable results with multiple and often nonproven approaches. And it explains why placebo (PBO) response is very high in emotional disorders, and especially with the mild and reactive disorders. This PBO response often occurs early and lessens with continued treatment, and it is not associated with age, sex, race, or education. Furthermore, true PBO response must be distinguished from spontaneous remission which occurs during the PBO period. Often the two are not separated.

3. *Comprehensive medical and psychiatric assessment.* A thorough psychiatric and medical assessment are indicated before a diagnosis can be established and treatment initiated. This often includes a review of past records, obtaining additional history from family members, a physical examination, and indicated laboratory tests. A careful mental status examination is also necessary as may be a period of observation.

The differential diagnosis may be complicated by the mimicking effects of unrelated syndromes. Also, the picture may be mixed as when trauma, substance abuse, and ill health are seen in individuals with apparent functional disorders.

DSM-III places emphasis on diagnostic precision and allows for diagnosis on five axes. Also, Axes I and II diagnoses must follow strict diagnostic criteria both for phenomena and duration of illness.

To assist in diagnosis, we find it helpful to pool data from six sources: delineation from other disorders, clinical description (course and phenomena), laboratory studies, response to treatment, family study, and follow-up. Delineation from other disorders includes identifying those cases which may arise from underlying biologic (e.g., CNS depressants and stimulants use, antihypertensive agents, hormones) origins. A careful history and mental status examination will best document the course and phenomena associated with the illness. Laboratory tests, special procedures (e.g., CT scan), and psychological testing are helpful in identifying etiologic factors. Treatment response provides some data on diagnosis and also for establishing a treatment plan. It is also helpful to identify self-treatment techniques (e.g., substance abuse, life style) for similar reason. Family study data is extremely important as some illnesses (e.g., bipolar affective disorder) are highly familial. At times it is necessary to interview family members to obtain additional historical data and to better assess family illnesses. Follow-up and a willingness to change the diagnostic impression are essential as monitoring is often necessary and the preliminary diagnosis may be incorrect.

4. *Target signs and symptoms.* Psychiatric disorders are basically syndromes and include a grouping of key signs and symptoms. Therefore, for precision in diagnosis and monitoring of the treatment course, it is important that the clinician identify and monitor cardinal signs and symptoms. In fact, their presence or absence is more important than the diagnosis itself when presenting the case to colleagues, establishing a treatment plan, and evaluating treatment. Many clinicians find it helpful to monitor the treatment course by rating target symptoms, such as with the Brief Psychiatric Rating Scale (BPRS).

Target signs and symptoms include: schizophrenia (cognitive disorganization, idiosyncratic responses, auditory hallucination); mania (pressure of speech, euphoria, flight of ideas, increased psychomotor activity); depression (depressed mood, insomnia, anorexia, guilt, agitation or motor retardation); and anxiety (apprehension, tension, autonomic changes).

5. *Avoid combination therapy and polypharmacy.* Polypharmacy refers to concurrent use of a number of agents, belonging either to the same or different groups. An extreme example for a psychiatric patient is the co-administration of one or more neuroleptics, one or more antidepressants, a sedative hypnotic, an antiparkinsonian/AP agent, and a benzodiazepine. Unfortunately, polypharmacy is much too common.

Yet arguments remain both against and for polypharmacy. The strongest argument against it is that it is impossible to determine which agent is therapeutic and which is producing adverse effects. Possible interactional effects may also be present increasing adverse lability risk. Finally, there is probably no sound clinical evidence which demonstrates that two or more agents within a drug class (e.g., neuroleptics) are more effective than a single agent. In general, polypharmacy tends to increase adverse effects without increasing efficacy. An important guideline is to try one agent at a time. Then after an adequate trial, substitute if necessary.

Nonetheless, combination therapy is indicated on some occasions and common examples as cited below. First, due to the lag period of lithium, a brief trial on a neuroleptic is often necessary to rapidly control acute manic symptoms. Second, delusional depressed patients often require a neuroleptic along with a tricyclic antidepressant (TCA). Three, the sedative effect of a TCA may be insufficient to improve sleep so a sedative-hypnotic may be temporarily indicated. In this latter case, it is best to add a benzodiazepine or chloral hydrate (vs. a barbiturate hypnotic) to avoid enzyme induction and increased TCA metabolic breakdown. Four, some depressed schizophrenic individuals require a low dosage TCA in combination with their neuroleptic. Five, up to 50 percent of patients started on neuroleptics will require an AP agent during the first two months of treatment for control of extrapyramidal symptoms (EPS). After adaptation occurs (normally within two months) only about 20 percent of the patients on neuroleptics will require an AP agent.

6. *Importance of avoiding adverse effects.* Toxicity seldom presents when psychotropic agents are taken in recommended dosage and when routine precautions are followed. Nonetheless, mild adverse effects are extremely common early in the treatment course and present in most cases. Despite this most patients are willing to tolerate mild discomfort especially if they are assured that the adverse effects are benign, and that the agent will be effective.

We find it helpful to discuss common adverse effects before initiating drug treatment. This reduces worry, greatly increases compliance, and allows the patient to separate adverse effects from psychopathologic symptoms. The physician, in turn, should take steps to minimize adverse effects. Starting with a low dosage and close patient monitoring are helpful. On other occasions, adjusting dosage, switching to another agent, or adding contra-active therapy are in order. Finally, openly encouraging the patient to report adverse effects creates an atmosphere of concern which has a positive effect on the treatment outcome as well as on compliance.

7. *Importance of correct dosage.* Psychotropic dosage schedules vary considerably and need to be highly individualized. A titration model is helpful with psychotropic agents. Namely, balancing drug dosage against symptom response and adverse effects. In general, it is helpful to begin with a conservative and divided daily dosage to establish response. If response is positive and immediate, there is no need to increase dosage. However, if the agent is well tolerated and the clinical picture unchanged, then the dosage should be increased within a day or two. And if significant adverse effects present, then the dosage should be reduced or the agent discontinued.

Lag periods or the delaying of clinical effects following initial administration are common with psychotropic agents. A positive response seldom occurs within the first 2-3 days with peroral neuroleptics. However, response with IM neuroleptics often presents within hours. With lithium and TCA therapy, the lag period normally is 3-10 days, and up to three weeks, respectively. With benzodiazepine antianxiety agents and the sedative-hypnotics effects normally occur almost immediately.

Underdosing is commonly seen, especially with TCA. Package insert guidelines are helpful for predicting dosage requirements, but individualization of the dosage schedule is essential. A two-phase dosage scheme is indicated for all psychotropic agents. Once the illness has moved into remission, the agent should either be gradually discontinued or the dosage slowly reduced to a maintenance level. Failure to do so will increase risk of adverse effects, and in some cases long-term toxicity (e.g., possibly TD with neuroleptics) might present. Serum levels (e.g., lithium) can assist with better determining the dosage requirements. The average maintenance levels for lithium, neuroleptics and TCAs are about one-third to one-half the dosage required to control acute symptoms.

8. *Adequate treatment trial.* Patients require an adequate treatment trial

before being considered refractory, and new treatment strategies initiated. Adequate treatment trials for a neuroleptic, TCA, and lithium are 2-4 weeks, 3 weeks, and 2-3 weeks respectively. Also, a prolonged trial will separate the slow-responders from the non-responders.

If the patient has not successfully responded within the trial period, diagnosis and dosage schedule should be reviewed. Despite this, about 25 percent of both manic and depressed patients will be non-responsive to initial treatment. But less than 10 percent of schizophrenic patients will be non-responsive to neuroleptics.

Backup treatments for mania include neuroleptics and ECT. Those for depression include other TCAs, trials on MAOIs, neuroleptics, lithium, and ECT. And those for schizophrenia include another neuroleptic or possibly trials on lithium or ECT.

9. *A consolidated bedtime dosage.* Administering psychotropic agents initially on a divided dosage schedule assists in establishing treatment response. Then within a few days the dosage can be consolidated to a single bedtime dose. The agents of exception are lithium where GI irritability may result and the short-acting antianxiety agents (e.g., oxazepam, lorazepam) which provide brief coverage. A single bedtime dosage greatly increases compliance through convenience while often reducing adverse effects. Moreover, if sedative effects are present they will assist sleep.

10. *Active patient participation.* It is helpful to engage patients actively in their drug treatment programs and to individualize the treatment approach. Reviewing the indications for drug and alternate treatments and the duration, potential risks and merits of treatment will better insure active participation. If maintenance drug therapy is required and added risks are possible (TD with neuroleptics, renal lesions with lithium, habituation with anxiolytic agents), the patient should be informed. In some cases, a signed informed consent form is essential.

Patients should also become aware of the prodromal symptoms of their illness so that exacerbations can be promptly identified and treated. In general, treatment outcome improves once a patient accepts his illness and assumes a responsibility for ongoing treatment.

STRATEGIES FOR ADMINISTERING PSYCHOTROPICS

Antianxiety Agents

The use of antianxiety agents has rapidly grown over the past 15 years and now they are the most frequently prescribed agents among the psychotropics. Concern now is on overutilization, especially since dependence (both psychological and physical) with benzodiazepines has been reported. The anxiolytics are effective predominantly in neurotic and anxiety states and have no established value in treating psychoses.

Recently our understanding of the action of benzodiazepines on anxiety states has increased.[1] First, there is now strong evidence that benzodiazepine receptors are present in the brain and that therapeutic potency may reflect the affinity of the agent to binding sites. The presence of the receptors suggests that an endogenous benzodiazepine type substance may occur naturally in the brain. Still none has yet been identified. Second, interaction with gamma-aminobutyric (GABA) increases the affinity for the binding sites. In turn, the benzodiazepines enhance the inhibiting neurotransmitter effect of GABA, which might explain some of the anxiolytic effects of the benzodiazepines. Three, the anxiolytic effects of the benzodiazepines may be secondary to their action on the locus ceruleus in the brain.

Adequate treatment of anxiety states requires a careful assessment of the nature of the psychiatric illness. This includes ruling out medical conditions which commonly underlie anxiety. A physical examination, medical history, and laboratory tests assist in the differential diagnosis. Lab tests may include a thyroid panel for possible thyroid-induced anxiety symptoms, adrenal assay for hyperadrenalism, and an EKG to determine the possible existence of arrhythmias. Also, "mitral-valve-prolapse syndrome" may present with symptoms very similar to anxiety states.[2]

DSM-III categorizes anxiety disorders into three subgroups: *phobic disorders, anxiety states,* and *post-traumatic stress disorders.* The phobic disorders include agorophobia, social phobia, and simple phobia. In general, phobic anxiety is a feeling of fear or panic experienced by a person in a certain situation or exposed to a specific object. Imipramine and phenelzine are more effective than the benzodiazepines in treating phobic states. Systematic desensitization and psychotherapy may also be effective.

Anxiety states include panic disorder, generalized anxiety disorder, and obsessive-compulsive disorder. Psychotherapy and drug treatment are indicated for the more severe and disabling disorders. Benzodiazepines are effective for the panic and generalized anxiety disorders. They are also highly effective with anticipatory anxiety, where the individual becomes anxious by merely contemplating exposure to the fear object. If significant depression is associated with anxiety, a sedating antidepressant (e.g., amitriptyline or doxepin) may be indicated. Panic associated with psychotic decompensation is best treated with neuroleptics. Finally, severe obsessive-compulsive disorders may respond optimally to TCAs and psychotherapy, but some cases do well with the benzodiazepines.

Post-traumatic stress disorders include acute, chronic or delayed, and atypical anxiety disorder. The clinical picture includes anxiety, nightmares, recurrent and intrusive recollection of the event, hyperalertness, and exaggerated startle response. Benzodiazepines may be helpful when given short-term. The ideal treatment program also includes psychotherapy and rehabilitation.

The benzodiazepines' popularity rests also on their established efficacy and their low incidence of adverse effects, drug interactions, and serious dependency problems. Clinical studies have shown little differences in their neuropharmacologic profiles. Administration is best peroral as when given intramuscularly, absorption is slow, erratic, and sometimes incomplete. Duration of administration should normally be brief as anxiety is typically an episodic disorder and maintenance therapy may lead to dependency. For clinical purposes, the benzodiazepines can be divided into two groups: short and longer-acting. The former includes oxazepam and lorazepam, while the latter includes diazepam, chlordiazepoxide, clorazepate, and prazepam. The short-acting agents may be given more than twice daily and cumulative effects are not a problem. The long-acting agents, in contrast, may have active metabolites and cumulative effects may occur with continued administration. Therefore, they should be given once to twice daily with closer monitoring of the dosage schedule.

Non-benzodiazepine alternative drug treatments for anxiety are available. Ethyl alcohol is the most common antianxiety drug taken by self-prescription and its adverse and toxic effects are well documented. The long-acting barbiturates, especially phenobarbital, were commonly recommended for the control of anxiety until the benzodiazepines first became available in the 1960s. Also, meprobamate was successfully marketed after its introduction in 1955. Meprobamate has several disadvantages when compared with the benzodiazepines and there are few indications for its use today. Disadvantages include reduced efficacy, and increased abuse and suicide potential. Antipsychotics are occasionally recommended as antianxiety agents. However, their potential short and long-term adverse effects are serious problems and limit the indications for their use in anxiety. TCAs should be considered as the single agent of choice if a significant depression is present in combination with anxiety. Benzodiazepines typically do not reduce depression, and may make it worse. Finally, beta blockers may be effective in anxiety disorder. Typically they reduce the psychophysiologic manifestations of anxiety but are less anxiolytic than the benzodiazepines.

Antidepressant Agents

Psychiatrists often find that the antidepressants are the most gratifying of the psychotropic drugs to prescribe. This is because major depressive disorders are extremely common, and the suffering associated with depression normally rapidly remits with medical treatment. Surveys report that at least 15 percent of the population will have one major depression in a lifetime, and that 50 percent of these patients will have recurrent episodes. Treatment response with TCAs normally occurs within three to four weeks following administration and with 70-75 percent of patients. Only shock therapy is more efficacious.

Much research has been focused on the psychobiology of affective disorders in recent years. In general, the unipolar depressed group is considered to be highly heterogeneous in contrast to the bipolar (manic-depressive) group where strong genetic influences are suggested. The pharmacologic actions and the differential effects that the various TCAs have on the re-uptake of serotonic and norepinephrine neurotransmitters have become better established. Numerous agents have been marketed since imipramine and the MAOIs were first introduced, but no agent has been found to be more effective than imipramine in the treatment of depression. And even today, agent selection is determined predominantly by clinical adverse effects, profiles, e.g., sedating (amitriptyline, doxepin) agent for the agitated; non-sedating agent (amoxopine, desipromine, imipramine) for the retarded depression; low cholinergic lability (e.g., desipramine) for the elderly, etc. The MAOIs are less frequently used in the treatment of depression. This is due to reduced efficacy, dietary restrictions, and concern for severe adverse effects, including hypertensive crisis.

In addition to the TCAs and MAOIs, a variety of new compounds have been investigated in recent years and many have unique chemical structures and pharmacologic properties. These new agents are commonly referred to as second generation antidepressants and include the tetracyclic derivatives (e.g., maprotiline) which has recently been marketed in the United States. Many of these agents act differently than the tricyclic agents on central monoamine metabolism. This, in turn, challenges our current theory on the mechanism of action of the tricyclics and indeed, our current understanding of the psychophysiology of affective disorders.[3]

Careful clinical assessment is indicated before beginning the depressed patient on tricyclics, for biologic conditions mimicking affective disorders must be ruled out and patients at risk identified. A thorough medical and psychiatric history should be obtained. The "endogenous" type of depression is more likely to respond optimally than other depressive states. The main contraindications to tricyclics are combination MAOI therapy, hypersensitivity, and early recovery from an acute myocardial infarct. Those at increased risk include geriatric patients, and others who experience pregnancy, cardiovascular disease, increased intraocular pressure, hyperthyroidism, seizures, and guanethidine therapy.

DSM-III lists major affective disorders as bipolar (mixed, manic, and depressed) and major depression (single episode, recurrent). TCAs are the agents of choice for the major depressions and may be more effective than lithium with depressed bipolar patients. With the psychotic depressed (e.g., hallucinations, delusions, cognitive disorganization), neuroleptics may be more effective than antidepressants. MAOIs may be more effective for the atypical depressions.

Drug administration best begins with a small divided dosage to establish tolerance. Most patients will experience minor adverse effects initially. Typically there is a lag period lasting up to three weeks before the depression remits. However, the sedative effects normally appear within days and help reduce insomnia and dysphoria. It is also helpful to consolidate the dosage to a single bedtime dosage early in the treatment course. This will help increase compliance and reduce adverse effects. Most patients require about 150 mg (or equivalent) of imipramine daily although dosage schedules must be highly individualized. Injectable TCAs are seldom used as adverse effects are more common than with peroral administration. Single episode depressions normally require three to six months of medical treatment.

Recently, serum assay findings have increased our understanding on kinetics, interactional effects, and the relationships between serum levels and clinical response. Of clinical importance is that only a small percentage of medication is circulating freely in the serum as the rest is fat soluble and lipid bound. Interactional effects with TCAs are numerous and are listed elsewhere in the text. Finally, serum level-response curves vary for the different agents, and a curvilinear shaped curve for nortriptyline and a sigmoidal shaped curve for imipramine have been proposed.[4]

Two additional issues are of clinical concern with TCAs, the refractory depressed patient and maintenance therapy. With the non-responsive patient, diagnosis, compliance, adequate trial, and underdosing are at suspect. If these have been excluded it is helpful to switch to another antidepressant. If unsuccessful, switching to a MAOI, lithium, or a neuroleptic might prove effective. For the endogenously depressed refractory patient, ECT remains a highly effective treatment.

Many depressed patients suffer from a recurrence of their illness. Patients with frequent episodes and those with exacerbations when off antidepressants are candidates for maintenance therapy. Often the dosage can be relatively small, in contrast to the higher dosage required for most acutely depressed patients. Maintenance therapy is normally well tolerated. Studies strongly document the effectiveness of antidepressants over PBO in preventing relapse. It also appears that maintenance tricyclic therapy is a relatively safe treatment strategy as long-term toxic effects have not been reported.

Psychotherapy is also effective in depression. Perhaps it is the treatment of choice in reactive depression and even in the more severe case once the patient has responded to medication. It is also well documented that PBO response is high in mild and reactive depressions but is low with major depressions.

Antipsychotic Agents

The list of antipsychotic agents has rapidly expanded since the introduction of chlorpromazine. Nonetheless, controlled clinical trials document that none of the newer agents are more effective than chlorpromazine in the control and prevention of psychotic symptoms. However, adverse effect profiles vary considerably and some patients respond best to a particular agent. The newer agents tend to be more potent, less sedating, but with a greater tendency to produce EPS.

All marketed neuroleptics have a dopamine-blocking effect and this property may explain their clinical effectiveness. This dopamine-blocking effect is also responsible for EPS and elevation of the serum prolactin level with its mild feminizing effects. Pimozide, a recently marketed neuroleptic, is an extremely potent dopamine-blocking agent with minimal if any norepinephrine-blocking action. Thus it appears that novel pharmacologic properties (other than dopamine-blocking effects) must be introduced before an agent is discovered that will be more effective than chlorpromazine in the treatment of schizophrenia.

Careful clinical assessment is indicated before administering neuroleptics. This includes ruling out medical and psychiatric (e.g., affective disorder, fictitious disorder, psychedelic-induced, etc.) disorders which can mimic schizophrenia. The FDA has approved neuroleptics in the medical management of psychotic disorders and the manic phase of manic-depressive illness. Neuroleptics are also approved for nausea and vomiting, intractable hiccups, presurgery sedation, acute intermittent porphyria, and as an adjunct in the treatment of tetanus. More recently, the APA Task Force on Tardive Dyskinesia recommended only short-term (less than six months) use of neuroleptics for schizophrenia, paranoid states, mania, certain cases of toxic or organic psychosis, and childhood psychoses.[5] They also recommended only short-term treatment for agitation in acute and chronic brain syndromes plus a limited number of nonpsychiatric conditions. The Task Force emphasized low dosage treatment whenever possible and long-term maintenance therapy only when definitely indicated for control of illness exacerbations.

DSM-III lists five subtypes of schizophrenia and neuroleptics are the medical treatment for control and prevention of each. The efficacy of neuroleptics in schizophrenia is well documented. Many studies have demonstrated superiority over placebo and other psychotropic agents. Also it is well documented that risk of relapse is significantly increased if the neuroleptic is discontinued.

Two recent concerns with neuroleptics are their long-term adverse effects, including TD, and their failure to greatly alter the natural history of schizophrenia. The association of involuntary movements, especially of the tongue, face, mouth, and jaw and neuroleptic administration is well documented. About 10-15 percent of patients on neuroleptics will develop TD. Often the movement disorder will subside and even completely remit after the neuroleptic is discontinued. Some cases move on to become severe and with progressive involuntary movements of the trunk and extremities. There is no known treatment for TD. Emphasis is placed on prevention and often with conservative utilization of neuroleptics.

Neuroleptics do not prevent residual effects from psychotic exacerbations nor do they prevent progressive deterioration. And despite maintenance neuroleptics, most chronic schizophrenic individuals function at a very low social economic level. Neuroleptics seemingly have limited effects on the natural history of the illness.

The typical pattern of administration begins with a low daily dosage. If response is delayed the dosage can be gradually increased until efficacy or troublesome side effects occur. With peroral administration reduction of psychotic phenomena often occurs within three days, but some patients may respond much more slowly. As EPS are common, it is helpful to anticipate their appearance and treat immediately with an AP agent. EPS may be distressing to the patient and therefore interfere with drug compliance and rapport. For the patient who responds slowly to neuroleptic treatment, switching to another neuroleptic, higher dosage strategies, and IM preparation may prove helpful. Finally, some psychotic patients refractory to neuroleptics may respond to lithium or ECT.

A rapid neuroleptization method is helpful when it is necessary to quickly control acute psychotic episodes. The safety and effectiveness with haloperidol has been most widely investigated. Reports document that both peripheral (e.g., agitation, belligerence) and core (e.g., hallucinations, idiosyncratic responses) psychotic signs can be reduced within hours.[6] Drug dosages recommended are 2.5-10 mg IM every hour until the acute illness is controlled. Normally 1-4 injections are required.

The benefit of neuroleptic maintenance treatment in schizophrenics is well documented. The key issue is identifying which patients require maintenance. In general, it is clinically prudent to gradually reduce the dosage in all patients to establish minimal dosage requirements and need for continued treatment. If the agent can be safely terminated, the patient should be monitored as risk for relapse is high. In contrast are the patients who definitely require maintenance treatment, but where compliance and motivation for follow-up care are problems. These difficult patients may benefit if switched to a long-acting injectable neuroleptic, especially if rapport is present.

There are no major drug alternatives in the treatment of schizophrenia. Reserpine has some antipsychotic effects but is slower in action, has more adverse effects, and is less effective than the neuroleptics. The beta blockers, lithium, and benzodiazepines have been tried but with limited success. ECT may be helpful, especially with the acute psychotic patient. Insight oriented psychotherapy may also have some beneficial effects, especially with patients who have had the more "reactive" type psychotic episode.

Mood Stabilizing Agents

Lithium is the only known mood stabilizing agent although the neuroleptics have some, yet reduced, similar effects. Lithium's contribution to psychiatry is not only an expansion of the therapeutic armamentarium, but also it has forced greater precision in the differential diagnosis of psychotic states while expanding our knowledge on the psychobiology of affective disorders.

The mechanisms of action for lithium, nonetheless, remain poorly understood. Kinetics studies show that lithium is completely absorbed from the gut within eight hours and that the peak serum levels occur one to three hours after administration; also, that lithium is not protein bound or metabolized to other compounds. It is excreted almost entirely by the kidneys and the biologic half-life is 18-24 hours.

As with all psychotropics, there are no trivial or by-demand indications for lithium administration. Overutilization and concern for long-term toxic effects are currently being debated. Due to favorable media coverage some patients request lithium for treatment of non-affective related disorders. Also, physicians pleased with the response of their mood disordered patients may prescribe it for non-related clinical states. In truth, lithium probably is underutilized in general and many candidates for lithium still go untreated. Careful diagnostic assessment is crucial as is the pre-lithium medical evaluation. Currently, lithium is approved only for the treatment and prevention of mania. It has also been used with some success in bipolar (and unipolar) depression, schizo-affective disorders, cyclothymic personalities, aggressiveness, and a subgroup (perhaps affectively disordered) of alcoholics. Medically, it has been used with some success in hyperthyroidism and cluster headaches.

In manic states it is clearly the agent of choice. However, due to a lag period of 3-10 days, combination therapy with a neuroleptic, often haloperidol, is in order. Of note, the acute manic patient often requires considerably more neuroleptic medication than does the schizophrenic patient for rapid control. In mania, the neuroleptic normally can be discontinued in 1-2 weeks, but some patients require maintenance low dosage in combination with lithium.

Typically lithium is well tolerated in divided dosage and the dosage can be rapidly elevated to the average daily dosage, about 1800 mg/daily. Serum lithium levels should be obtained 10-12 hours after the last dosage. Serum levels require 3-4 days after dosage changes to establish a new steady state. It is helpful to obtain 2-3 lithium serum levels during the first treatment week, and less frequently with continued treatment. Once the illness has remitted, dosage should be reduced to maintenance, which averages 300 mg/three times daily. Clinical response and adverse effects may not correlate with serum levels and daily dosage, therefore, should reflect the clinical picture. Lithium is available in both tablet (carbonate) and liquid (citrate) preparations.

Lithium is typically well tolerated biologically although symptoms of tremor, polyuria, polydipsia, and GI irritability are common early in the treatment course. Concern for weight gain and a return to a hypomanic state may present later. However, the area of most concern is the possibility of long-term toxic effects. Little is known about which patients are at highest risk. Renal lesions are a major concern, but currently limited information is available. For these reasons long-term monitoring of patients on lithium therapy is essential. Finally, it is now recognized that lithium has teratogenic effects, with a frequency of about 10 percent of lithium babies (first trimester on lithium) having anomalies, especially of the heart.[7]

Alternative treatments for bipolar affective disorders include no-treatment, other somatic therapies, and psychotherapy. These are important considerations as it is now readily apparent that only about 75 percent of manic patients respond successfully to lithium. Also, some patients are not candidates for lithium or prefer drug termination because of concern for adverse effects.

A hallmark of bipolar disorders is their episodic nature. The initial episode typically presents in young adulthood but exacerbations may be infrequent, last only for a few months, be only partially disabling, and have no residual cognitive effects. Thus, no-treatment is a viable choice, especially for the patient with a more benign form of the illness.

Other somatic therapies are available for the refractory or non-lithium candidate patients. The choices are predominantly neuroleptics and ECT. Prior to the lithium era, neuroleptics were the treatment of choice. Even today, neuroleptics remain the superior agent for rapidly controlling acute manic symptoms. But lithium is more effective with the long-term control of bipolar illness and is better tolerated by patients. This plus the concern for tardive dyskinesia has forced neuroleptics into a backup role. ECT is highly effective in treating both mania and depression in bipolar patients. A concern is its lack of prophylactic benefits unless given on a maintenance basis. Also, it may be less cost-effective if added hospitalization time is necessary.

The controversy continues over the long-term effectiveness of psychotherapy as a single treatment. It may have little effect on the natural history of the bipolar affective disorder. Nonetheless, it may reduce some of the disabling effects. Psychotherapy in combination with drug treatment may be the preferred approach. This will assist the patient in identifying possible "triggers" for the onset of their illness, help with identifying early evidence of exacerbation, and reduce recurrent episodes.

REFERENCES

1. Bunney Jr WE: Current biologic strategies for anxiety. *Psychiatr Ann* 11:21-29, 1981
2. Wooley CF: Where are the diseases of yesteryear? *Circulation* 53:749-751, 1976
3. Shopsin B: Second generation antidepressants. *J Clin Psychiatry* 41:45-56, 1980
4. Glassman AH, Shostak M, Kantos SJ, et al: Antidepressant plasma levels. *In*: Fann, Karacan, Pokorny et al. *Phenomena and Treatment of Depression,* New York, Spectrum Publications, 1977, pp. 267-271
5. Task Force on late neurological effects of antipsychotic drugs: Tardive dyskinesia: Summary of a Task Force report of the American Psychiatric Association. *Am J Psychiatry* 137:1163-1172, 1980
6. Donlon PT, Hopkin J, Tupin J: Overview: Efficacy and safety of rapid neuroleptization method with injectable haloperidol. *Am J Psychiatry* 136:273-279, 1979
7. Jefferson JW, Greist JH: *Primer on Lithium Therapy.* Baltimore, Williams & Wilkins, 1977, pp. 181-187

12

Neuroleptic Induced Extrapyramidal Syndromes

PATRICK T. DONLON, M.D.

Introduction
Clinical Diagnosis
    Pseudoparkinsonism
    Akathisia
    Acute Dystonic Reactions
    Tardive Dyskinesia
Determinants of Extrapyramidal Syndromes
Incidence
Treatment and Prevention
Neuroleptic-Antiparkinsonian Combination Therapy

Extrapyramidal syndromes (EPS) are frequently associated with neuroleptic therapy. Their origin is thought to be an extension of the antidopaminergic-anticholinergic pharmacologic actions of the neuroleptic on the striopallidal areas of the brain. There are five main problems related to EPS. First, they may go unrecognized and untreated. In fact, they may be incorrectly misdiagnosed as an exacerbation to the illness, resulting in an increase of the neuroleptic dosage with a further worsening of EPS. Second, because the involuntary motor movements, restlessness, and rigidity of EPS may be subjectively distressing, embarrassing, and may interfere with overall social and occupational productivity, the patient on neuroleptic therapy may not take his prescribed medications to avoid the troublesome EPS, perhaps resulting in an exacerbation of psychotic symptoms. Third, the contra-active treatment may be inappropriate and the EPS may persist. Four, the contra-active treatment may be administered or maintained unnecessarily. And five, neuroleptic induced involuntary movements may be irreversible in some patients. These problems, however, can be avoided or minimized with proper diagnosis and with proper administration of neuroleptic agents and indicated contra-active treatment. This chapter discusses the diagnosis of the

239

four general forms of EPS: *pseudoparkinsonism, akathisia, acute dystonic reactions,* and *tardive dyskinesia.* It also describes their incidence, determinants, and treatment, with a section on the uses and limitations of combination neuroleptic and antiparkinson (AP) therapy.

CLINICAL DIAGNOSIS OF EXTRAPYRAMIDAL SYNDROMES

The course and severity of the different types of EPS vary greatly. Dystonic and akathisia symptoms may wax and wane in course, while those associated with pseudoparkinsonism and tardive dyskinesia (TD) are more continuous. All symptoms disappear during sleep and none impair consciousness. All tend to increase during periods of tension, such as interviews and social gatherings, but may decrease during periods of intense voluntary efforts. All forms are reversible with the exception of some cases of TD which may persist despite neuroleptic discontinuation. In our experience about 45 percent of patients on neuroleptics will develop one or more forms of EPS during their course of drug therapy.

The following discussion of the four different forms of EPS include a description of their signs and symptoms, their appearance and course, and the differential diagnosis. Table 12–1 outlines them for convenience.

EPS may occur separately or in combination and may mimic other striopallidal symptoms, which originate from other causes, or other medical conditions. Proper clinical diagnosis is essential in outlining the most effective treatment. To assist in the differential diagnosis, the workup should include a complete physical and neurological examination, clinical observation, complete drug and medical histories, and indicated laboratory tests and clinical procedures.

Pseudoparkinsonism

This syndrome tends to progress rapidly, in contrast to the insidious onset of Parkinson's disease. Four signs characterize pseudoparkinsonism: akinesia (muscle fatigue and weakness), rigidity, alternating resting tremor, and autonomic nervous dysfunction. Presenting symptoms may be unilateral or bilateral. Both akinesia and rigidity produce decreased physical activity. The relationship between the two is unclear, although marked akinesia may be seen clinically in the presence of little or no rigidity. With advanced akinesia, the patient may complain of aches and pains in the musculature of the affected limbs or joints, most often about the shoulders. Clinically the patient may appear apathetic and in a psychomotor retarded state. Furthermore, anticholinergic agents frequently are more efficacious in controlling rigidity than akinesia. Another chief symptom, a regular rhythmic 4–8/second alternating resting tremor, is found characteristically in the hands and fingers but may also be found in the trunk, legs or perioral ("rabbit syndrome") areas. Deep tendon reflexes are normal unless interferred with by muscular rigidity, and muscle atrophy is absent. The dysfunction of the autonomic nervous system is characterized by drooling, hyperhidrosis and heat tolerance, sialorrhea and seborrhea.

Table 12-1. Extrapyramidal Syndromes (EPS).

Form	Common Clinical Differential Diagnosis	Onset	Age and Sex Predominance	Dose Related	Antiparkinsonian* Drug Contra-Active Treatment Efficacy
Reversible					
1. Pseudoparkinsonism	Parkinson syndromes, apathy, retarded depressions, tremors of other origins	Days to weeks	Geriatric F M 3:1	Yes	0 to 4
2. Akathisia	Psychotic agitation, restless leg syndrome	Days to weeks	Middle F M 3:2	Yes	0 to 3
3. Acute dystonic reactions	Psychotic posturing, hysteria, tetany, meningitis, tetanus	First 72 hours	Youths M F 2:1	Yes	4
Potentially Irreversible					
1. Tardive dyskinesia	Huntington's chorea, levodopa treatment, other involuntary movement disorders, transient neuroleptic withdrawal dyskinesias	Long-term neuroleptic administration	Geriatric F M 2:1	Unknown	−2 to 0

*Treatment Response:
 4–marked improvement
 2–moderate improvement
 0–no improvement
−2–worse

Pseudoparkinsonism may progress and develop into classic Parkinson's syndrome, which includes immobility, ("zombie") stiffness and slowness of voluntary movements, mask-like immobility of facies, shuffling, festinating gait, cogwheel rigidity, slow monotonous speech, micrographia, and symptoms of autonomic nervous dysfunction, such as drooling and skin changes.

Pseudoparkinsonism normally presents weeks to months after the initiation of neuroleptic therapy but may present earlier, especially if patients are started on higher dose medication or are biologically sensitive. Patients on long-acting depot neuroleptics may have a transient increase in symptoms immediately after parenteral administration. If untreated, pseudoparkinsonism symptoms will often spontaneously remit six to eight weeks after first presenting. Rarely will they continue for months after neuroleptic discontinuation.

Differential diagnosis includes idiopathic and post-encephalic Parkinson's disease, heredofamiliar tremor, tremor secondary to drug withdrawal (e.g., alcoholism, sedative hypnotics) and drug administration (e.g., lithium carbonate, TCA, nicotine), anxiety with tension, corticodentatonigral degeneration, striato-nigral degeneration, pseudobulbar palsy, the rigid form of Huntington's chorea, progressive supranuclear palsy, apathy, and retarded depressions.

Clinical evaluation of the tremor is particularly helpful in the differential diagnosis. Senile tremors have a predilection for the head, and when the extremities are affected, the tremors are increased by volitional movements, and rigidity is mild to absent. The heredofamilial tremors, in which rigidity is absent, are more rapid and are increased by voluntary movements. Tremors of hyperthyroidism, dementia paralytica, acute alcoholism and other drug poisoning are differentiated by their more rapid rate and lesser amplitude. Tremors of anxiety are associated with subjective distress.

Akathisia

Akathisia is the subjective desire to be in constant motion ("jitters") and is associated with the inability to sit still, hyperactivity, continuous agitation, restless movements, rocking and shifting of weight while standing, tapping of the feet while sitting, and a resultant disturbance in sleep with initial insomnia. Because of its subjective nature, it is often difficult to quantify clinically.

Although it may present early, akathisia usually presents weeks to months following neuroleptic therapy. It is frequently seen in combination with pseudoparkinsonism but may appear alone. Symptoms may temporarily increase after administration of long-acting depot neuroleptics. Akathisia most frequently presents with the more potent neuroleptics and is dose related, although it may be seen with relatively low doses.

Differential diagnosis is most common with that of psychotic agitation. It also includes painful neuropathies, restless leg syndrome, and "molimina crurum nocturna." Recognition of akathisia is essential, since an increased dose of a neuroleptic may potentiate the symptom.

Acute Dystonic Reactions

The syndrome is characterized by prolonged abnormal tonic contractions of striated muscle groups, especially those of the head and neck. Some patients experience mild symptoms such as a "tightness" of the throat or tongue, but spasms and cramp-like pain may be severe and more generalized. With masseter involvement, jaw movements are impaired. Overall, and in the severe classic form, there is exaggerated and unusual posturing of the head, neck, and jaw, which may present as torticollis or retrocollis; spasms of the musculature of the face or throat; protrusion and curling of the tongue; facial distortions and grimacing, oculogyric crisis with fixed upward gaze. Speaking, swallowing, but rarely respiration, may be compromised. Muscles of the extremities and back are less frequently involved, but may produce opisthotonos, lordosis, scoliosis, and bizarre gait. Dystonic symptoms may be accompanied by autonomic signs, such as profuse sweating, pallor, and occasionally fever.

Dystonic reactions are normally dramatic in appearance and acute in onset. Indeed, the muscle spasms can be most frightening to the patient and his family. Approximately 90 percent of the reactions occur within 72 hours of the initial neuroleptic treatment. And they occur most frequently in children and young adults, especially males. The course is characterized by waxing and waning of the symptoms, which usually remit within seven to ten days if untreated. Those occurring after months of therapy normally suggest that the patient has discontinued and then restarted neuroleptic drugs.

A variety of the dystonic reactions termed acute dyskinetic reactions may occur. Here involuntary movements are typically spasmotic and clonic in nature and may be either highly localized or widely distributed throughout the body. The course mimics that of the acute dystonic reactions.

Differential diagnosis includes tetany, tetanus, psychotic posturing, meningitis, seizure disorders, dystonias associated with neuronal storage disorders, post-encephalic states, hysteria, and levodopa toxicity. Incidence may be increased by hypoparathyroidism, dehydration, and other medical illnesses.

Tardive Dyskinesia

Tardive dyskinesia (TD) is also called "terminal extrapyramidal insufficiency," "persistent dyskinesia," and "complex dyskinesia." In adults, the early presenting signs include involuntary fine vermicular tongue movements, presence of ticks in the facial area, and abnormal jaw movements. Early symptoms are less frequently associated with involuntary movements of the extremities or bodily rocking. In children, where the course is typically more benign than with adults, the most frequent involuntary movements are choreiform in nature and involve the extremities. Involvement of facial musculature is much less common.

The advanced syndrome resembles Huntington's chorea and is characterized by repetitive, stereotypical, involuntary movements of the tongue, lips, facial musculature and mouth, and is occasionally associated with choreiform movements of the limbs and trunk. The most common symptoms are the "bucco-linguo-masticatory" (BLM) syndrome triad, which consist of sucking and smacking of the lips, moving the jaw laterally, puffing of the cheeks and more rarely thrusting of the tongue ("flycatching syndrome"). Rarer forms are associated with hyperkinetic and anterior-posterior bodily rocking, or ballistic movements.

In adults the symptoms may first present after weeks to months of neuroleptic therapy, but are normally associated with years of maintenance neuroleptic treatment. They may also first present when the neuroleptic is discontinued or when the dose is reduced. Movements become worse with stress and decrease with relaxation or sedation. Attempts to inhibit portions of the dyskinesia usually make it worse elsewhere (e.g., focusing on fine hand movements may increase BLM movements). TD is most frequently seen in elderly females and the relationship to possible underlying brain disease is unknown. Risk is increased with patients having previous histories of neuroleptic induced pseudoparkinsonism, and the two syndromes may occasionally occur in combination. In fact, if the dose of the neuroleptic is increased, the neuroleptic may temporarily mask dyskinetic movements, perhaps while concomitantly producing pseudoparkinsonism symptoms. TD symptoms may be transient (although occurring for months) or persistent. The course is most frequently established retrospectively.

Tardive dyskinesia must be distinguished from the transient dyskinesias which occasionally appear with neuroleptic withdrawal. From our experience these withdrawal dyskinesias most commonly present when neuroleptics, especially in combination with an AP agent, are abruptly withdrawn. This form of dyskinesia may be more common in children than in adults, and in children the most common form is involuntary movements of the trunk and extremities. No special treatment is required because of the transient nature. Readministration of neuroleptics will remove the involuntary movements. Any possible clinical or biological relationship between neuroleptic withdrawal dyskinesias and TD remains unestablished.

The differential diagnosis for TD also includes Huntington's chorea, Sydenham's chorea, dementia paralytica, hepatolenticular degeneration, psychotic posturing, hysteria, and levodopa toxicity. Physostigmine may temporarily reduce choreiform movement disorders and may, therefore, be helpful in establishing the differential diagnosis. Constitutional factors might also be considered. Because TD is also associated with sex, age and possible organic vulnerability, a debate continues about their importance in its origin.

DETERMINANTS OF EXTRAPYRAMIDAL SYNDROMES

EPS are related to biological sensitivity, neuroleptic molecular structure, dose, age, sex, and duration of neuroleptic treatment. Biological sensitivity is very important. Some individuals do not develop EPS regardless of the agent administered or the dose. The form of EPS also reflects biological determinants and is often familial. For example, TD more often occurs in older female patients and perhaps those with documented brain disease. Regarding molecular structure, the more potent, less sedating neuroleptics (e.g., piperazine phenothiazines, piperazine thioxanthenes, butyrophenones, diphenylbutylpiperidines) produce a higher incidence of EPS (TD?) compared with the less potent, more sedating aliphatic and piperidine phenothiazines. The different reactions may represent the relative anticholinergic-antidopaminergic potency ratios of the individual agents, for anticholinergic activity is contra-active for EPS. The dose also affects the incidence of EPS; very high doses (with the exception of akinesias and possibly TD) reducing it. For example, in patients receiving massive doses of neuroleptics (e.g., 300–1200 mg daily of fluphenazine), EPS are reportedly less common. The reduction of EPS at high doses may reflect the increased anticholinergic balance at such doses. Age and sex also affect the incidence of EPS. For instance, acute dystonic reactions occur more frequently in younger individuals, especially males, and pseudoparkinsonism is more frequently associated with an older population. Among females, pseudoparkinsonism, akathisia, and TD occur more frequently. A critical determinant of EPS is the duration of neuroleptic treatment. Continued neuroleptic therapy reduces the prevalence of akathisia, pseudoparkinsonism, and acute dystonic reaction; apparently a form of biological adaptation occurs. However, this adaptation is lost soon after neuroleptics are discontinued, and EPS may reappear, often in the same form and severity, with neuroleptic readministration. Prolonged neuroleptic administration appears to increase the prevalence of TD, although the syndrome may present after a few months of neuroleptic therapy. The contributing roles of neuroleptic molecular structure and dose in producing TD remains unclear.

INCIDENCE

Reported incidence of EPS varies greatly and reflects methodology, recognition of mild, subtle, or transient symptoms, and the demographics of the population studied. For example, the reported prevalence of TD varied from 2.2–56.0 percent, although some authorities concluded that it did not exceed 30 percent with patients on long-term neuroleptic maintenance therapy. Ayd found that 38 percent of a population of 3,775 patients on neuroleptics developed EPS: 21.2 percent akathisia, 15.4 percent pseudoparkinsonism, and 3.3 percent dyskinesias. Freyhan reviewed 1,015 medical records of patients on phenothiazines and reported that 52.9 percent experienced pseudoparkinsonism and 12.5 percent had dyskinesias. Van Putten found that 45 percent of 110 patients developed akathisia during some period in their neuroleptic treatment course.

We have found it helpful when discussing studies of incidence to separate EPS into two treatment periods: those occurring with initiation of neuroleptic therapy, and those associated with maintenance neuroleptic therapy. For example, 175 of our hospitalized schizophrenic patients were started on neuroleptics without combination AP therapy: 41.7 percent developed EPS within a mean period of seven days: 52 percent dystonic reactions, 28.8 percent pseudoparkinsonism, 2.74 percent akathisia, and 16.4 percent a combination of dystonic symptoms and pseudoparkinsonism. Most certainly the incidence of these EPS would have increased further had the study period been longer. Moreover, pseudoparkinsonism, akathisia, and TD would have been more prevalent, for they present later clinically. Incidence was in general dose dependent to an equivalent dose of 20–30 mg daily of potent neuroleptic (e.g., PO fluphenazine HCL), and was reduced at higher doses. With maintenance therapy a biological adaptation for EPS presents and the overall incidence of EPS is reduced to about 20 percent. During this phase of treatment TD tpically appears and often when the neuroleptic dosage is reduced or discontinued.

DiMascio concludes that AP agents are of limited value prophylactically for reducing the incidence of EPS. Our experience suggests that AP agents are of prophylactic value in some patients and that the incidence of EPS is reduced in both initial and maintenance therapy by AP agent administration or other combination therapy with an anticholinergic agent (e.g., TCA, antihistamines, aliphatic phenothiazine). AP agents may worsen TD.

Thus, the incidence of EPS with initial neuroleptic administration may range up to 65–70 percent depending on variables discussed above and prevalence is normally less than 20 percent for maintenance therapy. Frequencies for both periods are reduced by contra-active AP agents (except TD) and probably by prophylactic AP therapy.

TREATMENT AND PREVENTION OF EXTRAPYRAMIDAL SYNDROMES

Neuroleptics with their antipsychotic actions are the agents of choice in schizophrenia. They have also been found to be effective in treating other clinical disorders. Thus potential risks and merits must be weighed before administering neuroleptics. Furthermore, EPS should not be used as a guideline for establishing a therapeutic dosage of neuroleptics as formerly assumed, for EPS may occur at subtherapeutic doses of neuroleptics and may be absent in patients experiencing clinical response. This wide difference in response to the drug makes EPS of limited value clinically when establishing neuroleptic dose requirements for symptomatic patients.

In the striatal neurons, there theoretically exists a balance between the dopaminergic and cholinergic systems. Parkinsonism is considered to be associated with decreased dopamine levels. Studies have shown that a relative decrease in dopaminergic activity or cholinergic dominance may produce Parkinsonism or pseudoparkinsonism. Therefore, treatment of these two disorders is directed toward either increasing dopaminergic activity (e.g., levodopa, amantadine) or decreasing cholinergic activity through administration of various synthetic anticholinergic ("antiparkinsonian") agents (e.g., trihexyphenidyl, benztropine, biperidin). Levodopa, however, has limited effectiveness in treating neuroleptic induced EPS and may indeed exacerbate schizophrenic symptoms. Here the AP agents and the less potent anticholinergic agents (e.g., antihistamines) are the best choice.

AP agents, antihistamines, and diazepam are very effective for treating acute dystonic and dyskinetic reactions and response is immediate if given parenterally. Pseudoparkinsonism traditionally responds favorably to AP agents although in some cases may be refractory, and akathisia, especially late onset, may be persistent. Neuroleptic dose reduction, if clinically permissible, is often helpful. If EPS continues despite contra-active medication, and reduction in neuroleptic dose, substitution of another neuroleptic is recommended. Thioridazine, a piperidine phenothiazine, for example, produces a considerably lower incidence of EPS (except TD) and should be considered in substitution therapy. Diazepam and low dose sedative-hypnotics frequently rduce akathisia symptoms.

TD conversely is considered to be associated with dopamine receptor hypersensitivity in the basal ganglia. Attempts to correct the cholinergic-dopaminergic imbalance in TD through the administration of dopamine depleting agents, dopamine blocking agents, dopamine competing agents, and parasympathominetic agents have been ineffective. Levodopa and AP agents are not effective for treating TD and may potentiate the syndrome. Thus definitive prevention and treatment for TD remain unknown. The treatment of this form of EPS may place the clinicians on the horns of an insoluble dilemma, because many patients require maintenance therapy to prevent an exacerbation of schizophrenic symptoms. Nevertheless, TD may be possibly minimized if patients are maintained on the lowest efficacious dose required and if periodic attempts are made to discontinue the medication under close supervision. Drug holidays may help reduce the overall dose of neuroleptic and limit pharmacological effects. Fine vermicular movements of the tongue may be an early sign of TD, and, if neuroleptics are clinically stopped at this point, the syndrome may not develop. However, with neuroleptic withdrawal the dyskinesia may temporarily increase in severity. Following this some patients gradually improve and recover completely. If psychotic symptoms appear, readministration of the lowest possible dose of neuroleptic to control psychopathological symptoms seems indicated. The agent given should be different from the one which produced the movement disturbance. Occasionally, an antianxiety or sedative agent can be satisfactorily substituted for neuroleptics.

NEUROLEPTIC—ANTIPARKINSONIAN COMBINATION THERAPY

Indications—Limitations

AP agents tend to be overutilized in both initial and maintenance neuroleptic treatment and are probably contraindicated with TD. Conversely, they may be underutilized especially in subtle cases of akinesia and akathisia. Except for patients who are at high risk for developing EPS, it is best to administer AP agents only contra-actively, and not prophylactically. However, in patients with histories of recurrent EPS (except TD) on neuroleptic readministration, it is helpful to co-administer an AP agent. Hospitalized patients can be started on AP therapy at the first indication of EPS to minimize discomfort. Ambulatory patients can be prescribed a small supply of AP agent and instructed to take it if EPS present. Contra-active AP agents should be discontinued 1–3 months after first administration to demonstrate their continued usefulness. Patients requiring continued AP medication normally demonstrate EPS within 2–4 weeks of AP withdrawal. Nonetheless, the clinician must be constantly aware that EPS can present late in neuroleptic therapy, requiring adjustment in neuroleptic and/or contra-active therapies.

Following are 5 limitations in the routine administration of combination neuroleptic and AP therapy:

1. There is no reason to prescribe a medication that is not required. Cost, inconvenience, unnecessary pharmacological actions and drug interactions can be avoided. Furthermore, potential for abuse through intoxication has been well documented. AP agents, therefore, should be used predominantly contra-actively, except in patients starting neuroleptic therapy and who are at high risk for EPS.

2. AP agents are predominantly anticholinergics; thus they produce unpleasant atropine-like side effects including blurring of vision, dryness of mouth, constipation, etc. The anticholinergic effects may be additive in patients on combination therapy (e.g., neuroleptics, TCAs), producing serious medical complications (e.g., urinary retention, paralytic ilius, organic brain syndromes).

3. The margin of safety for AP agents is small. Toxicity, including organic psychotic symptoms, autonomic imbalance, fever, etc., may result from additive anticholinergic combination therapy, overdose or prescribing large doses of AP agents in attempting to reduce EPS.

4. Because AP agents affect the balance of acetylcholine and dopamine in the brain, they may play some casual role in the origin of TD. This remains speculative and presently undocumented, requiring further investigation.

5. Recent evidence suggests AP agents may produce an antagonistic interactional effect with neuroleptics. Clinical studies suggest that patients receiving combination therapy have a lower mean serum level of neuroleptic and also require a higher mean dose of neuroleptic for clinical response perhaps increasing the risk of adverse effects in neuroleptic therapy.

SUGGESTED READING

American College of Neuropsychopharmacology—Food and Drug Administration Task Force, Neurological syndromes associated with antipsychotic drug use. *Arch Gen Psychiatry* 28:463–467, 1973.

Ayd, Jr. FJ: Neuroleptic-induced extrapyramidal reactions: incidence, manifestations and management. The future of pharmacotherapy—New drug delivery systems. *Int Drug Ther Newsletter,* Baltimore, 77–88, 1973

Ayd, Jr, FJ: Do antiparkinson drugs interfere with the therapeutic effects of neuroleptics? *Int Drug Ther Newsletter* 9:29–31, 1974

Baldessari RJ, Tarsy D: Tardive dyskinesia. *From:* Lipton MA, DiMascio A, Killiam KF (eds): *Psychopharmacology: A Generation of Progress.* New York, Raven Press, 1978, pp. 993–1004.

DiMascio A: Towards a more rational use of antiparkinson drugs in psychiatry. *Drug Therapy* 1:23–29, 1971

Freyhan FA: *Extrapyramidal Symptoms and Other Side Effects in Trifluperazine— Clinical and Pharmacological Aspects.* Philadelphia, Lea and Febiger, 1958

Raskin DE: Akathisia: a side effect to be remembered. *Am J Psychiatry* 129:345–347, 1972

Sovner R, DiMascio A: Extrapyramidal syndromes and other neurological side effects of psychotropic drugs. *From:* Lipton MA, DiMascio A and Killiam KF (eds): *Psychopharmacology: A Generation of Progress.* New York, Raven Press, 1978

Tardive dyskinesia: Summary of a Task Force Report of the American Psychiatric Association. *Am J Psychiatry* 137:1163–1172, 1980

Van Putten T: Why do schizophrenic patients refuse to take their drugs? *Arch Gen Psychiatry* 31:67–72, 1974

Van Putten T: The many faces of akathisia. *Compr Psychiatry* 16:43–47, 1974

13

The Doctor-Patient Relationship

KAY BLACKER, M.D.
DON A. ROCKWELL, M.D.

Today's young physician has grown up in an age of science. The physician has watched astronauts walk on the moon, has been educated in gleaming biophysiological laboratories, and has been taught by computers. In hospital rooms, space-age technology assists in the treatment of patients. Despite awesome scientific and technical knowledge, the new physician is often caught unprepared in the maelstrom of powerful social and emotional currents that envelop the doctor-patient relationship. These forces may determine the effectiveness of prescribed physiological and pharmacologic treatments.

A knowledge of the contexts and parameters of the social and emotional flux of the doctor-patient relationship is vital to the medical care of each patient. It is the basis of effective humane medicine. Ignorance or misuse of these aspects results in treatment failure or worse. In this chapter we review the social and emotional aspects of the doctor-patient relationship, describe its genesis and describe its elements.

The power of the doctor-patient relationship has been recognized since antiquity and acknowledged explicitly in the Hippocratic Oath. A physician about to enter practice swears that he or she will not misuse the relationship.

"In every house where I come I will enter only for the good of my patients, keeping myself far from all intentional ill-doing and all seduction, and especially from the pleasures of love with women or with men, be they free or slaves. All that may come to my knowledge in the exercise of my profession or outside of my profession or in daily commerce with me which ought not to be spread abroad, I will keep secret and never reveal."

What constitutes this special relationship?

SOCIAL PARAMETERS

The key to good practice is the development of a good relationship. Without it all the knowledge and skills mean little. With a good relationship, even the death of a patient can be a mutual triumph of humanity. You will have some control over one side of the dyad, less control of the relationship process and little control over the patient's attributes.

Being a doctor is, among other things, a social role—a pattern of expected behavior. A role has inherent rights and duties regulated by cultural norms. Whether we like it or not, a role is routinely associated with a status position in a hierarchy. The student physician notes as time goes on in medical school that people outside and inside of medicine accord him/her different treatment and have different expectations from premed days. Some rights and duties are apparent.

Doctor's Role—Overt Functions

As a physician you have *confidential access* to extraordinary intimacies of the patient's social, physical and emotional experience. The patient gives you this right in the expectation it will be dealt with confidentially.

As a physician you are our culture's sole *legitimizer of illness.* Physicians serve in some sense as a social control agent through their legitimizing or not legitimizing incumbents of the "sick role."

As a physician you are expected to keep your feelings out of the treatment process as much as possible. Often described as "affective neutrality," in reality it comes closer to *"controlled affectivity,"* where the monitoring of your own feelings is crucial and the expression of them remains in the interest of the patient.

As a physician you are expected to be *knowledgeable* and use *scientific standards.* The patient has the right to expect a competent person using science rather than idiosyncratic standards. Most of medical education is directed at meeting this expectation.

As a physician you are responsible for responding to the patient's needs rather than to one's own needs. This complicated issue will be dealt with more fully later.

The patient's role also has some overt privileges and obligations. To be ill is much more than a medical disease—in many cases the social or psychological aspects will overshadow the disease process.

The Sick Role

The "sick role" is a legitimated temporary role. The sick one is exempted from normal social role behavior and responsibilities. It implies—increasingly at variance with reality—that the person is not responsible for the illness, can't help the situation and needs to be cared for. The sick one has three obligations:

- To desire to get well
- To seek "competent" help
- To cooperate in the process of getting well

This cultural stereotype clearly applies more accurately to acute illness than to chronic conditions.

These are essentially the traditional overt functions in the doctor-patient relationship. Much of the relationship, however, rests on more controversial latent functions.

Latent Functions for Patients

Many patients come to you with hidden agendas. These agendas may be hidden not just from you but, indeed, even from the patient himself.

Important ones we have identified include:

Catharsis. Most ill persons have a real need to talk. All patients are anxious and frightened initially by their symptoms. They need to be encouraged to tell all of their story. Let the pain speak freely.

Failure. Patients (people) need to cope with threatened or real failure. Often illness is an attempt to cope with some social, economic or interpersonal failure.

Need for Social Integration. Being ill may help integrate or reintegrate a patient into a social milieu. It may serve as a peculiar sort of reaffirmation of one's membership in society and the human race.

Need for Revised Status. Patients (people) may need a respite—temporary or permanent—from other roles and statuses. Being "sick" establishes an acceptable revised status or role. In an action- and success-oriented culture being "sick" can be a justification for passivity or failure. In the face of high aspirations but limited opportunity, sickness offers a legitimate "out."

Latent Functions for the Physician

Being a physician has hidden agendas also. Self-awareness of these hidden agendas allows for modification of potentially destructive behaviors growing out of these covert functions. Possible hidden agendas of physicians include:

Quest for Omnipotence. Many physicians harbor a search for mastery over death or control over life. There is a potential seduction in medicine in this way, but repeated inevitable encounters with therapeutic failure and ultimate death leads to pessimism, nihilism and depression in such physicians. This in part leads to physician impairment from drugs, alcohol and depression.

Social Control Agent. As the expert professionals who legitimize illness we are agents of social control. In a sense we are "health cops" and society "uses" us in this way. Physicians may be attracted to this "control aspect."

Voyeurism, Power, etc. Other motivations, less than altruistic, move all or many of us. The key is not that these elements need to be "eliminated," but rather that we recognize the elements within ourselves and in our behaviors with patients. Being aware of your own motivations will facilitate your working with people.

THE RELATIONSHIP

Fostering the doctor-patient relationship takes into account the patient's expectations. The patient's expectations can include:

- A doctor who knows what he/she is doing.
- A doctor who takes an interest in the patient.
- A doctor who behaves in a thoughtful, sympathetic way.
- A doctor who tells the truth.
- A doctor who gives sufficient time.
- A doctor who is reliable.

Failure to meet these not unreasonable expectations leads to poor compliance, doctor shopping, and medical malpractice. Most patients expect their doctor to be a friend and advisor (80+ percent) and note that the doctor's job has a "spiritual side" to it. All of the scientific knowledge or training will not meet these needs.

Often in discussions of the doctor-patient relationship, we focus on the development of rapport. Rapport, that "spontaneous, conscious feeling of harmonious responsiveness," really is the starting point and in our experience is not "developed" so much as "inhibited" by faulty physician behaviors. The patient's baseline expectancies as listed below are most often quite positive.

- **Hope**   The patient anticipates success. Activation of placebo effect.
- **Trust**   The patient expects respect and responds with trust.

- **Freedom to respond** The patient anticipates telling his/her story. Activation of emotional catharsis.
- **Faith** The patient is convinced the physician will understand. Activation of suggestion effect.
- **Liking** The patient expects to like the physician. Activation of empathy effect.

They begin the contact anticipating rapport. We inhibit the development of the relationship when we forget some basic facts.

a. What is routine to the health professional is an emergency or unusual event to the patient. Always view the situation from the patient's perspective.

b. Doctors and patients hold differing conceptions of illness. Nearly every patient views his/her illness as "serious" and views it with strong feeling. The doctor may view the same illness as "commonplace" and may view it with little feeling. These discrepant views need explicit attention.

c. The doctor doesn't listen. Listening is an active process. It is unforgiveable not to listen.

d. The doctor has no knowledge of the patient's background or emotional life.

e. The patient is frightened.

f. The patient needs an understandable, acceptable, factual explanation of his/her illness, prognosis and treatment.

g. The patient uses the relationship for support and encouragement.

PSYCHOLOGY OF THE RELATIONSHIP

Besides the sociocultural context of the relationship, there is a crucial psychological context. In order to fully comprehend the relationship, it is necessary to have an understanding of the early stages of human development. These stages are recapitulated in times of stress in the patient's relationship to the physician.

Early Human Development

Initially the fetus and mother are physiologically interdependent. Survival of the newborn is dependent on feeding—of both a nutrient sort and a psychological sort—soothing, stroking and attention. In the early months the infant cannot differentiate self from the nurturant one. Later this differentiation occurs and ultimately the nurturant one becomes defined specifically. Stranger anxiety, at about eight months of age, indicates this differentiation. As development progresses the child gains more security and trust in the identification of separateness, yet yearnings of separateness and autonomy are counterposed with yearnings to be close and enveloped by the nurturing one. This counterplay persists throughout life.

Two to four-year-olds think in a primitive way. They view themselves as the center of the world and perceive all events as relating to self. The belief that all events in the world are caused by one's own thoughts—magical and omnipotent thinking—is the norm. The "terrible two's" arise when omnipotence clashes against unyielding external realities. The six to eight-year-old develops logical thinking supplanting the primitive thought. The primitive magical thinking remains in vestigal state to be reactivated under certain conditions. Omnipotent and magical thinking becomes attached to internal images of parents. The child, forced to forego his/her own omnipotence, imputes this power to parents.

Wilford Trotter, the famous nineteenth century English physician, clearly perceived some of these elements in his experience with patients. He advised his students:

> *The attitude of the patient approaching the doctor must always be tinged for the most part unconsciously, with distaste and dread; his deepest desire will tend to be comfort and relief rather than cure, and his faith and expectations will be directed towards some magical exhibition of these boons. Do not let yourselves believe that however smoothly concealed by education, by reason, and by confidential frankness these strong elements may be, they are ever in any circumstances altogether absent.*

Regression

It is useful to recall that the central nervous system is comprised of a series of hierarchical organizations, one laid atop another. Older phylogenic structures are overlaid by newer ones. The newer systems comprise the more sophisticated portions of the brain. Diseases, which affect oxygenation and nutrition of the brain, selectively compromise or destroy the newer structures while older ones survive because of their greater adaptability; also, the newer portions of the brain are particularly sensitive to the effects of medications. Impairment in brain functioning produces confusion, emotional lability, and primitive thinking.

Pained or stressed patients regress psychologically from adult levels of emotional and cognitive functioning to earlier developmental levels characterized by omnipotency and magical thinking. The impairment of functions by anesthetics, drugs, or pathological lesions also contributes to regression, and more primitive brain systems gain ascendency as higher ones become dysfunctional. These two factors—psychological stress and impairment of physiological functioning—interact and combine in determining important parameters of the doctor-patient relationship.

Patients hospitalized for minor trauma or medical testing may be only slightly stressed and have little or no impairment of brain functioning. Some patients might be highly stressed and fearful and have no physiological impairment. Others, severely ill, will be both highly stressed and impaired. A physician or student physician must carefully assess these factors which intensify and shape the doctor-patient relationship.

Too often, physicians overlook subtle confusional states produced by side effects of one of the average of seven medicines which a hospitalized patient receives. Another common error physicians make is to underestimate the amount of stress and fright that patients experience. This false assessment arises from two sources: clinicians, working every day in hospital settings, may become insensitive or hardened to a patient's distress; and patients often have their own inner needs to deny their fears to themselves and to those who are taking care of them. This denial is superficial, however, and deeper fears still significantly affect a patient's attitudes and behavior. Physicians must be aware of this need to disguise and deny.

To the patient lying in a strange bed inside the maze of a modern hospital, the doctor is the center of the world. A physician's warmth, sensitivity and empathy are necessary to support a patient in this foreign environment. Behind each technical procedure and therapeutic intervention, a patient perceives the doctor as a parent caring for him/her—a distressed child. Even the physical examination, for example, has the meaning of being attended to, stroked, and soothed.

Transference

Important aspects of the doctor-patient relationship were accidentally discovered by Sigmund Freud while treating a young woman brought to him by her father because of neurological and emotional difficulties. Freud conducted his therapeutic interviews in 1900, in the style of a careful internist or detective. He worked diligently with this young woman to uncover the memories of the significant traumas in her life which had led to the development of her symptoms.

Dora refused to cooperate in the treatment. Rather than perceiving her physician as kind and helpful, she reacted to him as though he were her father, with whom she was angry and wished to defeat. Freud did not recognize that Dora was transferring feelings and attitudes that she held toward her father onto him during the course of the treatment. Only in retrospect, while examining the wreckage of the attempted treatment process, did Freud make the discovery of Dora's misperceptions of him. He called this transference of attitudes, which arise from a patient's relationship with parents onto the figure of a treating physician, *transference.* He later learned to identify the appearance of transferences and to utilize the transferences as a major factor in psychotherapeutic and psychoanalytic treatment.

The usefulness of Freud's discovery of transference is as important to a physician on a general medical or surgical service as it is to a physician on a psychiatric service. We need to remember that a patient's response to the physician is made up of two major elements: first, a patient responds to the "real" attributes and characteristics of the physician. Second, a patient will transfer onto the physician—an individual in authority over him or her when ill—feelings and attitudes held toward the important people of the past, i.e., parents, siblings and family. If these attitudes and feelings are positive, the doctor-patient relationship is affected in a positive fashion, and a patient's treatment is facilitated. If they are predominantly negative, they may defeat the most expertly conceived and carefully carried out treatment efforts.

Countertransference

The intensity of transference is increased by the degree of regression present in a patient: the deeper the regression the more powerful the transference. The frequency with which the doctor and patient meet and length of time they know each other also affect the intensity of transference. If a doctor and a patient meet several times a week, over a period of weeks, months, or years, the transference becomes much more powerful than if a doctor and patient meet infrequently and for brief time periods.

The following is an example of a strong transference which appeared during a brief surgical treatment of a slightly injured young man. As his bandages were being changed, he spontaneously spoke of his fear of the charge resident. He described this physician as six feet tall and "mean as hell." In reality, the resident was short, about 5'5" in height, innocuous and mostly ineffective. Further conversation with the young man revealed that his father was six feet in height and was a tyrant. He had transferred his attitude toward his father to his physician. The intense transference had distorted his view of the treating physician, even to the point of distorting the perception of the physical dimensions of the physician.

Placebo Effects

The *placebo response* reveals another parameter of the doctor-patient relationship. Sugar capsules are 25 to 40 percent effective in relieving moderate to severe pain in patients who have been told by their physicians that they have received an effective analgesic. The placebo response is not a response of a "kooky" patient. The placebo effect is most powerful in normal, trusting individuals and it is least powerful in suspicious, disturbed, unhappy people.

Perhaps the strongest and most flamboyant example of the placebo effect is the phenomena of hypnotism. A hypnotized patient can alter normal physiology to please the physician. For example, the physiological response to histamine can be prevented and bleeding can be decreased by a patient's response to the physician's suggestions.

Relationship Impact on Treatment

The power of the doctor-patient relationship is also seen in the capacity of a relationship to modify, amplify, and guide the active effects of drugs. In a famous experiment, a small amount of epinephrine was slowly infused intravenously into a resting volunteer subject. During the infusion and at the end of the test period, the subject filled out an adjective check list describing subjective experiences.

Actually the experiment was designed to asess the interaction between altered physiology and the conditions under which the drug was given. Under one set of conditions, the clinician who sat by the bedside while the drug was infused was jovial, light-hearted, told jokes and worked to create a warm, friendly environment. Under the second set of conditions, the clinician by the bedside was irascible, caustic, negative, and irritating to the subject.

Those who had been attended by the jovial clinician felt the drug produced a sense of excitement, well-being and euphoria. Those attended by the irascible clinician said the drug produced feelings of fear and depression. The same physiological effect was interpreted in a totally different fashion depending on the nature of the patient-clinician interaction.

A further demonstration of the power of a context to alter perception of a drug's action can be seen in this series of experiments: a subject was given a barbiturate and placed into a group of subjects who had been given amphetamines. When asked to describe the effects of the drug received, the barbiturate subject described amphetamine side effects. When the experiment was reversed and a subject who had been given an amphetamine was placed into a group of subjects who had been given barbiturates, the amphetamine subject described barbiturate side effects. The ambience in which a drug was administered determined the perception of its side effects.

One half of the doctor-patient relationship is the doctor. The doctor's past history and expectations, as well as the patient's, enter into the doctor-patient equation. Some information suggests one of the motivations to become a physician is the motivation to heal oneself through healing others. Physicians tend to come from childhoods in which there was more emotional trauma than in the childhoods of their peers. This tendency is strongest in primary care physicians, those who are most involved in the direct, continuing care of their patients. Binding one's own wounds by aiding in the healing of others may be a useful sublimation; however, it can create serious problems, and we must guard against their intrusion into the care of the patient.

It has happened that physicians, angered by their patient's seeming refusal to heal, have neglected or deserted them. A physician with frustrated omnipotent feelings may mistreat the patient. He/she must be aware of this possibility and guard against such an occurrence.

Dealing with Countertransference

A physician reacts to a patient in two ways: first, the physician experiences those common feelings one individual has for another. For example, if a patient is angry or bellicose, it would be expected a physician would have the usual emotional reactions of fright or anger; if a patient were provocative and seductive, a physician might well experience sexual excitement. Of course, physicians must be able to recognize and monitor these emotions and maintain a professional approach while treating all types of patients. Second, the physician experiences towards patients emotions and perceptions generated by the clinician's past history and development, personal experiences which are unique. These reactions, called *countertransferences*, are the mirror image of a patient's reactions (*transferences*), which were described previously.

Countertransferences are often unconscious and are intensified by the same factors that influence transference: the degree of regression present and frequency and duration of contact. Stress, lack of sleep, alcohol, or other drugs are among the many factors which can contribute to the degree of regression in the clinician.

Countertransferences can significantly alter a physician's treatment of patients. A brilliant young female house officer repeatedly quarreled with her middle-aged and older-women patients. When a woman patient would make a request, this house officer would experience it as a demand. She would either do a slow burn or explode angrily. She could not maintain a professional attitude and care for such patients.

Talking with the physician, it was found she had been reared by a caustic, demanding, psychotic mother. The mother, never hospitalized, had wreaked havoc on her husband, son and daughter. This house officer could not treat a demanding woman. In her mind, each such patient became intertwined with the image of her angry, psychotic mother. These countertransference feelings had not affected her medical career until the deepened clinical responsibility of a house officer had made continuing impossible for her. She transferred into a non-clinical field where she is a successful and contributing physician.

Everyone lives within a family, a culture, and a community, and each is helped or injured by the support or lack of support received. A physician can help organize these resources for the patient's benefit. By counseling and instructing, the physician can enable those close to the patient to support him/her and participate in treatment. Health education is an important facet of a doctor-patient relationship, for it enables a physician to multiply the numbers of those assisting in the case of the patient.

A hospitalized patient also lives within the context of a second family, i.e., a hospital family—those nurses, technicians, ward attendants, etc.—the professionals who comprise the health care team. If a physician is an effective leader, if nurses and others on the team like and respect him/her, they will provide support and excellent care to patients. If team members distrust a physician, find him/her shallow or ineffective or are angry at him/her, orders may be ignored or mis-interpreted and the patient may not gain their attention and support. The quality of the relationship of a physician with the health team members may determine whether a patient lives or dies.

SUMMARY

The doctor-patient dyad is a complex and powerful interrelationship. It is composed of many elements. It takes place in a complex social milieu. It derives its power from the regressive forces present as a distressed patient (child) seeks aid from a powerful authority (parent). Its life and manifestations recapitulate early developmental stages. When a patient and a doctor meet in a room, each is accompanied by ghosts from past developments and experiences. These ghosts, these transferences and countertransferences, affect the outcome of the medical treatment in either positive or negative ways. Technical procedures and desired drug actions can be facilitated by the doctor-patient relationship, and undesired side effects tempered.

Central to a physician's capacity to heal is wise utilization of the doctor-patient relationship in the best interest of those served.

REFERENCES

Blacker KH: The development of psychological impairment and drug abuse in physicians. *Impairment Newsletter, CMA*, Issue #5, August, 1978

Blacker KH: Drugs in the social setting. *Clin Toxicol* 2(2):201–207, 1969

Greenson RR: *The Technique and Practice of Psychoanalysis, Vol 1*. New York, International Universities Press, Inc., 1967

Rockwell DA: Social and familial correlates of antisocial disorders. *In* William Reed (ed): *The Psychopath*, New York, Brunner/Mazel, 1978

Rockwell DA, Pepitone-Rockwell F: The emotional impact of surgery and the value of informed consent. *Med Clin North Am* 63(6):1341–51, 1979

14

Special Patients
and Problems

PART I: OVERVIEW—Special Patients

DON A. ROCKWELL, M.D.

Problem Patients
   Crocks
   Complainers
   Criers
   Uncooperative
   Seductive
   Angry

"Special patients" come in several different forms. In this section the focus will be on a variety of people, patients and situations that may or may not be perceived as "psychiatric" but all of whom will be encountered by the primary care clinician. The common theme running throughout this section is that some patients we encounter and some situations we find ourselves in evoke in us certain feelings. The correct recognition, and perhaps even management of, these feelings is an absolute prerequisite to successful treatment of the patient or situation. Self-awareness of one's response is thus the focus of this section. Sometimes this is discussed as "countertransference," but we consider it to be above and beyond the issues of neurotic countertransference. Countertransference correctly used is a much narrower response to a patient. Here we are concerned about prejudice, sexism, anger, erotic feelings, fear, etc. in the clinician. We hope to sensitize you as to where and how to look for your own blind spots and to ferret out irrational but fully human feeling responses to certain patients and certain situations.

PROBLEM PATIENTS

While we may easily argue at some level that there are no problem patients, just problem doctors, this is not a particularly helpful approach. There are people who in interaction with the usual physician will evoke a response in the clinician that is counterproductive. Each clinician is likely to have strengths and weaknesses in dealing with patients. Noting patients that one dislikes or sees infrequently can be used to gain insight into the generic type of patient who will be problem patients for you. Noting nonverbal cues when with patients may also alert you to potential problems. Physically moving away from the patient (subtle), spending less time with a patient, writing atypical prescriptions (drugs or amounts unusual for you), being late for or missing appointments with certain patients, dreaming about patients, or noting displacement activities after seeing certain patients (angry at nurse, visible relief, etc.) are tipoffs to problem areas. Outright anger, fear or erotic feelings are much less common than the subtle and more pervasive responses. The recognition of the subtle interference in the doctor-patient relationship is the key to its management. In some ways identification of the clinician's feelings by the clinician is both diagnostic and therapeutic. It assumes that having identified a feeling in yourself (anger, fear, detachment, etc.) gives you the option of *not acting on it immediately.* This is not to say that the "feeling" is to be neutralized—a common idea—but rather temporized and, whenever possible, used diagnostically and therapeutically. For example, some patients regularly evoke annoyance in physicians. When this annoyance goes unrecognized, it may be manifest by the prescription of more medication than is appropriate—a nonverbal expression saying in essence, "please go away and don't come back as soon as my other patients." In some cases annoyance-dependence is directly related to the patient's depression. The annoyance in the physician may lead to the prescription of a lethal overdose of hypnotics.

The following is a brief list of what have been widely recognized as "problem patients." Following the "diagnosis" is a brief explanation as to why we sometimes experience these patients as problems and, in some cases, a treatment plan to assist in working therapeutically with these patients.

Crocks

These are patients who evoke anger in us because of our impotence in effectively removing their multiple symptoms ("positive review of systems," "positive serum porcelain," etc.). Crocks turn out to be interesting people who are 1) depressed and/or suffering from 2) somatization disorder. Refer to Chapters 6 and 7 for specific treatment of these disorders. The tipoff comes when we use pejorative descriptions of patients. When you do use a pejorative in talking about a patient, please take a look at whether your frustration/anger button is pushed by your apparent failure to successfully cure or treat this patient.

Complainers

These are patients whose complaints may be about symptoms (see above) or about "having to wait so long," etc. These patients may be suffering from depression or somatization disorders, or their complaints may represent a need for a particular kind of interpersonal transaction. Complaints have a content aspect, but with chronic complaints look for the process or interpersonal aspect. Again this requires the clinician to focus first on self and then on the interaction.

Criers

Patients who cry easily or loudly or profusely make many clinicians apprehensive. Allowing the patient expression of their tears is crucial and healthy in grief/loss situations. It is diagnostic in some depressive disorders. A simple device to encourage further diagnostic and therapeutic purposes is to inquire "what do the tears say," or "give the tears words" thereby encouraging translation of non-verbal behavior into verbal behavior with more opportunity for shared communication.

Uncooperative or Noncompliant

The noncompliant patient is the patient of a doctor seeking an active/passive relationship rather than a cooperative, consultative or covenantal relationship with patients. Uncooperative patients are very often patients (and their physicians) who haven't communicated. Running down a brief checklist of communication problems common to uncooperative patients will reduce the number to a bare minimum irascible few.[1]

1. Do I fully understand the patient's reasons for refusal? Often doctors will focus on the power struggle (do it my way, or else) rather than the patient's perspective. Listening to the patient's reasons will often reveal areas where he/she needs more information (or where you need more).
2. Do I have all the necessary diagnostic information? Sometimes refusal of procedures or uncooperativeness reflects a subtle organic brain syndrome with impairment in judgment. The brain syndrome may be acute or chronic and quite subtle.
3. Does the patient understand what is wrong and what is proposed to correct it? Exploration of this issue with the patient reveals educational and communicative gaps *or* reveals procedures that may not have a meaningful potential impact on patient care.

4. Does the family know what is going on? Enlisting the family in supplying diagnostic data and in enhancing therapeutic efforts may overcome problems in many patients.

5. Is there agreement among the medical/nursing staff as to optimal treatment for a patient? A split social field, especially if covert, will foster confusion in patients and their families and lead to refusal of cooperation.

6. What is the social or philosophical context in which the patient has refused a procedure or treatment? Some patients, for religious, philosophical, personal or even economic reasons may refuse proposals. Here respect and understanding may be appropriate where value systems clash. It is worthwhile investigating a patient's religious reasons for refusal to the extent of contacting his/her religious leader. Often you will discover a religious leader supporting a needed medical intervention.

7. Is there some need for change in approach to the patient? Many patients will need to maintain or reassert control over their lives and resist on this basis. Again the power struggle proves pointless. The patient needs information and control in order to make decisions. No one else has as much at stake.

8. Can I reconsider the need for the treatment or procedure? Some reasonable treatment compromises may be needed. Holding out for the ideal or right approach may lead to a correct physician and an untreated patient. Compromising and contracting with a patient are not always bad medicine.

Seductive/"Social Role" Patients

Some patients may "come on" in ways that fit a social role of "date" or potential mate or potential friend. This is a difficult problem since the physician—especially early in one's career—is open to and sometimes ready for an altered relationship. Being uncomfortable with the physician role, the student physician may seek a more informal, less professional relationship. It is important when faced with an erotic/seductive/friendly patient to remember that the doctor-patient relationship is a complementary one. Failure of the patient to play that role drastically alters the doctor's role. Moving from a professional relationship to a friendly or erotic one destroys the needed objectivity to make hard decisions. One has trouble being objective with a friend and it is impossible with a lover. In addition, there is inherent in the doctor-patient relationship the potential for taking advantage of the patient due to power or status differentials. Patients may be unconsciously or even consciously influenced in ways ultimately counter to their best interests.

Once again the awareness of friendly, warm, or erotic feelings for a patient should be used diagnostically. Is this something the patient is communicating for a purpose (often unconscious) and will it affect my treatment? Caution and consultation are in order before even thinking about stepping out of a professional relationship. A basic rule that if followed would prevent many problems—

don't have a nonprofessional relationship with a patient until you and the patient have terminated the professional relationship and six months have passed.

Having erotic or friendly feelings is inherently human but does need to be examined carefully rather than actualized. Patients may appeal to our rescue fantasies (I'll save you from your evil . . .), to our sense of omnipotence (those four previous doctors were not as good as I am), or our sexual prowess (I can satisfy you). People that flatter you, "turn you on," are unusually friendly or get you to do things (medical and social) that make you vaguely uneasy should alert you to possible problems.

The Angry or Hostile Patient

The angry or hostile patient is a difficult problem for many clinicians. When the anger has no apparent cause, as with the patient carrying a chip on the shoulder, it is often responded to with counter anger or irritation and an unhappy, untherapeutic interaction.

Again, a checklist of things to do and avoid will often lead to a more successful exchange.

1. Recognize the anger. Note the direction of the anger. Is the patient angry (irritated, annoyed, etc.) at you or at himself/herself? Is its expression "socialized" or "antisocial?" Is the intent serious or just bluster? Is the patient's control good or poor? These questions will separate the serious, poorly controlled, antisocial, dangerous patient from the usual upset patient.
2. Allow ventilation of the anger. Encourage the patient to talk about his/her anger. Check out the situation that may have caused anger. Obviously some patients will have good reason to be angry. In others you may find the anger has been displaced from a dangerous target to a safer one. Anger is usually related to a) a barrier in the pathway of gratification, b) deprivation, or c) conflict in principles or drives. Exploration of this may allow for successful ventilation or catharsis and a reduction in anger. Look for a long-time history of trouble with authority figures. As a physician you become for these patients—regardless of what you do—an authority figure. Don't cut the patient short in the narration. Don't necessarily agree with the patient but do acknowledge his/her feelings. Elicit information with sympathetic interest but provide an objective analysis for yourself. Go over the discussion several times as repetition may allow for working through of the problem.
3. Avoid several things. Don't criticize the patient either directly or in an implied way. Also don't criticize the object of the patient's anger. To err on either side is unproductive. Never provoke anger in angry patients. Take a professional stance, but do not avoid the patient's anger. These patients will evoke anger in the clinician. The key to coping with this is the ability to tolerate your own anger for brief periods. Counting to ten before acting or speaking may be crucial.

PART II: The Tired Patient

DON A. ROCKWELL, M.D.
WILLIAM BURR, M.D.

History
    Physiologic Fatigue
    Acute Fatigue
    Chronic Fatigue
Workup
Diagnosis
    Hysteric
    Depressed
    Situational Exhaustion
    Stress

One of the most challenging diagnostic problems that comes into the physician's office is the patient who complains of "being tired." It can prove to be a frustrating experience for the physician (especially if the physician is also tired) and to the patient. We propose a two-pronged systematic approach to the patient that can increase the probability of a satisfying outcome for both physician and patient. Our approach assumes the "complaint" of every patient has both informational value ("I think there's something wrong"), and transactional meaning ("Please take care of me"). Tiredness, fatigue, exhaustion need to be seen simultaneously as information and need. Both aspects require simultaneous workup.

The vagueness of the nonspecific complaint of tiredness covers a host of possibilities from brain tumor through incipient diabetes to being up all night with a sick child. Crucial to the differential diagnosis is a careful history. Detailed information on the following items is needed:

1. Onset of symptom; relationship to known factors (i.e., starting medications, increased activity, decreased sleep, important life changes such as job, new family member, etc.); duration; periodicity; intensity; associated symptoms.
2. Careful family history of diabetes, anemia, endocrine disturbances, depression, alcoholism.
3. Full review of systems—perhaps using a self-report or automated history taking.

4. Oral intake history—*anything* the patient puts into the mouth both in terms of nutrition and in terms of drugs. Careful inquiry of daily use of some over-the-counter or prescribed medication may be especially rewarding.

Having elicited the above history, we consider into which subgroup of fatigue the patient falls.

PHYSIOLOGIC FATIGUE

Patients and physicians are prone to ignore the fact that fatigue is reasonable to expect in the following circumstances:

1. Prolonged physical exertion without adequate rest.
2. Inadequate amount or restless sleep: drugs may interfere with REM sleep, such as many of the hypnotics and some tranquilizers. Drugs which have less effect on REM sleep are flurazepam (Dalmane) and doxepin (Sinequan).
3. Acute severe dieting or chronic moderate dieting: ketosis, negative nitrogen balance.
4. Sedentary life style: poor cardiopulmonary reserve.
5. Pregnancy: pre and postpartum.
6. Prolonged mental stress.
7. Advancing age: decreased physiologic reserve.

ACUTE FATIGUE

Lassitude or tiredness of recent or sudden onset should direct your attention towards:

1. Prodrome or sequelae of acute infection. Among the worst offenders are the meningitides, cerebral abscess, mononucleosis and most viral infections.
2. Metabolic disturbance. Any fluid or electrolyte imbalance—especially with extracellular fluid deficiency whether naturally occurring or iatrogenic—is associated with fatigue. Hyponatremia and hypomagnesemia are most notable although hypokalemia is most common.
3. Circulatory failure and/or digitalis toxicity.
4. Hemolytic anemia and acute leukemia.

CHRONIC FATIGUE

Longer, more insidious causes are found here and the differential diagnosis includes:

1. Chronic infection: among the possibilities include SBE, TB, brucellosis, parasitic infestations, and chronic pyelonephritis or osteomyelitis.
2. Anemias: megalobastic and iron deficiency anemias are most common but consider also polycythemia and hemoglobinopathies.

3. Nutritional dysfunction: any deficiency in diet—calories, protein, vitamins, etc.—may be fatigue inducing. A careful nutritional history is important since a "normal" diet may mean the patient is a vegetarian or macrobiotic "freak." Pellagra and cerebral beri-beri have not disappeared. Exogenous obesity also is exhausting.

4. Chronic exogenous intoxication: careful attention to common chronic intoxicants, alcohol, barbiturates, minor tranquilizers as well as less common ones such as heavy metal, gasoline, carbon monoxide and insecticide/pesticide poisoning is in order.

5. Chronic endogenous intoxication: here we encounter uremia and hepatic insufficiency most commonly.

6. Endocrine disorders: the following are associated with fatigue: diabetes mellitus, hyper and hypopituitarism, hyper and hypoadrenal function, hyper and hypothyroid function, hyperparathyroidism.

7. Malignancies: fatigue may be an early sign and is a common accompaniment of middle and end stage malignancy.

8. Iatrogenic fatigue: the following drugs have fatigue as a side effect in some or many people:
   All sedatives, hypnotics
   All tranquilizers
   All antihistamines
   Most anticonvulsants
   Most analgesics and salicylates
   Nicotine
   Tetracyclines
   Colchicine
   Cycloserine
   Adrenocorticosteroids
   Progesterones (and hence many birth control pills)
   Ergot alkaloids
   Insulin
   Mild digitalis toxicity
   Mild Vitamin A toxicity
   Mild Vitamin D toxicity

9. Neuropsychiatric dysfunction: intracranial neoplasia, sub and extra durals, amyotrophic lateral sclerosis, narcolepsy, Sydenham's chorea, depression and hysterical characters.

Having explored the specific differential with the patient, we move to a complete physical exam and related appropriate laboratory and x-ray examinations. Special exams are done when indicated by history or by age of the patient. In the physical, special attention is paid for evidence of muscle wasting, organomegally, lymphadenopathy, and skin changes. Laboratory examination routinely includes a CBC with differential, urinalysis and a chemistry panel with blood sugar and liver function studies. Other studies are done as indicated by clinical status and age. In spite of its lack of scientific status, we rely heavily on the clinician's intuitive sense that "something's up" and will pursue this. Trust in intuitive skills is important in the workup of the "tired patient," since chronic fatigue may precede positive physical and laboratory findings. In our experience a careful history and physical will uncover 80-85 percent of causes, the screening lab an additional 5 percent and the remainder will require more time and repeated evaluation. We often use a threshold model to explain chronic fatigue to ourselves and to our patients, since in many cases the causes are multiple and additive. For example, chronic fatigue may be precipitated by a minimal anemia in a patient already at threshold as a result of chronic minimal sleep loss (baby in the house) and minimal increase in usual physical activity (toddler in the house). For many patients such a reality orientation is both reassuring (i.e., there's nothing seriously wrong) and educational (i.e., maybe I can alter one aspect of the pattern and feel better). In addition we, therefore, often avoid a fruitless search for esoteric explanations. However, in the team setting, we are particularly wary of snap "psychiatric" or "organic" explanations of fatigue. Invariably the "organically" caused fatigue has an emotional reaction associated with it that requires attention. The patient who becomes depressed as a result of being on reserpine is no less a suicide risk! Thus while running down the organic causes (i.e., the informational aspect of the complaint), we also attend to the transactional or need side of the complaint. A psychiatric explanation of fatigue is never a diagnosis of exclusion. If we find no positive evidence of psychiatric disease using conservative diagnosis, then we conclude that the etiology is still unknown and necessarily continue to explore with the patient sources of fatigue. Just as a diagnosis of anemia requires significant change in red cell indices, so a diagnosis of depression or "hysterical character" requires significant positive evidence. The skilled clinician never makes a diagnosis purely by exclusion.

TIREDNESS AND PHYSICAL COMPLAINTS

There are two major categories of patients who manifest a primary complaint of tiredness plus multiple other physical complaints.

The first of these is the so-called *hysteric.* Woodruff and Guze[1] have developed a diagnostic pattern characteristic of the hysteric. This includes:

- A complicated or dramatic medical history
- A minimum of 25 symptoms in nine of 10 symptom groups
- A minimum of 25 symptoms in nine groups without medical examinations

If a patient meets Guze's criteria, there is a 90 percent chance that the clinical condition will remain stable and that other *serious* medical and psychiatric illnesses will *not* develop. This can be explained to the patient and also has an effect on management of these patients.

These patients represent a very small proportion of medical practice. It is crucial that the diagnosis be limited to those patients meeting Guze's criteria, since we otherwise get into a sophisticated kind of name calling. No one denies the existence of these patients, but the etiology has been hotly debated. It seems important to us that we not deny the presence of this life style, but rather maximize the possibility of a positive outome. This includes 1) not putting the patient through the pain and expense of a nonproductive workup; 2) recognizing the transactional nature of the complaint; 3) recommending appropriate treatment which can include suggesting that the patient re-examine his current role in view of changing sex roles; 4) allowing the physician to recognize the common countertransference problem of frustration, anger, undue interest and therapeutic impotence in dealing with these patients.

The second group of tired patients is *depressive* patients and patients with depressive equivalents. A developmental appreciation of depression is important since depression is manifested in quite different ways according to age, sex and socioeconomic status.

Infants and children rarely manifest depression by the typical "lowered mood." Infants and children manifest depression when they are hyperactive, run away, withdraw, have school, eating or sleeping problems and when they have vague physical complaints.

Adolescents likewise may frequently "act out" depressive conflicts with the result that depression manifests in boys as antisocial behavior or poor school performance; in girls as sexual misconduct, running away, and poor school performance and in both by "doing drugs," drinking and through psychosomatic problems.

Young adults more frequently somatize or act out depression than evidence a classic picture.

By middle age we see more typical "textbook" depressive pictures, but you need also to be aware that depression continues to manifest often via acting out behaviors—particularly sexual and drug—and in somatic problems.

At all stages "accidents" may be depressive unconscious self-destructive equivalents. A close look at the antecedents of "accidents" is worthwhile.

Somatization is a theme that also pervades the life cycle of depressive equivalents. Gastrointestinal symptoms lead the way as an arena for the expression of depression. The irritable colon syndrome is the most common equivalent, but remember that other functional or organic syndromes such as peptic ulcer, ulcerative colitis, etc. can be "symptoms" of depression and certainly are commonly accompanied by depression. While any organ system may be involved, skin disorders and pain syndromes (headache, backache, residual pain) lead the list after the GI tract.

Depression

Tiredness is a very common symptom of depression. The signs and symptoms of depression vary not only by age but also by sex and socioeconomic status. This is important to recognize.

Among males depression is more commonly manifested by lowered mood, pessimism, guilt and a sense of helplessness. Comparable early signs in women are insomnia, headache and social withdrawal.

The following points out the variation in the presentation of depression according to the patient's background.*

Low	*Middle*	*High*
AFFECTIVE		
Hopelessness	Loneliness	Decreased social life
Self-accusation	Helplessness	Pessimism
Crying	Guilt	Dissatisfaction
Dissatisfaction	Crying	Anxiety-tension
Guilt	Anxiety-tension	
Depressed mood	Depressed mood	
SOMATIC		
Palpitation	Decreased sex drive	Fatigue
Headache	Urinary complaints	Insomnia
Anorexia	Trouble falling asleep	
Waking early	Headache	
	Anorexia	
	Waking early	

Having diagnosed depression we then attempt to decide whether it is normal (as in grief), typical, or atypical. A practical classification of depression follows Hollister et al.[2] A brief summary of their work is in Table 14-1. On the treatment side of the equation rely heavily on both the relationship with patient (frequent brief visits) and an aggressive psychopharmacological approach. Once having selected an appropriate psychoactive agent, one should stick with that agent for three to six weeks and push the total daily dosage to near "toxic" levels. If the patient is not having side effects the "treatment" is not likely to be effective. We often attempt to involve the family in the treatment program having found as Cammer [3] did that the family can greatly facilitate progress or sabotage treatment. Once having even merely entertained the possibility of the patient having a depression, whether as a primary source of tiredness or secondary to other "organic" illness, a direct inquiry into the patient's potential for suicide is mandatory. Continued attention to this risk is necessary throughout the treatment course of the depressed patient. (See Section V following.)

Situational Exhaustion

There are other causes of tiredness that need attention. The first of these is "situational exhaustion." This is a form of physiologic tiredness but common

---

*Adapted from Schwab[7]

Table 14.1. Classification and Treatment of Depression.

Retarded Depression	Anxious Depression	Hostile Depression	Hypochondria
Deeply depressed.	Much "unworthiness" and guilt.	Paranoid and projective.	Little guilt.
Psychomotor retardation evident. Lacks environmental reactivity. Loss of interest in life.	Agitated. Reactive to environment.	Hostile belligerency. Hopelessness.	Moderate depression. Agitated. Feel "abandoned and unloved."
Visceral symptoms. No self pity. No sense of humor.	Reports anxiety. Self-pity. May have sense of humor—teasing in character.	Angry. Sense of humor is often sado-masochistic in character.	Multiple somatic complaints.
No precipitating stress. (it came over like a black cloud) Tend to be older.	Precipitating stress. Prior history of neurotic or behavioral problems.	Prior history of neurotic or behavior problems common.	Lifelong history of disturbances.
Weight loss common. Early morning or middle of the night awakening. Suicidal.	Trouble falling to sleep. Tend to cling to M.D.	Provocative.	Demanding. Psychopharmacologic agents likely to associate with many "troublesome side effects."
Best psychopharmacologic agents: Imipramine (Tofranil) Amitriptyline (Elavil) plus supportive psychotherapy; if no response after adequate dosage over three weeks consider electroconvulsive treatment.	Best psychopharmacologic agents—Phenothiazines like Perphenazine (Trilafon) plus psychotherapy. May use Doxepin (Sinequan) as alternative agent.	No best psychopharmacologic agent—often need a combination of tricyclic and phenothiazine.	

enough to merit special comment. These are situations where being tired is an appropriate response and symptomatic because of lack of rest, relaxation and sleep. This common sense diagnosis needs only two caveats. Be aware that in spite of all labor-saving devices many people continue to have too much to do. Also be aware that many "workaholics" are appropriately tired as a result of their being driven internally. The "workaholic" needs to be advised of the diagnosis and sometimes given the prognosis of his/her condition. Hard work or overwork often is a symptom of underlying personal or family problems. The person must be educated to appreciate that chronic overwork a) is a symptom; b) may well be detrimental to long-range physical and emotional health and happiness; c) is treatable using reality[4] and family therapy techniques. The physician's role in treatment may be to involve the patient's family, and together with the patient and family, realign health priorities and responsibility.

Stress and Exhaustion

Be attentive to chronic stress or a recent increase in stress upon a patient. We are well aware that life changes are additive and can lead to increased illness and accidents.[5] There is evidence to indicate that chronic overwork plus a sudden recent work increase is a cardiac "drain" and often antecedes an acute myocardial infarct.[6] An "enforced" vacation may be in order for these patients and certainly a "prescribed" change of pace is in order. The examples of this are innumerable, but keep in mind several practice-related situations:

1. Families with chronically ill or dying members (especially if the patient is a child).
2. Families in considerable emotional conflict often manifested by sexual problems.
3. Upwardly mobile young men and women.

The tired patient presents the physician with an informational problem ("Tell me what is wrong with me") and a transactional problem ("I'm scared about . . . and need you to take care of me"). Careful attention to both sides using all of the basic skills of the physician and his or her team will result in effective successful intervention in all cases.

REFERENCES

1. Woodruff RA, Clayton P, Guze S: Hysteria: Studies of diagnosis, outcomes, and prevalence. *JAMA* 215(3):425-28, January, 1971
2. Hollister L, Overall J, Shelton J, et al: Drug therapy of depression. *Arch Gen Psychiatry* 17:486-493, October, 1967
3. Cammer L: Family feedback in depressive illness. *Psychosomatics* 12:127-32, March, 1971
4. Glasser W: *Reality Therapy.* New York, Harper and Row, 1965
5. Liljefors I and Rahne R: An identical twin study of psychosocial factors of coronary heart disease. *Psychosom Med* 32:523-42, 1970

6. Bruhn JG, McCrady KE, du Plessis A: Evidence of emotional drain preceding death from myocardial infarction. *Psychiatr Dig* 29:34-40, April, 1968

7. Schwab J, Bialow M, Brown J, et al: Diagnosing depression in medical inpatients. *Ann Intern Med* 67:695-709, October, 1967

PART III: Crisis Intervention—Overview

DON A. ROCKWELL, M.D.

In addition to problem patients there are patients with problem situations. These are situations—common or uncommon—that evoke symptoms of distress in normal persons. They may not meet the criteria for a specific psychiatric diagnosis yet may benefit from psychiatric management. The generic approach for these patients is one of various forms of *crisis* intervention.

CRISIS INTERVENTION

The stress reduction techniques noted in Chapter 7 were used to promote positive mental and physical health. They may be adjunctive to crisis intervention which is essentially a secondary preventive technique. Put simply, a crisis is the emotional response of a person or a family when their usual coping style is overwhelmed by some problem. There are "normative" crises—turning forty, getting married, first baby—and "nonnormative" crises—divorce (barely nonnormative statistically), sudden death of a child, accidents, etc. Faced with a normative or nonnormative potential crisis, an individual will experience it as a crisis *if* it is perceived as threatening *and* usual problem-solving techniques don't work. Families or other close knit groups can be put into crisis when the homeostatic family system is threatened.

Four phases in the evolution of a crisis have been identified.[1]

1. The initial phase in which the individual uses habitual problem-solving techniques.
2. Tension increases when habitual techniques fail and the person feels upset and ineffectual. Functioning becomes disorganized and attempts at solving the problem become trial and error.
3. Tension increases further and emergency, novel, or bizarre problem-solving measures are attempted. This may mean denying or ignoring parts of the problem or forcing the problem into a presently unworkable but previously successful model.
4. If the problem is not solved, denied or avoided, tension mounts beyond the breaking point and emotional upset and disorganization ensues. Often the clinician will be able to identify a "last straw" that sets off the emotional storm. The last straw often is of symbolic importance reflecting the basic conflict in the crisis situation.

It is important to note that as a crisis evolves, a common way of dealing with the increased tension in phase three is either directly through help-seeking by way of the physician or more indirectly by developing physical symptoms and then secondarily, making a health care contact as a result of the symptoms. In either case the physician is seen at some point in the evolution of a crisis. Recognition of this fact allows the clinician to intervene early and effectively to prevent phase four disruption.

BENEFITS OF CRISIS INTERVENTION

Crisis intervention skills are an extension of the basic stress reduction skills discussed earlier with the addition of some basic counseling skills. The importance of crisis intervention is three-fold. First, early intervention prevents further spreading of the person or systems disorganization and allows for a return to normal functioning. Secondly, and perhaps more importantly, it offers the person or system a real opportunity for positive growth and change. Previously fixed and sometimes dysfunctional individual and family patterns may be permanently altered for the better by effective intervention. Finally, the experience and lessons learned by the patient during one experience with crisis intervention allows him/her to use this experience and education on his/her own in future crises and hence gives him/her control in dealing with future stressful periods before they get out of hand.

BASIC PRINCIPLES OF CRISIS INTERVENTION

Immediacy

Of importance to effective intervention is immediate availability of intervention. Crisis intervention needs to be done "now" as the crisis unfolds and not scheduled for "later." It requires the clinician to be available and to be flexible in terms of time for the patient.

Systems Perspective

It will be useful to involve family (or other involved social systems) in the treatment process. Enlisting others on the behalf of the patient (with the patient's approval) and serving an advocacy role is important.

Present Problem Perspective

The initial focus is on the present problem. The interventionist needs to find the answer to the question of why this problem appears now in the patient's life. Exploration of "the straw that broke the camel's back" is mandatory. This precipitant usually will have taken place within a week of the patient's seeking help.

Reality Orientation

The focus is on the reality of the present situation. Essential tasks include:

- Developing with the patient a clear, correct perception of the situation.
- Enabling the patient to view his/her role in the creation of the situation.
- In a context of support and understanding, confront the patient with maladaptive aspects of his/her lifestyle while communicating a belief in his/her ability to change.
- Provide the patient with information.
- Acknowledge and encourage the expression of the patient's feelings about the situation.

Brief and Behavioral

Crisis intervention contains within it the notion that short-term intervention—one to eight contacts—will be sufficient in most cases to resolve the crisis. Many problems initially appear to need "long-term therapy," yet by setting a short-term, time-limited contract, this will in some sense encourage the patient to work maximally on the problems and often achieve solution. The focus is not so much directed at intrapsychic understanding, but rather on behavioral change. Intrapsychic insight often accompanies behavioral change, but will not be a primary goal of the intervention.

CRISIS INTERVENTION PRACTITIONER

Ideally the interventionist would be a person skilled in traditional psychotherapy. In the real world this is unlikely to be the case. The next best thing, then, is to have available a psychiatrist for consultation and supervision as one learns "on the job." By its very nature crisis intervention takes place at unexpected times and in unexpected places. One cannot plan for a "crisis intervention" time in a primary care clinic. One can arrange a backup consultation and referral system. A basic rule is when in doubt, ask for help.

Baseline Requirements

There are two qualities of the interventionist that are mandatory. The first quality is that of "caring" for the patient. The cynical, cold, or technical health care professional will not be successful—nor likely to attempt—crisis intervention. The second quality is the ability to listen "with the third ear."[2] Caring is quite simply not enough. The caring "unhearing" interventionist will be unsuccessful. Listening with "the third ear" means the ability to a) hear the patient, b) hear what the patient is not saying, c) hear what goes on between the patient and the interventionist, and d) most important listen to and hear what is going on within the interventionist. If one is not able to monitor accurately one's own feelings, thoughts, and fantasies about the patient, then one ends up purely reactive and often not therapeutic.

Listening and hearing are facilitated by:

- Looking at the person as he/she speaks—pay attention to nonverbal cues.
- Provide feedback to the person—let the patient know what you heard and if what you heard is what the patient intended to say—summarize at times.
- Avoid interrupting—allow the whole story to unfold and don't be afraid of silences.
- Be nonjudgmental—don't take sides, don't judge, don't moralize.
- Empathize—try to get into the other person's experience and see what it feels like.

TASKS IN CRISIS INTERVENTION

Problem Focus

The initial task is to establish rapport. While easily stated, it may sometimes be difficult to establish rapport with the patient (see Chapter 13). In most cases allowing the patient to tell the full story in his/her own way, at his/her own pace while providing a nonjudgmental, safe environment will be sufficient. The task of finding a problem focus evolves from the establishment of rapport. Since most patients present without a discrete problem focus, it is useful to review with them the recent events in their lives. Looking carefully at the timing of physical or emotional symptoms and the events often reveals an association that is usually not coincidental. A frequent "last straw" turns out to be a recent loss or an addition to the patient's social circle. Once the interventionist suspects a problem focus, it is useful to explore this with the patient—who may accept or reject the suggested problem as the central issue. This problem focus may bring out one or several areas that need problem-oriented attention.

Prior Coping Efforts

Assess with the patient what efforts have been made to deal with the crisis. Be sure to find out about previous health contacts or mental health contacts, since in crisis some patients will make multiple contacts and these need coordination. Evaluate how the patient dealt with previous life stresses. This may often serve to shore up the patient's confidence (since he has "coped" before) and remind him of other coping techniques he has used successfully. A history of recurrent and severe stresses will imply a more massive intervention and advocacy than a prior high level of function recently disrupted.

Exploration of Feelings

The patient needs to express whatever feelings come up. Catharsis is often useful. In patients who are acutely anxious, specific relaxation techniques may be helpful to calm them enough to continue their story. At some point discussion of how the patient feels about discussing his problems may be useful. Frank discussion of this issue is important since "the match" between patient and interventionist is a good predictor of outcome. If it isn't "clicking" it may be helpful to ask another interventionist to join you to try and determine why it isn't clicking.

These tasks essentially will represent for most situations the first intervention and, in many situations, the only intervention needed. The expression of feelings and the verbalization of problems to another in a safe setting will lead to renewed and successful efforts to deal with the crisis. The ending of the first contact comes when the patient feels in better control and there are no pressing reasons to go further (such as suicide risk or severe disorganization).

At that point it is appropriate to set up plans for the next contact and provide information about appropriate resources to help the patient in the interim. These resources will vary with problems of the patient (social, economic, legal, educational, housing, protection, etc.). Knowledge of community resources is vital, and utilizing a patient advocate role will facilitate the connecting with resources in often very complex systems. These reality-based steps accomplish two things. They provide the patient with needed resources or information *and* they foster a working relationship.

Crisis Intervention Contracting

At the end of the first session, you should note some relief in the patient, have provided support, education and access to appropriate resources, defined problem areas and set up a time and place for the next visit.

At the next visit many interventionists set up an explicit contract. The "contract" meets several overt and several covert purposes. The overt purposes of the contract are:

1. To specify in behavioral terms what it is they want to change in order to solve the problem. Specificity is a must. "I want to change my life, marriage, etc." is impossible. "I want to be more assertive with my spouse" is more workable.
2. To specify the limits of the contract. Here ask the patient to determine how many sessions he/she desires within a narrow range such as two to eight. Decide on the duration of the sessions—20 minutes being a minimum and 50 minutes a maximum—and the frequency—every day, once a week, etc.
3. To specify as clearly as possible what you want the patient to do within the session:

   - "I'd like you to talk as honestly as possible about your feelings."
   - "I want you to observe what we are doing as clearly as possible."
   - "I want you to talk about your feelings about how a session is going."
   - "I'd like you to meet your appointment even if you don't feel like it so we can discuss why you didn't want to come," and as a corollary what you will do:
   - "I'll listen carefully to what you say."
   - "I'll work actively to help you understand your problems and potential."
   - "I'll make observations about behavior—yours and mine."
   - "I'll work with you to develop realistic solutions."

The covert messages in the contract are:

1. Behavioral change is our goal and you can make such changes in a short time.
2. The patient has a good idea of what he or she needs or fears.
3. The process of what goes on between us is to be discussed.
4. Both parties are here to work.

INTERVENTION TECHNIQUES

In the subsequent sessions there is no single usual pattern. There are a variety of intervention techniques that will be used in some or all subsequent sessions.

Listening

Listening to the patient each time and allowing him to present his agenda and secret agendas without imposing your plan on a session is in and of itself therapeutic.

Confrontation

The judicious use of confrontation about self-defeating patterns done in the context of a working relationship can be helpful. Pointing out how certain behaviors seem repetitive and maladaptive while supporting adaptive behaviors is necessary.

System Management

Involving other family members, friends and so forth in the sessions themselves will both reveal the nature of problems and assist the patient in developing a support system. Often the crisis patient feels alone and isolated. The discovery that others care may be important. The interventionist needs to "check out" statements like "my parents, spouse, friend, etc. don't care." Sometimes this is the case, most often it is not.

Information/Education

The provision of specific information and educative efforts are often helpful when the patient operates on the basis of faulty information or common mythology. We often forget that patients don't have the level of physiologic, psychologic, etc. sophistication necessary to good decision making. An extension of this is in terms of providing information about alternative resources. Often this fosters hope as well as providing practical solutions.

Direct Intervention

In some situations direct intervention with some system or person is appropriate and mutually informative. With the client's permission, contacts with schools, jobs, family may resolve communication problems quickly and effectively.

Advice and Suggestion

Direct advice—"common sense" should be used infrequently. The patient will have most often already used the advised approach and found it wanting. Suggestion is inherent in the situation—the overriding suggestion is that you anticipate resolution. This powerful force operates without much specific suggestion.

Behavioral Homework

Fairly often "homework" assignments can be made for behavioral tasks. These tasks do several things. They encourage the patient to work on the behavioral contract. They extend the therapy situation into the patient's real world. When they remain undone or fail they are the source of important information about either the patient or the homework assignment. Again, specificity of the task is important. "I'd like you to approach one person tomorrow in an assertive, non-aggressive way and report on it at our next session." Assertiveness versus aggressiveness would need to be discussed in behavioral terms.

Monitoring of Progress

The specific contract for change needs to be monitored at each session. It may need refining or alteration but, again, the patient needs to be consciously working on a specific self-defined behavior change.

Modeling and Rehearsal

In many situations the interventionist serves as a model for clear communication and as a broader model of competence. In addition, it is often helpful to role play with the patient situations that he/she finds problematic. This practice can then be carried out to the real situation and subsequently reported on.

Paradoxing

Paradoxing is a more complicated technique that is sometimes striking in its effects. One example is to ask the patient to become more symptomatic while with you. By doing so the patient discovers that control—in either direction—of symptoms is possible. Giving the patient a choice as to when he/she will do a previously difficult task is another form of a paradoxical communication. Predicting a negative outcome or predicting that the patient will be reluctant to attend a particular session often has a paradoxical effect.

Encouraging the Aerial View

Asking the patient to view his actions at a distance, for example, to imagine himself watching as a "Martian" might, may facilitate the development of a self-observing ego. Each may discover recurrent patterns in interpersonal conflict situations as a result.

Humor

Spontaneous humor may be valuable in sessions. Obviously it should not be at the patient's expense. Being able to laugh at oneself turns out to be a very valuable way of gaining perspective. With some patients, where the crisis involves recurrent arguments with spouse or parent, we have suggested that they cassette tape record their next argument. We have yet to receive a tape but have innumerable reports that the assigned task broke up a pattern of recurrent fights—often by getting the people involved to laugh at the "absurdity" of most fights.

SOME WARNINGS

Crisis interventionists need to be well aware of their own feelings and limits. The intensity of some situations may require the use of a co-interventionist. Some patients may develop a dependency on the interventionist or the clinic and in those cases consultation is obligatory. However, with supervision and experience, a great deal of crisis intervention can be done by the primary care clinician.

REFERENCES

1. Caplan G: *Principles of Preventive Psychiatry*. New York, Basic Books, 1964
2. Gill M, Newman R, and Redlich FC: *The Initial Interview in Psychiatric Practice*. Chicago, University of Chicago Press, 1980
3. Ewing CP: *Crisis Intervention and Psychotherapy*. New York, Oxford University Press, 1978

PART IV: Grief

DON A. ROCKWELL, M.D.

Grief is an incredibly common life experience—in some sense a quite normative crisis. Grief is a response to a significant loss. That loss can be a clear "objective" loss such as loss of parent to death or loss of spouse to desertion or divorce. One normally anticipates that these losses will be followed by a grief reaction. However, equally as important and much more common are losses that are purely subjective—losses that the individual patient considers major but may be less apparent to the health care worker. For example, the loss of a pet by an older and otherwise "alone" person or the loss of a fantasy relationship by an adolescent may be viewed by the individual as a major calamity. Likewise, a loss or threatened loss of health or loss of some physical function may precipitate a grief reaction. Therefore, it behooves the alert clinician to inquire routinely about losses to the patient over the past year. There are three major reasons for this routine inquiry.

GRIEF AND HEALTH

Grief-stricken individuals are at a high risk for deleterious health changes. The bereaved have an increase in mortality from all causes (40 percent higher) and from heart disease (67 percent higher). They increase their visits to health centers and are hospitalized four times as frequently as expected. In some studies as many as 28 percent report "a marked deterioration" in health during the year following a major loss. In terms of mental health consequences, an abnormally large proportion of widows and widowers enter psychiatric treatment and are at high risk for suicide. Loss of a child has similar serious consequences for the surviving parents and children. On the basis of health consequences alone, concern for the grief-stricken is quite appropriate.

GRIEF AS "A PROBLEM"

Unexpressed grief after a loss is like an unpaid debt that gathers compound interest over time. While minor losses may evoke a mild reaction that is temporary and easily managed, many losses will evoke a grief reaction that needs work. In many people's lives grief work that goes undone, for whatever reason, serves as a chronic emotional drain causing a subtle interference with psychological function. The mild depression, impaired spontaneity and altered interpersonal relatedness serves to leave the person less than fully able to love, live, and work. There is no question that the psychological work of grief needs to be done and that often people need help in accomplishing the work.

NORMAL GRIEF

Thirdly, a major deterrent to doing "grief work" is the cultural pattern of grieving very privately. As a consequence of this, many people do not know what is normal in grief and are reluctant to express their feelings and experiences out of fear that they are "odd" or "crazy." The astute clinician then needs to understand grief and its pathological variants in order to help the grieving client express himself/herself and to complete necessary grief work. "Normal" grief is a relatively new area of understanding. The notion that "grief work" can be done in a short period of time has recently been laid to rest. Grief after a major loss of an important other due to death or separation takes a minimum of 12 to 15 months and in many cases well beyond that. When grief has been inhibited, it may take much longer and extract an enormous toll on the individual. Helping someone to talk about all the feelings following a loss is the first step in facilitating grief work and reducing the risk for a pathological grief reaction.

Of comparable importance to offering an empathic ear is providing reassuring information about grief. What follows is overly simplified and does not take into account subcultural and religious aspects that can alter grief but is a baseline description of the "typical" grief reaction in a "typical" patient. We recognize that the "typical" rarely ever happens in medicine, yet most grief-stricken persons will have some or all of the following experiences.

Loss

The first step in a grief reaction is the intellectual appreciation of the loss. This happens when one is told a person has died or has left and one appreciates the intellectual truth of the statement. A common first reaction is denial; "No, it can't be," followed by acute severe psychic pain. This pain may be so overwhelming that it is countered by "numbness"—the reduction or elimination of all feeling.

This protective device allows some minimal function for the first few days but should break down in the first few days to be replaced by the second common reaction.

Alarm

The alarm reaction is a fairly total psychological and physiological storm. The onset of a clinical depression starts with an acute emotional outburst, often associated with profound stress, loud wailing and weeping. All too often this "breakdown" is inhibited by family or health care personnel who are made uneasy by the very visible emotional display. Unless *the patient* asks for sedation themselves, they should not be routinely sedated or tranquilized. Sedation blunts the reaction and delays the grief work which is an essentially healthy, normal, and necessary response to loss. The alarm reaction persists for days or weeks and has associated physiologic changes probably responsible for many symptoms and for the increased morbidity and mortality of the bereaved. Closely associated with this phase is the presence of:

Pangs—episodes of intense psychic distress that come on unexpectedly and without provocation, are intensely painful, and render one unable to function. They are, if you will, the other side of pangs of love—the reverse painful side of the exciting, euphoric experience of being newly in love. The person needs to be reassured that over the next weeks the pangs will become less frequent and less intense, and after the first few weeks can be delayed and "scheduled" so as to not seriously interfere with psychological, social or work place functioning. This is often crucial, since these functions are critically important to long-term psychological and economic survival. Encouraging the patient to take some grief time daily and when it is convenient facilitates progression through this phase.

Pining—preoccupation with the lost person and memories of that person is universal. Intrusive images of that person are commonplace. Again, this serves a healthy function both in terms of solidifying the bittersweet memory and regularly confronting the person with the reality of the loss.

Depression—the grief-stricken person now has all the characteristics of a clinically depressed person. They look and feel sad; they lose all appetites such as for food, work, sex, life; they have trouble sleeping; they may be anxious and/or slowed down; they withdraw from social contact; and they may become passively or actively suicidal. The essence of treatment here is to allow the patient to "give sorrow words," to use Shakespeare's advice.

Searching

Associated with "pangs," which peak at five to 14 days after the loss, is the development of "searching" behavior. This behavior is especially distressful to the individual because it makes no logical sense. The searching takes place at all behavioral levels. It is an attempt to recover the lost person and probably represents a primitive survival mechanism. The animal example can be seen when puppies are separated from their mother—the pup searches for its mother in ever-widening circles while giving off plaintive cries while the mother similarly searches for the lost pup. The survival value stems from this behavior increasing the likelihood that the two will be rejoined as a result of their searching behavior. The human animal is not much different. My sense is that an intellectual awareness of a loss far precedes a true appreciation of the loss, and the searching behavior represents a sort of biologic imperative that serves the grief reaction precisely because it meets inevitably with consistent failure. It thus progressively reinforces the fact of the loss. The experience of searching often leaves grief-stricken individuals to conclude that they are "losing their mind" or that they "can't cope." Being given the intellectual information about their behavior is often enormously reassuring. The behaviors are at several levels.

1. Motor behavior—here we see a characteristic restlessness, an inability to sit still, pacing through the house, and so on. This is a repeated attempt to locate the lost person.

2. Perceptual behavior—because of the intense drive to find the person, the bereaved perceptually scans the environment to find the lost one. This leads to misperceptions that are startling, such as catching a glimpse of what seems to be the lost one at a distance, or misreading environmental cues, such as sounds as evidence that the lost one is coming. The full extension of this is the production of hallucinations, usually auditory, of the lost one calling one's name or speaking to you. These hallucinatory experiences occur in large numbers of profoundly grief-stricken individuals—in some series as high as 80 percent. They may be intensely anxiety provoking, since hallucinatory experiences in our culture are rare and associated in many people's minds with frank madness. Reassurance that this is common and, in fact, useful to working through the grief, may allay the very considerable anxiety the person has about "breaking down."

3. Interpersonal behavior—the searching can have untoward effects if a too early attempt is made to search out a replacement. This replacement person rarely turns out in the long run to be what he/she appears to be since the bereaved imbues him/her unrealistically with qualities of the lost person. Advice to the bereaved (or divorced) may include the suggestion that they wait for a period before they remarry or start a new relationship or have a child to replace the deceased or departed. Another pathologic variation is to overidealize the lost one or to develop a "shrine" of sorts for the lost one. This usually represents an unproductive way of dealing with grief and when noted the patient may need encouragement to seek mental health assistance.

4. Psychological searching—this takes the form of retracing the relationship with the lost person even going so far as embarking on an extended journey through the country to revisit old places and old friends. This has healthy

aspects if the reminiscences incorporate all aspects—positive and negative—of the lost relationship. Almost universally the bereaved will have the sense that the lost person is present with them in some way. Again, this can be a healthy aspect to a transition to full acceptance of the loss.

Anger

The searching and its failure confronts the person on every level with the fact of the loss and often evokes anger. The anger response is evidenced when the bereaved becomes increasingly irritable, short tempered, difficult to be around and is most often in evidence four to eight weeks following the loss. It is of critical importance since the effect of the anger is to push the social support system away and people begin to be less solicitous and less frequently supportive. It is compounded, since many persons will react to the anger with anger. Further it is not culturally acceptable to express anger about the death of a loved one. Skillful clinicians will do two things: They will be able to accept the anger and encourage its ventilation, and having done that will help the bereaved peel away the layers of anger in an accepting way. The anger is often directed first at the health care system that failed to keep the patient alive. If one can listen to this expression without becoming defensive, the patient often goes on to the deeper layers. The deeper layers are not often spoken to anyone close to the patient because they represent culturally taboo feelings. The second layer is often directed at family and friends who have failed the bereaved in the mourning period or who failed the lost one. Again, ventilation of the feelings is helpful with the clinician not agreeing or disagreeing, but encouraging expression of the patient's views. The next layer down is anger of the patient for things done or not done that may have contributed to or helped to prevent the loss. Sins of omission and commission are universal and evoke anger and guilt in the bereaved.

Finally, the patient may be able to express, in many situations, anger with the lost person. Since this seems so "unfair" and "illogical," the usual person holds this private and views it as odd or crazy when, in fact, it is a normal human reaction to being "left." Many patients experience tremendous relief after verbalizing this anger and having it met with understanding acceptance. Peeling the angry onion away may mean crying with each layer, but it is an important step in the grief work.

Guilt

The angry feelings, the sins of omission and commission, plus the experience of surviving, regularly evoke guilt in the individual. The obsessive "if only I . . ." needs to be met with a reality based reassurance that 1) one does the best that one can do in most circumstances, and 2) feeling guilty is entirely normal. Everyone feels guilty following a loss. The guilt, if used in a healthy way, allows us to live differently in the future and is a clear sign that the grief is close to resolution.

Mutilation

By now, months have passed. If the grief work is moving ahead, there is now the experience of having been "scarred" or "wounded" and that the wound is very tenderly beginning to heal over. A positive sign is the report by patients that they feel as if "a part of them is gone" or that they feel as if they have been "torn up" or some similar statement that indicates a full level of appreciation for the loss and a sense that they are "scarred" in some way permanently but the acute wound has begun to heal. During this time most patients begin to reorganize their lives without the lost one, make tentative attempts to break out of the social withdrawal and hesitantly start new relationships. Here the physician encourages these patients to go slowly and expect setbacks. These setbacks are inevitable so that the prediction of them is paradoxically comforting. Consistently, however, the clinician encourages these steps back into a reorganized world.

Identification Phenomena

Occasionally in the course of grief we encounter identification phenomena. Here the bereaved takes on some characteristics of the lost person. This may be an interest the lost person had, a mannerism, a behavior, some characteristic. The clinician's interest in this is the fact that a common identification phenomenon is with the physical signs and symptoms of the person deceased. Sensitivity to this issue may prevent needless expense to the patient for workups of what are in fact identification reactions. However, remember that the person with grief is at high risk health-wise and careful evaluation of the symptoms may be quite appropriate. It is, indeed, possible to die of a broken heart—in a very literal sense. However, often the identification symptoms are not associated with any clinical signs or other evidence and may, at first blush, appear bizarre or out of context. An example might be a mother who develops symptoms that relate to the uniquely pediatric disease that killed her child. In these circumstances we often find that the grief over the loss was incompletely expressed. Going back to the time of death and encouraging the expresssion of grief and sorrow may lead to an outpouring of sadness and total remission of the somatic symptoms.

Anniversary Reaction

The person often experiences a minigrief reaction around important dates and especially around the annual time period when the loss occurred. The person may not make this association, especially if several years have passed. Patients presenting with a mild or moderate depression and no apparent precipitant in the recent past should be questioned about the possible significance of this particular time of year. Anniversary reactions are entirely normal and serve as a way of reminding us of the lost person.

To reiterate the essence of this brief discussion:

1. Grief is normal and healthful, but very painful.
2. Expression of grief is to be encouraged.
3. Understanding common grief experiences and reassuring the patient about their essentially useful quality may be enormously reassuring.
4. Depression is the persistent background throughout the 13 plus months of grief.

PATHOLOGIC GRIEF

Pathologic grief represents some inhibition in the grief work. It is more likely to occur when the loss is sudden or unexpected, when the person has multiple other stresses, when he/she has multiple losses or important losses early in life, and when there is a prior history of clinical depression and when the loss is of a child, a long marriage, or an ambivalent (love-hate) relationship.

Identification of a pathologic grief reaction means in most cases referral for professional counseling. About 2-3 percent of grief reactions following major losses will evolve into pathologic grief reactions.

The most common pathologic grief reaction is "prolonged" depression. Prolonged is a difficult time to define but for practical purposes, patients who feel disabled by their depression six to eight months after the loss should be carefully evaluated as to the progress of their grief work. If they appear "hung up" in their grief, then referral is appropriate. Sixty percent of pathologic grief reactions are prolonged depressive states.

The most immediately treatable pathologic grief reactions are 1) sudden onset of problem drinking following a major loss. Here the person often attempts to treat the depressing pain with alcohol (or minor tranquilizers) and becomes a temporary abuser. This grief equivalent is successfully treated by encouraging grief work and the use of TCAs. This is a "symptomatic alcoholism" that has an extremely good prognosis. It represents 15 percent of pathologic grief reactions; 2) development of phobic symptoms. The onset of a discrete phobia (bridge, hospitals, open spaces) in a patient with no prior phobic history following a significant loss is often a grief equivalent. It is again uniquely responsive to grief work and TCAs. This represents 10 percent of pathologic grief reactions.

The most difficult pathologic grief reactions are 1) the development of chronic hypochondriacal symptoms (10 percent), and 2) the development of a psychotic reaction (5 percent). These will require referral for treatment.

Finally, it is crucial to remember that grief reactions are commonplace. Allow the patient to tell you of these recent losses and you will discover many under-recognized grief reactions. The patient will present with fatigue, depression and vague somatic symptoms. The losses may sometimes seem trivial. Helping with grief work is both simple and worthwhile if one understands its expression.

REFERENCES

1. Parkes CM: *Bereavement: Studies of Grief in Adult Life.* New York, International Universities Press, 1972
2. Bowlby J: Pathological mourning and childhood mourning. *J Am Psychoanal Assoc* 11:500-541, 1973
3. Lindemann E: Symptomatology and management of acute grief. *Am J Psychiatry* 101:141-148, 1944

PART V: Suicide

DON A. ROCKWELL, M.D.
FRAN PEPITONE-ARREOLA-ROCKWELL, Ph.D.

Overview
Recognition
Diagnosis
Management

Patients who are potentially or currently suicidal are common in practice. A comprehensive study[1] reveals that at least 2.25 percent of patients have problems that are clearly or potentially of suicidal import. Incidence and prevalence studies are beginning to delineate the parameters of suicidal behaviors and a useful approximation of these behaviors is evident in Figure 14-1.

Of major interest to clinicians is the fact that in the course of any one year roughly one in 100 will threaten suicide, and one in 10 will have suicidal ideation. Figure 14-1 illustrates this suicide "iceberg" graphically. One percent of all deaths are reported as suicides and the true figure is two to three times as high.[2] It has been shown that 75 percent of suicides consult their physicians before acting on their impulses.[3] From 60[4]-74 percent[5] of suicide attempters have been treated recently by their physician. Perhaps as many as 10 percent see their physician on the day of or just prior to their suicide and are provided with the means for their attempt by the unsuspecting physician.[6]

Primary care clinicians, then, have a large number of suicidal patients in their practice. The failure to recognize these patients is related to a variety of reasons;[7] death denial, suicide as a taboo, suicide as an anxiety inducer, inadequate skills for managing suicidal patients, and inadequate information about recognition and management of suicidal patients.

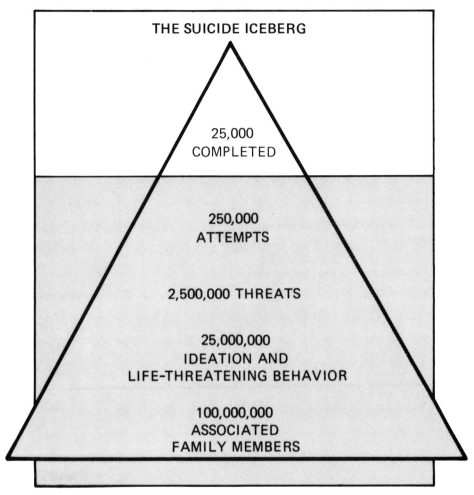

THE SUICIDE ICEBERG

25,000
COMPLETED

250,000
ATTEMPTS

2,500,000 THREATS

25,000,000
IDEATION AND
LIFE-THREATENING BEHAVIOR

100,000,000
ASSOCIATED
FAMILY MEMBERS

Figure 14-1. The Suicide Iceberg.

RECOGNITION OF THE SUICIDAL PATIENT

As in many problems in medicine, certain factors can be recognized as putting an individual at unusual risk for a disease process. The suicidal individual has certain characteristics that make suicide more likely.

A look at demographic factors below shows that the rates for male suicide increase progressively after the age of 35. At age 65 the rates for women begin to decline again while for men the rate increases precipitously. A recent marital disruption and/or job problem also contribute to significantly increased risk.

Sex:	Males complete suicide three times as often as females
	Females attempt suicide three times as often as males
Race:	White > black
Age:	Increasing risk with increasing age

Marital Status: Separated > divorced > widowed > single
Socioeconomic Status: Downward mobility
                        Unemployed
                        Retired

The theme of loss is of paramount importance in the patient's life. The loss may be one of a fantasy, e.g., the promotion which did not happen, the failure to develop an important relationship, as well as the loss of real things or people. The onset of a depression and a lightening or deepening of the depression are also high-risk periods. Evidence indicates that the nine to 15-month period following recovery from a depressive episode is a high-risk period. In the assessment of the individual patient, it is important to determine the patient's plans for suicide, vague or well thought out (intentionality), and the potential method, high-risk methods being guns and jumping and lower-risk methods being poisoning and wrist slashing (lethality). Finally, the factor of social isolation is crucial both diagnostically and therapeutically. Lving alone increases one's risk—especially if this is the result of a recent change in life circumstances. Reversal of this isolation is often possible through family or social agency intervention.

Past historical factors essentially point out that past behavior is the best predictor of future behavior. Persons with demonstrated problems in controlling impulses (the substance abuser, the violent or impulsive person) or with a prior model of suicidal behavior (personal, familial, or peer group) are at much increased risk.

Some patients constitute special risks even in the absence of demographic or other risk factors. The patient who reports being in some sense "already dead" is the first of importance in the truly emergent suicidal situations. This patient is likely to act quickly and effectively on impulses and immediate hospitalization is mandatory, possibly against the patient's will. The basis for all suicide prevention is the play for more time, as suicidal individuals have mixed feelings about their deaths.

Patients who are frankly psychotic are also at special risk, again because the momentary impulse is often acted on or even mandated by their psychotic state.

Until recently the potential for the family to participate in suicidal behaviors was poorly recognized.[7] Some families (or other close social systems) may collude to exclude a member. These excluded or scapegoated members are frequently adolescents or elderly members. The family often gives covert or even overt messages to the individual to in some sense "disappear." Direct messages spoken in anger to the adolescent include "get lost," "I can't stand you," "you're more trouble than you're worth," or similar rejecting messages. The susceptible adolescent then acts to meet their angry request with counter-anger and suicide— both as a response to the family anger and as a way to "get back at" the rejecting family. Similar dynamics are often found in families with an elderly depressed relative. The scenario is one in which the elderly person makes many demands or has many complaints ultimately generating anger in the other family members.

The covert wish is "I wish you'd go ahead and die," and this is communicated nonverbally—sometimes even directly. This leads the already depressed person to attempt to comply by suiciding. These families require immediate attention if a disaster is to be averted. Suicides happening in these contexts are frequently followed by severe pathologic grief reactions which are not readily treatable and prevention is much the preferred approach.

Finally, the depressed patient is to be considered at high risk. This category is mentioned last since it is well recognized that depression and suicide are coincident. In point of fact perhaps as many as one-third of suicides are not "typically" depressed. Nevertheless, the formula "depression = suicide potential" needs to be firmly fixed in every physician's mind. *Patients who are depressed, have early morning insomnia, and feel hopeless are especially at risk.* One way to assess hopelessness is to ask patients to discuss how they envision the next six months or year. If patients have difficulty in foreseeing the future, the physician should inquire further.

There are some populations such as the following whose risk is higher than would be expected on the basis of demographic or other factors:

Students
Young blacks
Indians-Eskimos
Gifted individuals
Physicians
Immigrants
Air traffic controllers
Police officers

These atypical populations can be generally characterized as being composed of individuals who are more intelligent than average and/or experiencing unusual change and flux in their lives. These groups illustrate Durkheim's thesis that high social integration reduces suicide while change increases suicide rates. One word about physician suicides: The high risk period is atypical in that it occurs in the 35-54 year old range. The major problem is the physicians' hesitancy to recognize their own and their colleagues' personal problems and to seek help for depression and drug dependency problems. These deaths are preventable.

As indicated previously, it is crucial to recognize that every depressed individual is potentially suicidal. Depression which extends over any length of time is a progressively painful and a horizon-narrowing experience. Inevitably, the patient wishes to be free of the depression, and death becomes one of increasingly fewer apparent alternatives. The signs and symptoms of depression are as follows:

Biological	*Psychological*	*Interpersonal*
Insomnia—especially early a.m. awakening	Loss of interests Fatigue	Troubled expression "Depressed" look

Biological	*Psychological*	*Interpersonal*
(continued)	(continued)	(continued)
Diurnal mood variation	Trouble concentrating	Slowed speech
Anorexia	Decreased libido	Lose sense of humor
Weight loss	Guilt feelings	Irritable
Psychomotor retardation or agitation	Pessimism-self-criticism	Dependent
Physical complaints, especially headache, musculoskeletal, gastro-intestinal and cardio-respiratory complaints	Unusual fears	More complaints
	Feel empty, deserted "Blue"	
Constipation		
Dry mouth		

All too frequently it is forgotten that depression, like suicide, is merely a final common pathway and can be approached from a variety of avenues. Physicians tend to see depression in "neurotics" and tend to see it as psychopathology rather than the common, often normal, human response that it is. People who are experiencing normal grief (bereavement, for example) are depressed *and* suicidal sometimes. Aspects of normal aging (turning grey, for example) may be interpreted negatively by the individual, initiating a feeling of deterioration leading to depression. The depression associated with anemia is understandable yet remains potentially suicidal. The list presented here contains a variety of "organic" illnesses which are frequently accompanied or followed by a depressive episode.

Infectious Diseases
    Most common viral illnesses
    Infectious mononucleosis
    Infectious hepatitis
    Encephalitis
    Chronic Pyelonephritis
    Brucellosis
    Tuberculosis
    Subacute bacterial endocarditis
    Parasitic infestations
Endocrine Disorders
    Diabetes mellitus
    Hypo and hyperthyroidism
    Hypo and hyperadrenalism
    Hypopituitarism
    Hyperparathyroidism

Metabolic and Nutritional Disorders
　　Anything causing metabolic acidosis
　　Increased blood urea nitrogen (BUN)
　　Hepatic or hypertensive encephalopathy
　　Pellagra
　　Hypervitaminosis D
　　Heavy metal poisoning
　　Iron deficiency, anemia
　　Nutritional deficiencies secondary to fad diets

Degenerative/Collagen Vascular/Neoplastic Diseases
　　Arthritis
　　Lupus erythematosus
　　Polyarteritis nodosa
　　Occult tumors (especially pancreatic)
　　Brain tumors (especially temporal)
　　Amyotropic lateral sclerosis
　　Huntington's chorea
　　Most dementing processes

Miscellaneous
　　Anemias (especially iron deficiency, aplastic, hemolytic and secondary)
　　Acute intermittent porphyria
　　Psychomotor epilepsy
　　Meniere's disease
　　Postoperative patients (especially following psychologically or cosmetically disfiguring surgery)

Depression in these situations, although organically "caused," is no less painful and is very real. It is helpful for these patients to know that the "blues" a) are expected and b) will not go on for long. This information reduces patient anxiety and prevents a vicious cycle of depression and anxiety.

Depression is a side effect of a variety of drugs. Again, even though the depression is understandable it may still lead to suicide. The list in its totality is startling. Most commonly prescribed drugs are included—birth control pills, minor tranquilizers, antihistamines, and so on. While not all patients taking these drugs will become depressed, a significant number will, ranging from 3-25 percent, depending on the specific drug. In most cases alternative treatment can be substituted for a depression-inducing medication. Patients with a family history of depression and/or alcoholism are usually susceptible to depression as a side effect. In any case, depression due to any cause cannot be ignored; depression is equally serious due to drugs or intra-psychic causes. Below are listed drugs which produce depression as a side effect:

Salicylates
Antihistamines

Antibiotics—especially sulfas and tetracyclines
Rauwolfia alkaloids-reserpine
Steroids—especially adrenocorticosteroids and progesterones—hence many
   birth control pills
Sedative/hypnotic/minor tranquilizers
Ergot alkaloids
Xanthines
Nitrates, nitrites
Sympathomimetics
Hallucinogens
Anticonvulsants
Digitalis
Levodopa
Methyldopa
Amantadine
Indomethacin
Propanolol
Cycloserine
Carbamazepine
Alcohol

DIAGNOSIS

The diagnosis of the suicidal patient can be made easily if the clinician is alert.
Patients presenting with complaints referrable to depression (especially insomnia, weight loss, and "fatigue") can be asked about the depth of their depression
and despair. If they feel the depression is out of control, then they are in fact suicidal. A series of questions such as the following taps the depth of the depression.

> Dr.: How bad are you feeling?
> Pt.: Pretty bad.
> Dr.: Can you tell me about how bad?
> Pt.: Oh, I don't know . . .
> Dr.: Do things look pretty grim (or hopeless)?
> Pt.: Yes.
> Dr.: Are you wondering if you can cope?
> Pt.: Yes.
> Dr.: Most people who feel bad for a time think about doing themselves in. Are
>   you thinking about suicide?
> Pt.: Yes, but I'd never do it.

The patient who is ambivalent about suicide is often eager to talk about it. Since
nearly everyone has considered suicide when highly stressed, the physician is not
going to suggest or cause a suicide by such a line of inquiry. There is a small
number of patients, usually older in age, who are unambivalent about committing

suicide. They will not directly or even indirectly cry for help. Often the cry for help in ambivalent patients is obtuse and indirect. The presenting complaint (fatigue, loss of appetite, insomnia, general malaise) is the ticket of admission to the physician's office and the hidden agenda can then be elicited by the alert physician.

MANAGEMENT

Diagnosis is the major step in management of the suicidal patient. Eliciting the thought or intent, making it overt, in and of itself serves to reduce the risk and raise the possibility of hope. Management is then as follows:

1. Assessment of "biologic" causes for depression, for example, replacing a reserpine-containing antihypertensive with another antihypertensive medication or replacing a birth control pill with an intrauterine device;
2. Evaluating intentionality, for example, does the patient have a well thought out plan requiring emergent intervention or is this a patient without a specific plan but a great deal of psychic pain requiring counseling and medication;
3. Evaluating lethality of intended method. This requires physician awareness of the commonest methods of completed suicide.

The differences between men and women in terms of means of suicide are striking.

| | Percent | |
Method	Males	Females
Firearms, explosives	47	18
Poisoning	33	65
Hanging, strangulation	12	7
Jumping	3	4
Cutting and piercing	2	2
Drowning	1	2
Miscellaneous	2	2

The two most common means, guns and poisoning (the latter usually being prescribed medication), are potentially accessible to patient and physician control. The suicidal patient, and the patient's family when possible, should be made aware of the danger and urged to reduce the available lethal resources in the environment. *It is worth remembering that not having access to a lethal method at a moment's impulse may be enough to prevent the attempt. The method chosen is often symbolic in some way to the individual and, if that method is not available, an alternative method is often not sought.* Thus, the physician through elimination of guns and medications from the patient's immediate environment will reduce the absolute chance of an attempt and will often mitigate any attempt being made. One final note about prevention that may be useful to the patient and the patient's family: alcohol is often involved in a suicide attempt. Drinking serves both to disinhibit and depress. While cautions about drinking are often not heeded the warning should, nevertheless, be given.

4. General management. General management takes into account several aspects of the suicidal patient. The patient identified as being suicidal—crying for help—has already opened the major treatment avenue—that of open communication. The physician's responsibility is thus to maintain a clear channel of communication with the patient through the crisis. Most patients' suicidal crises are short lived, a matter of hours or days. Being available through this period of labor is indeed life-protecting. One expedient often forgotten is the use of the telephone. Telephone therapy is readily available, time efficient and effective. Other crisis intervention strategies can be employed (see Section III). Involving the family and dealing with the "last straw" or system disequilibratory event can be done without great expenditures of time. Consultation by the physician with a mental health professional may provide the physician with a workable plan without having to refer the patient. Involving other members of the treatment team—nurse practitioner, office nurse, and aides is often useful to both patient and physician alike.

5. Specific management. Specific management is aimed at the specific system dysfunction. The depressed or suicidal person with a biologic etiology can be managed by:
   a. removal of organic causes (drugs)
   b. patient and family education as to the etiology and self-limited nature of the illness
   c. judicious use of antidepressant medication
   d. consideration of a urine and blood drug screen to evaluate use of other drugs, i.e., bromides, decongestants, and over-the-counter drugs.

The patient whose problems are more in the individual psychological system realm needs to be permitted expression and often acceptance of negative feelings about self and others. The empathic physician can, in most cases, offer brief (20 minute "hours"[8]) crisis intervention and assist the patient in reestablishing a satisfactory equilibrium.

Quite often the dysfunctional system is interpersonal (marriage, family) rather than purely individual. Family or marital counseling is then entirely appropriate. This is especially true for suicidal adolescents. Exploration of covert conflict and hidden agendas by the tactful physician may lead the patient to seek more extensive help from appropriate social and mental health professionals.

The physician can both highlight a chronic problem and effect an appropriate referral as the following illustrates:

Dr.: Things are kind of tough at home?

Pt.: Yeah, it's been hard.

Dr.: The boys are teenagers and John's working a lot.

Pt.: I don't know how to manage them and John's not available.

Dr.: Communication breaking down?

Pt.: Yes. We can't talk anymore without it breaking down into a fight.

Dr.: Maybe working on some family communication skills would help.

Pt.: That's for sure, but where can we do that?

Dr.: There are several possibilities (some church groups offer programs, some school systems, family service agencies, the mental health system, etc. Specific referrals depend on the community but nearly all communities will have some educational or mental health professional with special communication skills. A focus on a positive goal—learning communication skills is much more acceptable to most patients than a focus on "psychopathology"—i.e., there is something wrong or crazy).

Ultimately, then, the alert physician has the opportunity to prevent suicide. To do so requires a high index of suspicion and the willingness to explore with patients the depths of their depression and the risk of suicide. The major treatment parameters include:

- Understanding and eliminating the common means of suicide;
- Preventing or reducing the social isolation of the suicidal patient by involving the family and others in the treatment;
- Being available to the patient during the period of crisis;
- Treating the underlying problem;
- Consulting with mental health professionals as needed.

Treatment is inhibited primarily because of physician hesitation. That hesitation is often related to lack of information. The rewards for recognizing and effectively managing the suicidal individual are immense. There are few other situations where the opportunity for life saving is so clear and so immediate.

REFERENCES

1. Marshland D, Wood M, and Mayo F: Content of family practice: Part I: Rank order of diagnoses by frequency. *J Fam Pract* 3:37, 1976
2. Rockwell D A, and O'Brien W: Physicians' knowledge and attitudes about suicide. *JAMA* 225:1347, 1973
3. Motto J, and Greene C: Suicide and the medical community. *Arch Neurol Psychiatry* 80:776, 1958

4. Buckle RC, Linnane J, and McCarachy W: Attempted suicide presenting at the Alfred Hospital, Melbourne. *Med J Aust* 52:754-58, 1965

5. Litman RE: Acutely suicidal patients: Management in general medical practice. *Calif Med* 104:168, 1966

6. O'Brien JP: Increase in suicide attempts by drug ingestion. *Arch Gen Psychiatry* 34:1165, 1977

7. Richman J, and Rosenbaum M: The family doctor and the suicidal family. *Int J Psychiatr Med* 1:27, 1970

8. Castelnuevo-Tedesco P: *The Twenty-Minute Hour.* Boston, Little-Brown, 1965

PART VI: Rape

FRAN PEPITONE-ARREOLA-ROCKWELL, Ph.D.

Rape is the fastest rising violent crime in the United States.[1] With the advent of the women's movement, there has been a confronting of this phenomenon in terms of its mythology, public attitudes, occurrence, and prevention.

Early writings on rape centered around the rapist—his psychodynamics, and his rehabilitation prospects. Literature about the rape victim was lacking. As feminists became concerned with the distribution of power in interpersonal relationships, rape became the focal point: the rapist has absolute power. Metzger[2] says it well:

> *The rapist acts for society, concretizing certain ideas through his behavior. He is often marginally integrated into the society, and rape is the way he affiliates himself, if not through the act, then through the attitudes. Through rape he asserts power and possession in a common violent and spontaneous action. By choosing to assert himself against woman and her body, he—like church, state, schools, advertisers and the media—is simply asserting certain rights and prerogatives over woman, using her for his own purposes. He is translating cultural thoughts into action.*

Rape is socially seen as response rather than provocation—it is the desperate male response to powerlessness that is confirmed for him by the spectre of female identity.

RAPE DEFINED

Rape can be defined socially and/or legally, depending on one's perspective. Socially, rape has been defined as the act of taking anything by force. However, rape to one person may not be rape to another. Rape is seen as contingent on one's values and sexual experiences. That is, rape could be considered a logical extension of cultural values that sees men as possessors of women. The social definition of rape frequently is provided by the woman as victim.

All victims would agree that rape is an act of violence, most having felt certain that they would be killed by the rapist. Rape is perceived as a brush with death which accounts for the severity of psychobiologic responses in victims. Sex is the vehicle for this violent act. "Rape is a crime against the person, not against the hymen."[3] Burgess and Holstrom[4] have noted a consistency of symptom reporting by victims which they have named the *Rape Trauma Syndrome:* "The syndrome includes physical, emotional, and behavioral stress reactions which result from the person being faced with a life-threatening event."

The response to rape has been compared with war victim responses to traumatic situations. The degree of powerlessness and helplessness experienced by the victim no doubt sets rape apart from other life events. Notman and Nadelson[5] have compared rape responses to other situations of stress: "Since it is an interaction between an extreme environmental stimulus and the adaptive capacity of the victim, it is similar to other situations described in the literature on stress, including community disasters, war, surgical procedures, etc."

Another aspect of the social definition of rape is the fact that mutual consent to the act is lacking as the rapist displays his hostility and gratification-seeking.

Legally, rape is carnal knowledge of a person by force and against that person's will if there is sexual intercourse and force without consent. Force refers to the use of actual physical force to overcome a victim's resistance or by threat of great and immediate bodily harm. Excluded from this legal definition are acts of anal or oral intercourse, and homosexual assaults.

INCIDENCE OF RAPE

Rape is one of the most under-reported crimes because of the fear, embarrassment and humiliation experienced by the victim. In 1973, the FBI documented 51,000 cases of forcible and attempted rape, a rise of 62 percent over a five-year period compared with a 45 percent rise for other criminal acts. It has been said that only one in five rapes are reported.

VICTIM RESPONSES

Rape is a violent act which for most victims is a major and unforgetable crisis. The victim will state that she had an overwhelmingly frightening experience for which she feared for her life and paid for her freedom in the sexual act. The victim's life style becomes severely disrupted as well as those close to the victim: her family, friends, co-workers, etc. The victim's family and others may believe that "she asked for it" since they often believe that rape can only occur that way. Rather than support the victim emotionally, the family may withdraw, be openly critical or wonder how they failed as a family. The victim's social partner may feel that the victim is untouchable, dirty or no longer worthy of respect. Seiden[6] points out that when society, the family, police or psychotherapists assume that the victim contributed to the rape, that this contributes to the victim's own victimization. The rape victim already blames herself for the assault. Many women will ask: "What did I do to bring this on" which assumes that the woman could have avoided rape. This self-blaming process often serves as a means of controlling the unpredictable future. That is, if she could find out how she could have avoided rape, then she could control her future since obviously she feels out of control at the present. Paradoxically, a simultaneous seemingly universal phenomenon occurs, and rape victims will state: "I can't believe it happened to me." This phenomenon manifests in the sense of shock, bewilderment and trauma.

Phobic reactions are also common for the rape victim and represent a defensive reaction. Six major phobic reactions have been observed:

- Fear of indoors (especially those women raped in their beds)
- Fear of outdoors (women attacked outside of their homes)
- Fear of being alone
- Fear of crowds
- Fear of people behind them
- Sexual fears (especially victims who had no prior sexual activity)

Some rape victims feel suicidal. As a result of rape, the victim has most likely experienced an incredible degree of powerlessness and helplessness. Feeling suicidal is concomitant to feeling isolated due to the social stigmatization of rape, the inability to put into words the terror, and guilt, and the inability to find people who are genuinely empathetic. Many rape victims will say they feel like they are "going crazy" as they live a total disruption, a crisis unparalleled to any other life experience.

Interestingly, anger is not a primary or immediate emotion for many victims; it seems to be experienced later. In general women tend to be slower to anger than men. When rape victims begin to experience anger, it is apparent in dreams, or more specifically nightmares, in which the rapist is killed, maimed or otherwise put into a powerless position. Anger also is not a primary experience for the rape victim because she is so engrossed in trying to figure out how she brought it on. When she can stop her self-blame, she can redirect her energies to the man who violated her.

The responses to rape that a victim has are also contingent on the myths that most of us have grown up with, and to some extent share as a result of our relatively common socialization experiences. The stigmatization process is based on myths which essentially and subtly imply that women fabricate rape incidents.

Hilberman[7] points out that the notion of the "woman as a liar" typifies our attitudes about rape victims.

> *This image of women as liars is likely the explanation for the assumption that women often make false charges of rape against men, even men they don't know. Law enforcement personnel are aware that false charges of crime do occur, but it is only in rape that it is assumed that the usual safeguards in the system are inadequate to protect the innocent from a lying witness. Contrast a charge of rape with that of robbery, where it is understood that property is taken from the victim without his/her consent, and there is no need to prove that fear of death or grave bodily harm was at issue . . . the law grants more protection to property than to person, especially if the person is female.*

The myths which help to maintain the stigmatization process serve to depict the victim as responsible and not innocent. The myths are simply that—myths.

Myth: Most rapists see an attractive woman and are absolutely overcome by uncontrolled sexual impulses.

Fact: Rape is a violent, not romantic, planned aggressive act. Factors such as physical attractiveness of the victim, her age, do not deter rapists.

Myth: Rape is impossible if the woman struggles enough—rape can be avoided.

Fact: Most women are smaller and weaker physically than their attacker. Additionally, rapists may threaten a sleeping child in an adjoining room if the woman does not submit. Frequently, rapists have actual weapons, and may have already harmed or plan to mutilate, or kill the victim. A counterattack by the victim may not be protective.

Myth: Women provoke rape.

Fact: In a similar fashion, one might assume that bank tellers provoke bank robberies. This myth assumes that men have no responsibility, and that in essence women are responsible for men's sexual and/or aggressive impulses. The person who is robbed is not accused of asking for it.

Myth: Only "bad" women get raped.

Fact: All women are potential rape victims. To assume that "bad" women are the victims serves to further split women into the good/bad dichotomy and to help maintain a double-standard of sexuality.

Myth: Women cry rape when they are trying to retaliate against a man.

Fact: Rape is under-reported. Women already feel stigmatized and guilty, and are more likely not to report rape.

Myth: If you are going to be raped, you might as well relax and enjoy it.

Fact: This notion discounts the seriousness of rape as an aggressive, violent act, and assumes that women want to be raped. It suggests that a man should relax and enjoy being mugged and beaten—an unlikely enjoyable experience.

Myth: Rape occurs outside of the woman's home.

Fact: Over half of the rapes occur in the victim's home. Being in one's residence does not guard against rape.

Myth: Most reported rapes involve black men raping white women.
Fact: Most reported rapes are intraracial, not interracial. Rapist and victim tend to be of the same race.

COUNSELING THE RAPE VICTIM

Rape victims are a special group of people who require skilled, sensitive and empathetic helpers.

The victim needs to feel safe and that she has an empathetic listener to tell about her strong feelings as well as to describe what may seem to the victim to be unspeakable acts. The "controlled" victim appears to have a calm or subdued demeanor about her, unlike the "expressed" victim who demonstrates her feelings more clearly. To pressure the "controlled" victim to talk is to replay the rape experience of force. The victim must be allowed to choose this style of being; this style of expression is hers and must be respected as such. Medea and Thompson[8] discuss this need for control on the part of the rape victim:

> *At this time the victim has little or no desire for outside help. She may well resent it. Her emotional well-being depends on her believing that she has coped with the matter and she needs time to adjust.*

Rape victims have been shown to manifest a cluster of adaptive psychological responses now called the *Rape Trauma Syndrome.* These responses include such fears as fears of crowds and being alone, etc. Feldman-Summers, Gordon and Meagher[9] found that rape victims reported less enjoyment of sexual activities as a consequence of rape. "Rape obviously does not merely harm the victim—its impact is felt by the significant others in the victim's life. Indeed, the very fabric of human relationships is disrupted by the rape experience."[10]

In trying to provide emotional support to rape victims, the physician should be aware of guidelines to follow:

- Encourage the victim to talk about her feelings
- Do not try to determine the validity of the rape
- Provide information on police procedures, legal resources, medical facilities, victim of violent crimes information, and supportive community groups
- Assume that a wide range of emotional and behavioral responses are part of a major normative crisis
- If possible, and only with the victim's consent, enlist the support of her significant others

The physician will more likely be called upon to treat the physical manifestations of rape or help gather information to determine if in fact the rape did occur. This information-gathering process is the evidentiary examination, often initiated by the police. It should be understood, however, that rape is in actuality determined in a court of law, and *not* by the physician.

The physician's major responsibility to rape victims is to ascertain the levels of injury and to provide the appropriate treatment as for any patient. More specifically, the following duties have been identified:[10]

- Immediate care of physical injuries
- Prevention of venereal disease
- Prevention of pregnancy
- Proper medicolegal examination with documentation by evidence collection for law enforcement
- Prevention or alleviation of permanent psychological damage

Consent for examination and treatment should be obtained from the victim *before* the examination and treatment. The victim has the right to request medical treatment only and to refuse examination for the collection of legal evidence. However, many hospitals are required to report cases of suspected assault and battery to the local authorities. The patient should be made aware of this. Therefore, it is recommended that the collection of legal evidence be encouraged, since the alleged victim may decide to prosecute at some later date. No information gathered from the medical examination should be released by the hospital or physician unless the victim has signed an authorization for the release of this information.

History

The history and interview should be brief and need not be an interrogation. The physician should ascertain the nature of the assault which identifies those body parts involved. A brief inquiry about the victim's menstrual cycle should be made noting last menstrual period as well as present birth control methods. The victim should be asked if she bathed, changed clothes or used a douche since the assault.

Clothing

The victim's clothing should be noted and described on the report and retained for evidence.

Diagnosing Trauma

Bruises, lacerations and the general appearance of the victim should be noted. Any foreign materials such as dirt should be saved.

A gynecological examination using a water-moistened speculum is carried out. The physician should examine the external genitalia, perineum, cervix and vaginal wall for trauma and lacerations. The vaginal pool material should be swabbed for a wet mount, acid phosphatase, dry and fixed smears. Oral and rectal swabs and smears may also be collected if indicated. Other collections for legal evidence may include clipped and pulled pubic hairs, photographs, and fingernail scrapings.

Prevention of Pregnancy

Most rape victims are concerned about the possibility of pregnancy. Three possibilities exist which should be discussed with the patient:[7]

1. Administration of diethylstilbestrol (DES) usually 0.25 mgm, twice a day for five days, if the victim was not pregnant prior to the rape. Glover, et al.[11] found that 11 percent of rape victims discontinued DES because of nausea and vomiting, despite the use of an antiemetic. There is also controversy surrounding DES because of its association with vaginal tumors.
2. Menstrual extraction at the second or sixth week return visit.
3. Suction abortion at six-week check-up.

Prevention of Venereal Disease

Baseline information for the presence or absence of gonorrhea and syphilis as well as the less common venereal diseases should be obtained. Intramuscular procaine penicillin may be given prophylactically. Follow-up appointments at two or six weeks in the gynecological clinic should be given to assess GC cultures and the VDRL. Six weeks after the rape, the VDRL should be repeated.

The physician has the task of caring for the rape victim in a thorough and medically responsible manner. The victim may have been subjected to brutalization and be faced with numerous physical and psychological injuries. The possibility of an unwanted pregnancy and venereal disease are imposed upon a victim who has not consented to such abuse. Rape is a violent crime and most victims believe they had a brush with death.

REFERENCES

1. McCombie S, Bassuk E, Saritz R, et al: Development of a medical center rape crisis intervention program. *Am J Psychiatry* 133:418, 1976
2. Metzger D: It is always the woman who is raped. *Am J Psychiatry* 133:405, 1976
3. Hilberman E: Rape: The ultimate violation of the self. *Am J Psychiatry* 133:436-37, 1976
4. Burgess A, Holstrom L: *Rape: Victims of Crisis.* Bowie, Md., Robert J Brady, 1974
5. Notman M, Nadelson C: The rape victim: Psychodynamic considerations. *Am J Psychiatry* 133:408-13, 1976
6. Seiden A: Overview: Research on the psychology of women. I. Gender differences and sexual and reproductive life. *Am J Psychiatry* 133:995-1007, 1976
7. Hilberman E: Medical aspects of rape. In: *The Rape Victim.* Washington, D.C., American Psychiatric Association, 1976
8. Medea A, Thompson K: Psychological reactions. In: *Against Rape.* New York, Farrar, Strauss and Giroux, 1974
9. Feldman-Summers S, Gordon P, Meagher J: The impact of rape on sexual satisfaction. *J Abnorm Psychol* 88:101-105, 1979

10. Pepitone-Rockwell F: Patterns of rape and approaches to care. *J Fam Pract* 521-529, 1978

11. Glover D, Gerety M, Bromber S, et al: Diethylstilbestrol in the treatment of rape victims. *West J Med* Oct: 331-334, 1976

PART VII: Sex Role Stereotyping

FRAN PEPITONE-ARREOLA-ROCKWELL, Ph.D.
DONNA STRINGER-MOORE, Ph.D.

Why This Chapter?
Physician Differences
Women's Problems
    Depression
    Phobic Syndrome
    Role Confusion
    Self-Esteem
The Future: Treatment Options
    Consciousness-Raising Groups
    Assertiveness Training
    Peer Counseling
    Reeducation

WHY THIS CHAPTER?

The structure of our society with its arbitrary attribution of sex roles is a major source of women's oppression. Merely talking about "society" relieves each of us of individual responsibility. "Society" is all of us. Its very impersonality precludes positive action. The bulk of women's mental health needs is met by primary care practitioners, most of whom are male. It is ethically imperative that the physician for women's mental health recognize ways in which he/she may perpetuate rather than alleviate problems. Further, the physician must acknowledge that the potential for effective therapy may be significantly reduced without an understanding of sex roles and socialization, including recent and ongoing societal changes in those roles.

Historically mental health professionals have reflected cultural stereotypes of women. Occasionally they have presaged enlighted understanding but certainly many traditional forms of psychotherapy can be and have been used to reinforce stereotyped sex roles. Interestingly social scientists have been most enlightened regarding sex role stereotyping. Margaret Mead's work[1] with three New Guinea

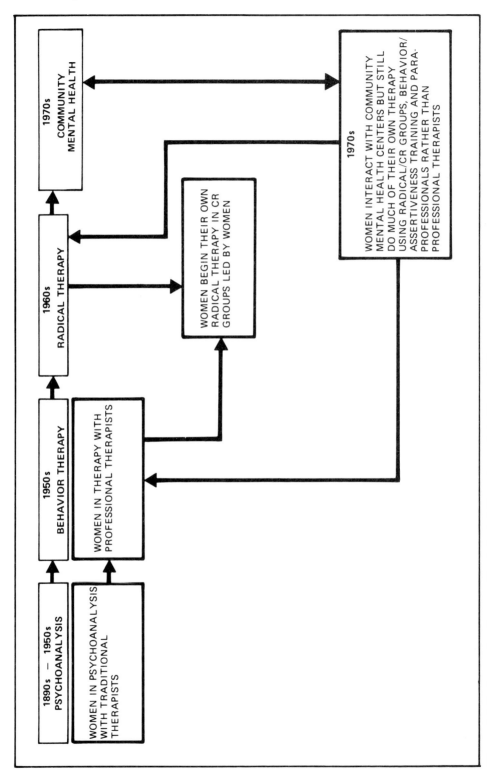

Figure 14-2. Interaction Between Psychological Therapies and the Women's Movement.

tribes provides evidence to show that among different cultures, sex roles are quite variable and are based on cultural beliefs. In essence sex roles are not biologically but culturally determined.[2] More importantly sex roles are often assigned quite separately from role competence. The Women's Movement in the 60's led to radically new perspectives on women's roles and the physical and mental health needs of women. The evolution of the interaction between psychological therapies and the women's movement is illustrated in Figure 14-2.

The male physician as part of our male-centered society has often perpetuated the stereotypes surrounding women by expecting women to adjust to their roles rather than appreciating the social context from which a woman emerges. It is crucial to recognize the social changes occurring for women and men, the stress this puts on them and how this stress can be dealt with.

The women's movement has opened up a multitude of options for women: it must also accept responsibility for acknowledging and addressing the conflicts which these options often create for women. We are suggesting that the women's movement and physicians have a responsibility to discontinue their antagonisms regarding who is doing what to/for women and join forces in developing new, innovative and non-sexist methods of helping women select from their array of alternatives those which fit *their* individual needs. Choices must be based not on sex role stereotypes, but on individual strengths and needs. This includes the right to consciously choose traditional roles. For many clinicians this will mean accepting the fact that the choice of nontraditional roles may be the healthiest alternative for some patients. Failure to recognize these options for women may be to accept responsibility for denial of the development of mental health in women.

In the words of Carol Nadelson:

We are not involved with sick or well people in the traditional sense, but rather with women experiencing conflicts and seeking to find a way of resolving these conflicts. There are many ways of doing this. One way is to seek psychological help or "treatment." While the psychologist (psychiatrist, etc.) is not in a position to make radical changes in society's attitudes, (s)he can help a woman move toward being able to make more conscious and deliberate choices.

In order to work toward these ends, the clinician's values cannot interfere. Indeed, at times a capitulation or compromise may be the solution for a particular individual. It may be a choice that is quite opposed to the clinician's values. However, it is the clinician's responsibility to accept this end and to remain objective, understanding, and supportive as the person searches for goals that might have been unattainable in the past. Those engaged in the various therapies must be aware of the impact of social change and of their own attitudes, and they must be open to change.

As the traditional medical model becomes less useful in this concept of mental health, so does the traditional view of the doctor-patient relationship. This concept implies the interaction of a "well" and a "sick" person in an activity designed to make the "sick" person well. Obviously, this model communicates a set of values and standards which do not apply to the people we have discussed and those like them. It also implies a firm definition of "illness" and "health" which may apply in only very specific situations.

Let's look first, then, at physician characteristics followed by a review of the female patients they will be working with.

PHYSICIAN DIFFERENCES

By and large physicians in the U.S. are male. Up to the late 60's males represented 90-95 percent of physicians. Even now the proportion of women in medical school has risen to only 30-35 percent. The bulk of American physicians then are male.

Many adhere to a double standard of mental health—one for men and one for women. In an important study[3] researchers administered a sex-role stereotype questionnaire to practitioners. They found that the clinician's attitudes reflected agreement about the definition of a healthy male adult, healthy female adult, and adults in general:

> *Thus, for a woman to be healthy, from an adjustment viewpoint, she must adjust to and accept the behavioral norms for her sex, even though these behaviors are generally less socially desirable and considered less healthy for the generalized competent, mature adult.*

Broverman, et al. conclude that their findings are microcosmic of society—that as clinicians confirm sex-role stereotypes, they encourage these stereotypes bound in culture. Furthermore, they raise an important issue.

> *Clinicians should be concerned about whether influence of the sex-role stereotypes on their professional activities acts to reinforce social and intrapsychic conflict.*

A common question arising in feminist and counter-cultures is whether or not a male clinician can be fair to his female clients. The issue of stereotyping (whether it be a sex-role, racial or ethnic) must be considered on the part of the clinician, and it may be a difficult process as Rice and Rice[4] point out:

> *A common result of a woman's increased awareness as to her traditionally expected role and 'place' in what she perceives as a male-dominated society is a sense of generalized hostility toward men. The male clinician is not likely to escape these feelings.*

An argument for female physicians working with female patients is that they can provide role models of successful women in a nontraditional profession. Nadelson suggests:[5]

> *This aspect may be particularly important if the clinician is a woman, since she represents an alternative, a woman who in some way, has transcended traditional values and norms and, in those terms, has succeeded. For a man in a therapeutic*

relationship with a woman, the horizon may be significantly widened by the experience of working, perhaps for the first time, with a woman in a nontraditional role.

This might be a particularly important issue for female patients who are having conflicts with regard to their career goals or abilities.

It might be true that the origins of many emotional issues are in the nuclear family, but our male-dominated society, of which the woman is a part, perpetuates the issues.

Labeling role conflict as psychopathological and interpreting it in intrapsychic terms underscores the basic failure of most clinicians to appreciate the social context that forces a subtle "schizophrenia of person" for a woman.[4]

A healthy redefinition on either a woman's part or on the part of the physician is one way in which sex-role biases can be lessened. The change in thinking and perceiving is not easy, as is witnessed by the uproar created when women request even the simplest changes, e.g., language changes from Miss or Mrs. to Ms.; chairperson rather than chairman, etc., ad nauseum.

Some of the ways in which physicians might be most effective with female patients are:

1. Acknowledging broad alternatives to the traditional family, career and achievement, child care, sexual behavior and marriage wherein egalitarianism becomes more of a reality.
2. Discontinue labeling of female behaviors as pathological against the norm of male behaviors. The male physician must be aware of the costs to both men and women of sex-role stereotyping.
3. Shifting gears as a nondirective clinician. The traditional blank-screen, silent style fosters passivity in women and increases the insecurity in women who have been so conditioned to depend on external sources (especially male) for their self-esteem and definition. The physician may need to openly encourage the female patient's "deviance" and become an advocate for social change.
4. To allow women to choose to remain in traditional roles if it becomes clearly their choice.
5. To discontinue perpetuation of the "one-down" position where the physician is the extolled expert which merely encourages "the fantasy that an idealized relationship with a more powerful other is a better solution to life problems than taking autonomous action."[6]
6. To set aside the double-standards of mental health for men (aggressive, competitive, logical) and women (passive, dependent, masochistic). This allows for more ranges of behavior for both men and women.
7. To perpetuate the notion that it must be "bad mothering" when disturbed children or adolescents are seen, again stereotypes women. It is not clear

that "schizophrenogenic" mothers are more responsible than "schizophrenogenic" fathers.

8. To avoid terms that suggest only a male could be considered, i.e., chairman versus chairperson, fireman versus firefighter, etc. Furthermore, the use of the word "girl" for a female past her teens, a regular occurrence, suggests she has not grown up and may never feel masterful if addressed by this word. Few people ever call adult males "boys."

9. To encourage women to learn about themselves so they can differentiate between what "I should do" versus what "I want to do." Women too easily become invested in pleasing others rather than themselves, thus blinding themselves to the variety of options available to themselves.

WOMEN'S PROBLEMS (Depression)

Generally speaking, it is clear that for men, marriage acts as an immunity against depression, while for women, marriage and depression may be synonymous. "The traditional female role may contribute to depression."[7] Married women rather than unmarried women are more apt to seek psychiatric help,[8] attempt suicide, report somatic symptoms demonstrating psychological stress,[6] seek out physicians more, get more prescriptions and use more psychotropic drugs.[7] Married women express unhappiness, seek marriage counseling and start divorce proceedings more often than do husbands. There are several reasons why married women may be more prone to depression.

> *Gove and others attribute the disadvantages of the married female to several factors: role restriction (most men occupy two roles, as household head and worker, and therefore have two sources of gratification whereas women have only one); housekeeping being frustrating and of low prestige; the unstructured role of housewife, allowing time for brooding; and even if the married woman works, her position is usually less favorable than a working man's.[7]*

Women who have never married or who are widowed report a lower incidence of depression than married women. Radloff[9] suggests that these women "have been less indoctrinated in the helplessness stereotype than those who marry."

Depression is notably higher in all women of all age groups and in all countries over all time periods. Chesler[10] explains this phenomenon:

> *Women are in a continual state of mourning—for what they never had—or had too briefly, and for what they can't have in the present, be it Prince Charming or direct worldly power.*

Similarly, Seiden points out that depression in women coincides with the stereotypical role expectations of females: Women are taught a "learned helplessness" model of vulnerability which is consistent with what has been expected of them. Seligman[11] argues that hopelessness, helplessness and low self-esteem are not the manifest symptoms of depression, but in fact are the cause of the depression itself.

With respect to depression and its relationship to physiology and hormones, Weissman and Klerman examined the literature in the areas of oral contraceptive use, postpartum and menopause. For oral contraceptive use:

> *In summary, the amount of female depression that could be attributed to the possible psychopharmacologic effects of oral contraceptives is small.*

For postpartum depression:

> *It must be concluded that women are at greater risk for psychiatric disorders, particularly depression, in the postpartum period although, if any specific endocrine abnormality is involved, the mechanism is not understood.*

For menopause:

> *In summary, there is no evidence that women are at greater risk for depression during the menopausal period or that depressions occurring in this period have a distinct clinical pattern.*

Phobic Syndrome

A second critical area of women's mental health is the phobic syndrome in women. Fodor[12] points out that animal phobias and agoraphobia are "the phobias of women." In general she states that there are "similarities between aspects of the phobic syndrome—the extreme superhelplessness, avoidance of mastery experiences, competition, and lack of assertiveness—and descriptions of stereotypic feminine behavior." She sees a way out of the struggle, but it is a big order:

> *Woman's biggest problem is overcoming dependency. Somehow, even most independent women hang on to a few phobic symptoms (often fear of driving or flying) as a last remnant of dependency. Some seemingly independent women are afraid of riding bikes, skating or skiing. Since they have only recently learned to stand on their own feet they fear what they can't control.*

Fodor advises us that men and women must (encourage each other, be encouraged to) come to terms with dependent/independent issues. If women change, then men cannot help but change too. In fact, we might begin to see more direct reporting of depression by men, rather than indirectly as in alcoholism which is more common in men.

Role Confusion

All women have probably been touched in some way by the women's movement—both positively and negatively. Women who may previously not have questioned their roles and goals are finding themselves in a new kind of dilemma with numerous options. The questioning of one's role and identity can be disquieting.

It might be said that women are going through an "identity crisis" not on just an intrapsychic level, but socially and intellectually as well.

Women are learning that their oppression, or "fear of success" does not necessarily originate in oneself, but may be anchored in the structure of our society. However, as much as many women would like to change their life styles, they are apt to be deficient in the necessary behaviors to evoke the new ways of relating: the experiences and role rehearsals accorded to men since birth are not in women's repertory of behaviors. Women may need to be resocialized—as if they were starting all over.

Nadelson classifies the conflicts women experience as falling into the following five areas. The first area of conflict for many women is that between her identification with her mother and life goals, which may be different from those her mother had chosen.

A second area in which role conflicts can occur is that between career and home life. Routinely, we have expected that women will become mothers and wives. Jane Doe is Johnny's mother or John's wife. Not only has she given up her personal identity, but she probably has also relinquished her maiden name (which was also a man's—her father's), thus indicating through her new name who she belongs to. If a woman chooses to be a housewife, then she is delegated to a second-class role both by virtue of her assumption of someone else's name and by the fact that she is unpaid.

Another difficulty with women who elect to be housewives and mothers is that which occurs when children have finally grown and leave home. Since the woman's identity has come largely through her husband and children, she is likely to feel lonely, rejected, and depressed when her children achieve independence. She has lost an important part of her identity, a part of herself.

On the other hand, women can choose to have careers. The risk here, of course, is that most careers are still male dominated so the women are never quite "normal." They are labeled, and often come to see themselves as "special," not quite like other women.

There is, of course, another option which Nadelson discusses as a third conflict for women. They can choose to carry out both roles. A woman can choose to be a wife/mother and a career person. The double-bind this puts her in seems obvious. She never has enough time to fulfill either role quite adequately—each half of her is constantly demanding more than 50 percent of her time, thus she is left feeling inadequate at both roles and most often resolves this through depression or intense bitterness and rejection of those around her.

A fourth conflict for women is that over achievement and competition.[13] Boys are socialized in such a way that their options are expanded. They are taught that being masculine means being competent and achieving. Girl children, on the other hand, are taught that they must not win too much if they want to be considered feminine; girls don't fight, girls can't be too strong, too smart, or too independent. The final result, then, is that adult women are afraid of success which might define one as masculine. A woman cannot be both feminine and successful at the same time. For women who want badly to succeed, this presents incredible stress—socialization as children runs too deep to simply throw off in favor of succeeding at adulthood.

A final conflict Nadelson discusses is that of dependence versus independence. The problems here are very similar to those involved in achievement vs. competition. Women have been socialized into dependence while males are expected very early in life to exhibit independent behavior. The woman who chooses independence, therefore, is labeled deviant.

In addition to those conflicts discussed by Nadelson, we see two additional ones—one signifying identification with new societal norms, the other a return to older norms.

As a result of more women being professional and active in their own public lives, in combination with growing concern regarding over-population and all of its inherent problems, women are now questioning whether they want to have children—and if so, when. If a woman chooses to remain single and childless she will probably be labeled deviant (e.g., "spinster," "old maid"), undesirable, or homosexual. If she chooses to marry but remain childless, the assumption is that she or her partner is "unable to have children." Should they make it public that they are childless by choice, they are then labeled deviant. But what if she chooses to marry and wants to have children. When should she have them? For women the conflict between career and childrearing is grave indeed. She can have children first and begin her career after her children are older, thus entering the career market at a later-than-average age and jeopardizing her ability to ever truly excel in a profession. On the other hand, she can choose to begin her career first and "drop out" to have children, which also jeopardizes her career. Additionally, women have been told repeatedly that having children "late in life" (usually meaning past 30!) endangers the physical lives of both mother and child. The battle rages internally, often without resolution, and often reaching the point of totally immobilizing a woman in her ability to successfully achieve either role.

A final conflict comes for the woman who chooses to live a traditional life style. She gets messages from the media, and often from women and men around her, that if she were really a "modern woman" (generally meaning "superwoman") she could do both roles and do them well—after all, other women do it. She is told that the housewife's role is dull, meaningless and statusless until she begins to think so herself, thus becoming depressed and feeling inadequate.

So what is the bottom line on all of these conflicts? It would appear that few women in today's society, full of expanded options without new role models, escape incredible amounts of intense guilt. No matter what they choose to do, they are made to feel guilty for what they are *and* what they are not doing! A brief examination of the self-esteem literature tells us what a heavy toll these processes take.

Self-esteem

As indicated in the previous section, women have been given a variety of double messages by society which must contribute to confusion, as stated by Rice and

Rice:[4]

> *A woman's self-image is deeply affected by societal programming of double-binding behaviors that tell her to be sexy, yet to be a virgin; strong, yet weak; subordinate, yet challenging; smart enough to get a man, yet needing to hide her intelligence; to achieve in school, yet to 'fail' in the world of work.*

While people are now recognizing that women's roles have broadened and are no longer based only in wife and motherhood, recent research yields the disheartening information that both men and women continue to stereotype acceptable female behavior in traditional ways.

Although the sources of self-esteem have been defined in many different ways, there seem to be four major contributors which all operational definitions might fit: treatment by significant others, history of successes, method of dealing with devaluation and a person's own values and aspirations.[14]

Treatment by significant others can be defined as the amount of respectful, accepting and concerned treatment persons receive from significant others in their lives. All of the above information regarding the value of female sex roles would lead us to believe that it might be significantly more difficult for a female to get respectful, accepting and concerned treatment from significant others if she chooses to depart from traditional role behaviors than if she chooses to maintain traditional behaviors.

A second factor in self-esteem research is "our history of successes and the status and position we hold in the world. Our successes generally bring us recognition and are thereby related to our status in the community. They form the basis in reality for self-esteem and are measured by the material manifestations of success and an indication of social approval." So once again we have a female in conflict: If she gets approval from significant others it is most likely to be for traditional sex role behaviors which denies her, by their very definition, success, status and social approval, except as they are attained from a male (e.g., father, husband's status). If, on the other hand, she chooses to attain significant social/career/public success, she is likely to not be given the approval and support of significant others in her life.

The third major factor contributing to self-esteem is the person's own values and aspirations through which the above history of successes gets filtered. It is within this factor that the issue of salience comes to the fore, and probably where the most difficulty in interpreting female self-esteem occurs. Physicians seeing an attractive woman who is, by all definitions, a good wife and mother OR a woman who is extremely successful in a career might wonder what brings her to the clinician: "What more could she possibly want!" But remember, when we discuss self-esteem, the most important word is SELF. If the successful homemaker really wants to be a career woman, she has not succeeded in her salient value/aspiration area and vice versa. Physicians must be very cautious, therefore, that they first allow patients to define their own significant others, perceived successes and failures, and values and aspirations. As soon as the physician begins judging a client from his/her value system rather than from the client's the groundwork has been laid for extremely ineffective therapy.

Finally, the person's method of dealing with devaluation becomes important to self-esteem. It is perhaps with depression, which has been discussed earlier, that most women respond to devaluation.

We can also, as true physicians, take our role as community educators more seriously by working with young women PRIOR to their parenting experiences to help them develop positive attitudes about themselves and their future children; by working within school systems to train educators and youngsters regarding positive aspects of both male and female roles; by working with the profession to see that the percentage of male/female physicians is more equalized in order that patients can see both female and male models.

THE FUTURE: TREATMENT OPTIONS

Male and female clinicians must attend to women's changing roles. Traditional psychotherapy may best be balanced with innovative therapies arising out of feminist concerns. Traditional psychotherapy alone may merely maintain the status quo which does not address the issue of sex-role bias.

Femininism incorporates the notion of change rather than mere adjustment to one's assigned sex-role. With this in mind, we will turn to the several forms of innovative therapies available for women. Typically, these are offered or become most viable through city and university women's centers, women's counseling centers, or women's professional organizations. Planned parenthood offices are another resource.

Consciousness Raising Groups (CR)

The goal of these groups is the need "to change the social structure and culture through the individual."[15] The CR groups are composed of women who have an opportunity to examine sex-roles and the attitudes and behaviors associated with these roles. Unlike traditional psychotherapy groups, there is often no leader. Many CR groups have definitive purposes, i.e., sexual issues, single-parenting, professional women, etc. and others are more vague in their goals. In general, CR groups provide incentive to "activity to change self, culture and social structure."

Assertiveness Training

Assertiveness training is founded on behavior modification principles and uses techniques anchored in learning theory. As with most behavior modification strategies, therapy is aimed at symptom removal, the extinction of old roles, and the learning of new ones. Hence therapy is relatively short. Procedures likely to be used include desensitization, modeling, role playing and role rehearsal.

Participants usually define their own goals and are helped through behavioral contracts and group support to enact behavior changes through the use of hierarchies, beginning with least threatening changes and working toward those considered by the individual to be most difficult. Leaders of these groups are sometimes professionals but most frequently are paraprofessionals, often self-trained, whose major objective is to help women change themselves in order to ultimately change the social milieu.

Peer Counseling

Another form of the paraprofessional which is becoming more visible and more acceptable is the peer counselor. Based on the model of self help, peer counselors are women and men who are usually given minimal skill training in counseling skills and then work with clients in cooperative problem solving around the client's specific concerns. Peer counselors also act, on occasion, as a consumer advocate by mediating between the client and his/her professional health workers.

Reeducation

Continuing education to change attitudes of the public is constantly ongoing at the college level. There is emphasis on vocational and sensitivity training, as well as an exploration of commonly shared stereotypic notions. This becomes a method for clinicians to keep informed regarding the populations they will be working with and new directions in demands of patients.

Reeducation has another important impact for women. Women are currently "reentering" school and work fields in ever-increasing numbers, preparing to have a career after families have grown or marriages dissolved. These women present special problems which often are brought to physicians.

It is hoped, as awareness and attention is paid to sex-role bias, that men too will be liberated. They too will be encouraged to experience and express a wider range of behaviors. They are victims in a system where no one wins. The cost of human oppression is felt by all.

REFERENCES

1. Mead M: *Sex and Temperament in Three Primitive Societies.* New York, Mentor, 1950
2. Weitzman L: Sex-role socialization. *In:* Freeman J (ed): *Women: A Feminist Perspective*, Palo Alto, CA: Mayfield, 1975
3. Broverman IK, Broverman DM, Clarkson FE, et al: Sex-role stereotypes and clinical judgments of mental health. *J Consult Clin Psychol* 34:1-7, 1970
4. Rice, J, Rice D: Implications of the women's liberation movement for psychotherapy. *Am J Psychiatry* 130:191-96, 1973
5. Nadelson C: Adjustment: New approaches to women's mental health. *In* McBee M, Blake K (eds): *The American Woman: Who Will She Be?* Beverly Hills, Benziger, Bruce & Glencoe, 1974

6. Seiden A: Overview: Research on the psychology of women. II. Women in families, work, and psychotherapy. *Am J Psychiatry* 133:1111-1123, 1976

7. Weissman M, Klerman G: Sex differences and the epidemiology of depression. *Arch Gen Psychiatry* 34:98-111, 1977

8. Gove W, Tudor J: Adult sex roles and mental illness. *In* Huber J (ed): *Changing Women in a Changing Society.* Chicago, University of Chicago Press, 1973

9. Radloff L: Sex differences in depression: The effects of occupation and marital status. *Sex Roles* 1:249-69, 1975

10. Chesler P: *Women and Madness.* New York, Avon, 1972

11. Seligman M: Depression and learned helplessness. *In* Friedman R, Kutz M (eds): *The Psychology of Depression: Contemporary Theory and Research.* Washington, D.C., V.H. Winston & Sons, 1974

12. Fodor I: The phobic syndrome in women: Implications for treatment. *In* Franks V, Burtle V (eds): *Women in Therapy.* New York, Brunner/Mazel, 1974

13. Block JH: Conceptions of sex role: Some cross-cultural and longitudinal perspectives. *Am Psychol* 28:512-26, 1973

14. Coopersmith S: *The Antecedents of Self-Esteem.* San Francisco, W. H. Freeman & Co., 1967

15. Kirsch B: Consciousness-raising groups as therapy for women. *In* Franks V, Burtle V (eds): *Women in Therapy.* New York, Brunner/Mazel, 1974

PART VIII: Consultation and Referral

DON A. ROCKWELL, M.D.

Consultation
Referral

The successful consultation or referral requires much more attention in psychiatry than in other medical specialties because of the sensitivity of the issues and attitudes involved. Patients and their physicians retain many cultural stereotypes about psychiatry and about "mental illness" that are patently stigmatizing. While we may wish that "mental illness is like any other illness," we have a long way to go attitudinally to accomplish this goal. Once one accepts that bias exists against referral to psychiatry then it becomes possible to deal with it.

CONSULTATION

The primary care clinician should be well aware of several different types of consultation that may be sought from the psychiatrist or other mental health practitioner. The usual medical model of asking the consultant to see the patient may not be best for all patients or practitioners. Before discussing aspects of asking for a usual consultation, it's appropriate to point out two other useful consultation models.

The wise clinician may seek advice from a consultant informally before asking the consultant to see the patient. This happens often in general medicine—the curb-side consult—but is especially useful with patients with psychosocial problems. In this model the clinician, when confused or uncertain about diagnosis or management, calls the consultant to discuss the case before or in place of a traditional consultation. This procedure will obviate many formal consultations and facilitate the clinician's own knowledge and skills while maintaining or improving his/her theapeutic relationship with the patient. Since the bulk of psychiatric treatment in medicine is carried out by the primary care giver, this model maximizes the effectivenss of this approach. The single requirement to carry out this form of consultation is the development of a comfortable working relationship with a competent psychiatrist. This relationship will be of mutual benefit to both practitioners and their respective patients.

A second form of consultation is a variation of the above model. In this approach the clinician invites the consultant to review his/her practice in a systematic way. The maximal variation is to have the psychiatrist (or other mental health professional) "sit in" on one's practice for a half day per week. This is an excellent way to have timely diagnostic and therapeutic skills under supervision. The less intense approach is to arrange a regular "consultation" with a psychiatrist to review "problem cases" in one's practice. Again one is using the consultant to augment one's skills but without the necessity of referring patients out.

In the usual model the physician asks the consultant to actually see the patient and assist with "consultative" advice about diagnosis or treatment. For this to be effective a number of matters must be attended to:

1. The physician and patient need to be clear as to the purpose of the consultation. The first point is that the physician must know why he or she is asking for a consultation. In other medical areas this is related to:

   - The need for help in making a diagnosis
   - The need for help in complex management
   - The need for confirmation of a diagnosis or treatment program
   - The need to assure the patient, self, family, insurance company, etc. that the diagnosis and treatment is correct and appropriate

All of these apply in the psychiatric consultation. In addition there are consultations that are requested out of countertransference reasons. The practitioner may be wishing to "dump" the patient or to "discount" the patient or the patient's symptoms. Thus the clinician needs to examine his/her own feelings about the patient to be sure the consultation request is not an acting out of angry or rejecting feelings toward the patient.

The patient needs to know why the consultation is being requested. Legitimate reasons along with those listed above include:

- Help with legal aspects
- Assistance in identifying community or other resources for patients

The patient needs to be told honestly and directly the purpose of the consultation and what the psychiatrist (or other mental health professional) expects of the consultation.

2. Exploration of ideas about and resistances to psychiatry need to be fully explored. Patients may have many misconceptions about psychiatry and these need to be talked out. Many people view a referral as:

   - An indication they are "crazy"
   - A prelude to being locked up
   - A sign they are weak willed
   - A sign their doctor doesn't believe them or believe in them
   - Evidence that they "can't handle their own problems"

3. Be clear with the patient about what will happen during the consultation. Paint a realistic picture of the consultation. Don't arouse unrealistic expectations.
4. Be sure the consultant knows what question you are asking and what you and the patient need.

There are some circumstances when the usual consultation is contraindicated. In acute emergencies with psychotic patients or acutely suicidal patients, it is important that contact with psychiatry be direct and immediate. Ideally this means literally having the crisis team come to your office or you or a staff member accompanying the patient to emergency psychiatric services. The direct contact insures no intervening disasters.

A second situation in which routine consultation is contraindicated is for patients with suspected factitious disease or Munchausen's syndrome. In these cases once the diagnosis is suspected, and, before the patient is confronted, informal consultation between clinician and psychiatrist is mandatory.

REFERRAL

The issues discussed under consultation apply equally to referral. The same cautions obtain and the same care is required in effecting a successful transfer of the patient. Referral is much easier after a consultation which recommends ongoing psychiatric treatment. The first step (consultation) has been taken, and the patient (if the consultation has been effectively accomplished) will be ready to proceed.

Some patients will ask for or be candidates for referral without the intervening consultative step. Here the key to appropriate referral is the clinician's knowledge of the patient's problem, the appropriate treatment and the variety of available psychiatric resources. There are a wide variety of such resources, and the clinician will wisely explore the various resources with the help of a consultant psychiatrist or an agency such as the Mental Health Association or local mental health program. Getting the correct match between patient and psychiatrist maximizes everyone's satisfaction and potential for therapeutic outcome. The most common problems and most emergent problems may go to different psychiatric "subspecialists" if you know them:

1. Family problems—including acting out children → refer to family therapist
2. Marital problems → couples/family therapist
3. Sexual problems → sex therapist
4. Profound depressions/suicidal patients → psychiatrists with inpatient access
5. Acutely psychotic patients → psychiatrists with inpatient access
6. Phobias → behavior therapist
7. Vague "life unhappiness" → psychotherapist

Many psychiatrists will have identified their subspecialty interests to their local psychiatric society. It then becomes possible, for example, to refer a patient with a specific phobia to a competent psychiatrist with both behavioral therapy expertise as well as broad psychodynamic skills.

15

Clinical Issues in Child Development

LENA K. ERICKSEN, PH.D.

This chapter presents common clinical issues associated with the childhood years. Both clinical manifestations and treatment techniques will be briefly stated. However, before these specific problems are discussed major landmarks in normal child development will be outlined. Such a perspective will aid the clinician in understanding the timing of the onset of various behaviors. A section including atypical child development (i.e., when most behaviors associated with normal development are late in onset or not at all evident) will also be presented.

LANDMARKS OF NORMAL DEVELOPMENT— THE FIRST YEAR

Physical Development and Motor Behavior

The growth rate is rather rapid during the first year of life. The infant gains around 15 pounds in weight and 9 to 10 inches in length (Watson and Lowrey, 1967). There is also a rapid development in musculature coordination and motor abilities. During this phase, "handedness" usually shifts around. The first muscles to be voluntarily controlled are around the head and the neck, and the last muscles to be voluntarily controlled are the leg muscles (Richmond, 1964). As can be seen in Table 15-1, walking alone is among the last of the basic motor skills to appear during the first year of life. Naturally, there are marked individual variations in growth patterns, in musculature coordination, and in motor abilities (Bayley, 1965).

Language

The newborn's earliest sounds are monosyllabic cries, but at the end of the first year the vocabulary usually consists of three to four words in addition to "mama" and "papa" (Caplan and Caplan, 1977). Around four weeks spontaneous vocalizations can be heard. The shift from these spontaneous vocalizations into words is dependent upon a variety of factors. They include maturation and voluntary control of the muscles involved in speech, normal cognitive development, an environment in which imitation of speech can take place, and reinforcement for vocalizations (Keppel, 1964). Deprivation experiences during the infancy period have been shown to irretrievably retard language development (Provence and Lipton, 1962).

Personal and Social Behavior

Distress and delight can be observed around three months. By six months the infant can display fear and disgust and by one year elation and affection appear. As an infant becomes better at distinguishing among people, his emotional repertoire also becomes more selective (Pikunas, 1969). For example, the development of attachment is a process that is now being established between the infant and his primary caretaker. Briefly, the theory of attachment holds that the infant becomes attached to the one person who mostly feeds, interacts, and plays with him (Ainsworth, 1964). As soon as attachment to the primary caretaker has developed, the child does not accept caretaking from anyone else (Bowlby, 1951). At this point in development the only signs of tension or anxiety in the infant should be the threat of losing the primary caretaker. Simultaneously with the development of attachment is the occurrence of fear of strangers and new situations. This fear usually peaks from the seventh to the ninth month (Schaffer, 1963). It usually holds true that the stronger the attachment is to the caretaker the more intense is stranger anxiety (Collard, 1968). Fear of strangers and new situations generally ends at the fifteenth month (Tennes and Lampl, 1964).

FROM THE FIRST THROUGH THE THIRD YEAR

Physical Development and Motor Behavior

The growth rate, having been very rapid during infancy, now slows down and the child gains four or five pounds and grows two to three inches per year (Bayley,

Table 15-1. *Landmarks of Normal Behavioral Development—The First Year.*

Age	Motor Behavior	Adaptive Behavior	Language	Personal and Social Behavior
Under 4 weeks	Makes alternating crawling movements. Moves head laterally when placed in prone position.	Responds to sound of rattle and bell. Regards moving objects momentarily.	Small, throaty, undifferentiated noises.	Quiets when picked up.
4 weeks	Tonic neck reflex positions predominate. Hands fisted. Head sags but can hold head erect for a few seconds.	Follows moving objects to the midline. Shows no interest and drops objects immediately.	Beginning vocalization such as cooing, gurgling, and grunting.	Regards face and diminishes activity. Responds to speech.
16 weeks	Symmetrical postures predominate. Holds head balanced. Head lifted 90 degrees when prone on forearm.	Follows a slowly moving object well. Arms activate on sight of dangling object.	Laughs aloud. Sustained cooing and gurgling.	Spontaneous social smile. Aware of strange situations.
28 weeks	Sits steadily, leaning forward on hands. Bounces actively when placed in standing position.	One-hand approach and grasp of toy. Bangs and shakes rattle. Transfers toys.	Vocalizes "m-m-m" when crying.	Takes feet to mouth. Pats mirror image.
40 weeks	Sits alone with good coordination. Creeps. Pulls self to standing position.	Matches two objects at midline. Attempts to imitate scribble.	Says "da-da" or equivalent. Responds to name or nickname.	Responds to social play such as "pat-a-cake" and "peek-a-boo." Feeds self cracker and holds own bottle.
52 weeks	Walks with one hand held. Stands alone briefly.		Uses expressive jargon. Gives toy on request.	Cooperates in dressing.

Source: Adapted from Chess M.D., S: In Eisenberg M.D.. L: 1975:2039. Printed with permission.

1965). There is little sex differentiation in height and weight during the childhood years. The rapid changes that do take place during the second and third year involve the child's increasing fine and gross motor coordination. Even before the second year, the child can manage complicated fine motor maneuvers such as partly feeding and dressing himself (Ryan, 1966). With regard to gross motor development, the child can ride a tricycle and alternates feet when going up or down stairs around three years of age (see Table 15-2).

Language

By the age of two the child may have a vocabulary of 250 words (Irwin, 1949). The child is also able to combine words into grammatically meaningful sentences. It is quite common for the child to continue to use infantile pronunciations throughout his fourth year (Bellugi and Brown, 1964). The young child often tends to ramble on in a loosejointed manner, as well as omitting key information when attempting to relay a story (Stone and Church, 1968).

Personal and Social Behavior

There is now an expanding awareness of self and others. During the second year a period of "negativism" may develop. This means that the child resists requests from adults (Hurlock, 1968). This does not mean, however, that attachments and affections have abated in strength. Instead it should be viewed as the child's strivings for autonomy in that the child is interested in exploring and manipulating the environment by himself (Erickson, 1959). Other plausible explanations of this phase include that the child is repeatedly confronted with novel situations, for which he has yet to develop complete cognitive comprehension, and that the child now seeks to do new things, for which he has not yet developed adequate motor skills (Strang, 1959).

One task demanded by others of the child is that he control his bowel and bladder in a socially prescribed manner. The learning of this behavior depends in part on maturational readiness and the child's appropriate reactions to internal cues. The timing of toilet training varies with each child, and usually ranges from fourteen or fifteen months to two and a half years. It often coincides with the maturation of the child's skill in walking. Furthermore, the child must be psychologically ready to delay the urge to release his stool as soon as he feels the impulse.

FROM THE THIRD THROUGH THE SIXTH YEAR

Physical Development and Motor Behavior

There are some significant changes in the child's bodily proportions during this phase. The child loses his top-heavy "sack-like" resemblance and begins to approach adult proportions. The most rapid growth rate is in the limbs, whereas head circumference growth is the slowest. During this period the child has not yet

Table 15-2. Landmarks of Normal Behavioral Development—From the First Year Through the Third Year.

Age	Motor Behavior	Adaptive Behavior	Language	Personal and Social Behavior
15 months	Toddles. Creeps up stairs.		Says three to five words meaningfully. Pats pictures in book. Shows shoes on request.	Points or vocalizes wants. Throws objects in play or refusal.
18 months	Walks, seldom falls. Hurls ball. Walks up stairs with one hand held.	Builds a tower of three or four cubes. Scribbles spontaneously and imitates a writing stroke.	Says 10 words, including name. Identifies one common object on picture card. Names ball and carries out two directions, for example "put on table" and "give to mother."	Feeds self in part, spills. Pulls toy or string. Carries or hugs a special toy such as a doll.
2 years	Runs well, no falling. Kicks large ball. Goes up and down stairs alone.	Builds a tower of six or seven cubes. Aligns cubes, imitating train. Imitates vertical and circular strokes.	Uses three-word sentences. Carries out four simple directions.	Pulls on simple garment. Domestic mimicry. Refers to self by name.
3 years	Rides a tricycle. Jumps from bottom steps. Alternates feet going up stairs.	Builds tower of nine or 10 cubes. Imitates a three-cube bridge. Copies a circle and a cross.	Gives sex and full name. Describes what is happening in a picture book.	Puts on shoes. Unbuttons buttons. Understands taking turns.

Source: Adapted from Chess M.D., S: In Eisenberg M.D.. L: 1975:2039. Printed with permission.

acquired highly complex, fine-detailed psychomotor skills, but these abilities ordinarily appear during the school years (Gutteridge, 1939). Instead, the preschool child seems to enjoy manipulating tools suited for him (such as blunt-edged scissors) as well as drawing and painting (Stone and Church, 1968). Dominant "handedness" is usually acquired by the third or fourth year. (See Table 15-3.)

Language

Language is now becoming an important tool for self-expression. It permits the child to initiate and carry on various social behaviors in addition to assisting in establishing his self-identity (Gardner, 1964). Ferguson (1970) drew a parallel between the development of motor skills and the development of language capabilities and stated that whereas the former allows manual exploration of the environment, the latter provides opportunities for symbolic exploration and mastery. This can be observed by the way preschool children are often thinking through their actions aloud (Bereiter, 1961). The rate of learning new words takes an immense upsurge during the third and fourth years, and then seems to taper off (Templin, 1957). By the age of four the child understands almost 1500 words, by the age of five almost 2100, and by the age of six almost 2600 words (Smith, 1926).

Personal and Social Behavior

The school-aged child is now striving to win recognition through achievement and seems to receive satisfaction from seeing his tasks completed. The six-year-old child may present behavioral problems because of his increasing preference for more independence than his parents are willing to give. The child may become secretive, which seems totally opposite to the open and frank discussions of his feelings just a year or two ago. It is usually at this point when the child turns away from the family in favor of being with his peers (Stone and Church, 1968). The methods the child is utilizing to acquire independence from his family are most likely to be the ones he will continue to use into and throughout adulthood.

CLINICAL ISSUES: ATYPICAL CHILD DEVELOPMENT

The term "atypical child development" was coined by Rank in 1949. This term refers to those children whose development has been arrested at a very primitive infantile level. Thus, the terminology of "atypical child development" is equated with the early onset of psychoses or infantile psychoses. That is, the onset of developmental arrest is manifest before the age of three. Moreover, this term refers to emotional delay and disorder in personality development and associated ego functions. It does not include brain deficiencies or subnormal mental functioning (APA Glossary, 1980).

Table 15-3. Landmarks of Normal Behavioral Development—From the Third Year Through the Fifth Year.

Age	Motor Behavior	Adaptive Behavior	Language	Personal and Social Behavior
4 years	Walks down stairs one step per tread. Stands on one foot for 4 to 8 seconds.	Copies a cross. Repeats four digits. Counts three objects with correct pointing.	Names colors, at least one correctly. Understands five prepositional directives: "on," "under," "in," "in back of," or "in front of," and "beside."	Washes and dries own face. Brushes teeth. Plays cooperatively with other children.
5 years	Skips using feet alternately. Usually has complete sphincter control.	Copies a square. Draws a recognizable man, with a head, body, limbs. Counts 10 objects accurately.	Names the primary colors. Names coins: pennies, nickels, dimes. Asks meanings of words.	Dresses and undresses self. Prints a few letters. Plays competitive exercise games.

Source: Adapted from Chess M.D., S: In Eisenberg M.D., L: 1975:2040. Printed with permission.

This section will list behavioral characteristics associated with infantile symbiotic psychosis, which was proposed by Mahler in 1952, early infantile autism, presented by Kanner in 1949, and childhood schizophrenia, presented by Kestenbaum in 1978. If the practicing physician recognizes any of the below mentioned characteristics, it is strongly advised that the child receive immediate referral for psychiatric treatment.

Infantile Symbiotic Psychosis

In 1952 Mahler outlined the clinical syndrome of infantile symbiotic psychosis, which she considered distinct and separate from early infantile autism. Utilizing a developmental psychoanalytic framework, she noted the following characteristic behaviors and symptoms:

1. Deviant behavior is not usually observable during the first year of life. However, low frustration tolerance and sleep disturbance are noted.
2. When growing independence and separation from the mother is expected around the second year, anxiety and frustration appear and emotional development stops. There is a strong clinging attachment to the primary caretaker, usually the mother. The child's body contours appear to "melt" into the mother—the symbiotic position.
3. There is excessive focusing on parts of the body (e.g., hands, hair, fingers, etc.).
4. The child exhibits magical omnipotence and attempts oneness with his mother through delusions and hallucinations.
5. The child insists on sameness in the environment. To control the presence of his mother, he learns to manipulate and throws temper tantrums.
6. The parent often feels confused since the child craves body contact and seems to want to crawl into the parent, but if such contact is initiated by the parent, the child screams in panic.

Mahler (1952) believed infantile symbiotic psychosis was largely environmentally induced but recognized these children's predisposed constitutional vulnerability.

Early Infantile Autism

In 1949 Kanner presented his detailed and carefully documented account of early infantile autism. The onset of the below noted behavioral categories are in early infancy or before fifteen or twenty-four months of age. Kanner's (1949) criteria have proven useful for diagnostic purpsoes and include the following:

1. In early infancy there is an inability or refusal on the child's part to form interpersonal relationships. However, development may proceed in a relatively normal pace until the second year. At this age regression occurs, which involves profound withdrawal from physical and emotional contact

with significant others. The child becomes more interested in objects than in people. Loss of a seemingly normal developing language function also occurs. If speech is present, it is usually imitative and echolalic in quality. Whatever timing of the onset, the child is often believed to be deaf because of his display of simulated deafness. The child stops smiling spontaneously and looks "through" a person rather than meeting a person's eyes.

2. There is an intense desire for the preservation of sameness (with distress at any change). The child often displays a repetitive, autoerotic activity (e.g., rocking, whirling, rubbing, and bizarre hand movements).

3. There is a fascination with a limited number of small, inanimate objects. These objects are usually handled with adequate motor coordination but are not used functionally. Manipulation has a ritualistic and perseverative quality.

4. The child gives the impression of having a higher intellectual and cognitive potential than the actual retarded level on which he is invariably functioning. This is so because, at times, the child gives the impression of being mentally alert. However, there is little motivation for learning and mastery.

Childhood Schizophrenia

This condition stands in contrast to infantile symbiotic psychosis and early infantile autism. In a more recent clinical usage and classification system, childhood schizophrenia has been assigned to the "late onset" psychoses of childhood. The schizophrenic child may have a formal thinking disorder, hallucinations, and delusions similar to adult schizophrenia. The onset is in about the fourth or the fifth year. Kestenbaum (1978) presented the British Working Party's [originally reported in Creak, 1961] diagnostic criteria for childhood schizophrenia as including the following characteristics:

1. One of the most distinguishing signs of childhood schizophrenia is that the child never develops language, or the little language function that has been acquired is lost.

2. The child exhibits gross and sustained impairment of relationships with people.

3. There is an apparent unawareness of self to a degree which is inappropriate for the child's age.

4. The child has an abnormal preoccupation with inanimate objects and they are handled without regard to their apparent function.

5. There is an intense sustained desire for the preservation of sameness in the environment.

6. The child exhibits an apparent abnormal perceptual function (in the absence of discernible organic abnormality).

7. The child has frequent, acute, excessive, and seemingly illogical anxiety attacks.

8. There is distortion in both fine and gross motor functioning.

9. The child is often seriously retarded but fractions of near normal, normal, or exceptional intellectual functioning or behavioral skill may be observed.

CLINICAL ISSUES—EMOTIONAL AND BEHAVIORAL DISTURBANCES

Childhood Depression

The problem with depressive affect in childhood seems to be that the clinical symptoms may not be readily indicative of manifestations of depression. These children have often visited their pediatrician for problems of somatic complaints, which most often include dizziness, nausea, abdominal pain, headaches and/or difficulty in sleeping. Moreover, anorexia, pruritus, and migraine headaches have also been found to have their origin in depression. Encopresis and enuresis may also be part of the symptom complex in childhood depression. Malmquist (1972) listed the following signs, among others, of childhood depression:

1. The child appears sad and unhappy-looking. The child may not verbally state that he is unhappy but his psychomotor behavior reveals sadness.
2. The child does not show any interest in any activities and appears bored. An observer often gets the feeling that there must be something physically wrong with this child.
3. The child often gives the impression that others, even the examining clinician, are responsible for his predicament.
4. The child exhibits low frustration tolerance and irritability.
5. The child complains of somatic symptoms: most frequently abdominal pains or headaches but also dizziness, nausea, insomnia and/or eating disturbances.
6. The child may mask his depressive feelings by clowning around or by being provocative, all in an attempt to detract from his assets or achievements. When asked if the child feels sad, there is a blatant attempt to deny these feelings.
7. The child exhibits passivity and seems to expect others to anticipate his needs.
8. The child appears obsessive-compulsive and enjoys magical activities.
9. Acting-out behaviors (e.g., showing anger) are also observed. These types of behavior are believed to be part of the child's defense mechanisms so that the child may avoid experiencing the painful feelings associated with depression.

Psychiatric treatment of the depressed child should involve both the parents and the child. It has often been recognized that a pattern of mutually reinforcing hostility exists between the parents and the child. The child's depressed feelings and anger affect the parents, who, in turn, feel justified in punishing their angry and frustrated child, who now, in turn, begins to experience shame, which furthers his depressed feelings. This process becomes more and more intense with a resulting increased distance between the child and his parents. Family and personal histories often reveal that one of the parents has suffered or is suffering from depression, too. Thus, both the parents and the child will benefit from psychiatric treatment.

Encopresis

Kanner (1966) defined encopresis as the act of involuntary defecation, which cannot be directly linked to organic disease or deformity. There is a surprising pathological similarity among family interaction with encopretic children and among encopretic children themselves. The family interaction often demonstrates the following pathology. These families tend to (1) withhold information; (2) miscommunicate about essential family and personal histories; (3) infantilize the child; (4) mishandle anger through repression and denial; and (5) utilize severe and traumatic bowel training (Baird, 1974). The encopretic children often display a high rate of language disorders, such as reading disorders and/or seem to be slow in acquiring language skills, as well as some degree of uncoordination and neurological immaturity. Furthermore, they often feel unloved, lonely, and depressed and long for acceptance.

Treatment of these children is often frustrating since they are usually resistant to abandoning their soiling. Bemporad (1978) stated that seeking symbolism for the child's soiling is virtually nonproductive. Instead, encopresis should be viewed as one of the few acts that the child performs that receives parental attention. Psychiatric treatment involving the entire family is strongly advised.

Enuresis

Kanner (1957) defined nocturnal enuresis as involuntary bed-wetting at night by children after three years of age. Diurnal enuresis is observed less frequently and is often associated with organicity. The incidence of nocturnal enuresis is higher in boys than in girls. Children suffering from nocturnal enuresis often also share other behavioral problems such as stealing, overeating, fire setting, stammering and thumbsucking. Indeed, enuresis should seldom be viewed as an isolated symptom, but rather as part of the child's overall psychological make-up. It may be recalled that the depressed child may exhibit nocturnal enuresis.

Treatment of the enuretic child should *not* entail fluid restrictions, punishment for bed-wetting, or awakening of the child during the night for urination. These techniques have not proven effective and may actually harm the child psychologically. Sometimes merely the clinician's interest in the child may suffice for some children. For other children behavioral modification techniques seem helpful (Yates, 1974). Poussaint and Greenfield (1966) showed that imipramine was significantly superior to a placebo in the treatment of enuretic children with a genetic-constitutional dysfunction. A careful family history may reveal that the father of these children also suffered from this condition as a youngster. If enuresis persists, child psychotherapy is strongly recommended.

REFERENCES

Ainsworth MD: Patterns of attachment behavior shown by the infant in interaction with his mother. *Merrill-Palmer Quarterly* 10:51-58, 1964

American Psychiatric Association. *A Psychiatric Glossary.* Washington, D.C., American Psychiatric Association, 1969

Baird M: Characteristic interaction patterns in families of encopretic children. *Bull Menniger Clin,* 38:144-153, 1974

Bayley N: Research in child development: A longitudinal perspective. *Merrill-Palmer Quarterly* 11:183-208, 1965

Bellugi U, and Brown R (eds): The acquisition of language. *Monographs of the Society for Research in Child Development,* p. 29, 1964

Bemporad JR: Encopresis. *In* Wolman BB, Egan J and Ross AO (eds): *Handbook of Treatment of Mental Disorders in Childhood and Adolescence.* New Jersey, Prentice-Hall, pp. 161-178, 1978

Bereiter C: Fluency ability of pre-school children. *J Gent Psychol* 98:47-48, 1961

Bowlby J: *Maternal Care and Mental Health.* Geneva, World Health Organization, 1951

Caplan F and Caplan T: *The Second Twelve Months of Life.* New York, Grosset and Dunlap, 1977

Collard RR: Social and play responses of first-born and later-born infants in an unfamiliar situation. *Child Dev* 39:325-334, 1968

Creak M: Schizophrenic syndrome in childhood: Report of a working party. *Br Med J* 2:889-890, 1961

Eisenberg L: Normal child development. *In* Freedman AM, Kaplan HI and Sadock BJ (eds): *Comprehensive Textbook of Psychiatry, II.* Baltimore, Williams and Wilkins Company, 1976

Ferguson LR: *Personality Development.* Belmont, Brooks-Cole, 1970

Gardner DB: *Development in Early Childhood,* New York, McGraw-Hill, 1968

Gutteridge M: A study of motor achievement of young children. *Arch Psychology* 44, 1939

Hurlock EB: *Developmental Psychology.* New York, McGraw-Hill, 1968

Irwin OC: Infant speech. *Sci Am* 18:22-24, 1949

Kanner L: Problems of nosology and psychodynamics of early infantile autism. *Am J Orthopsychiatry* 19:416-426, 1949

Kanner L: *Child Psychiatry.* Springfield, Illinois, Charles C. Thomas, 1957

Kanner L: *Child Psychiatry.* Springfield, Illinois, Charles C. Thomas, 1966

Keppel G: Verbal learning in children. *Psychol Bull* 61:63-80, 1964

Kestenbaum CJ: Childhood psychosis: Psychotherapy. *In* Wolman, BB, Egan J and Ross AO (eds): *Handbook of Treatment of Mental Disorders in Childhood and Adolescence.* New Jersey, Prentice-Hall, pp. 354-384, 1978

Lewis, M: *Clinical Aspects of Child Development.* Philadelphia, Lea and Febiger, 1973

Mahler MS: On child psychosis and schizophrenia: Autistic and symbiotic infantile psychoses. *In* Freud A (ed): *The Psychoanalytic Study of the Child.* New York, International Universities Press, pp. 286-305, 1952

Malmquist CP: Depressions in childhood and adolescence. *New Eng J Med* 284:887-893, 1971

Pikunas J: *Human Development: A Science of Growth.* New York, McGraw-Hill, 1969

Poussaint F and Greenfield R: Epilepsy and enuresis. *Am J Psychiatry* 122:1426-1427, 1966

Provence S and Lipton RC: *Infants in Institutions: A Comparison of Their Development With Family-Reared Infants During the First Year of Life.* New York, International Universities Press, 1962

Rank B: Adaptation of the psychoanalytic technique for the treatment of young children with atypical development. *Am J of Orthopsychiatry* 19:130-139, 1949

Richmond JB: Observations of infant development: Clinical and psychological aspects. *Merrill-Palmer Quarterly* 10:95-101, 1964

Ryan MS: *Clothing: A Study of Human Behavior.* New York, Holt, Reinhart, and Winston, 1966

Schaffer HR: Some issues for research in the study of attachment behavior. *In* Foss BM (ed): *Determinants of Infant Behavior.* New York, John Wiley and Sons, 1963

Smith ME: An investigation of the development of the sentence and the extent of vocabulary in young children. *University of Iowa Studies in Child Welfare* p. 3, 1926

Stone LJ and Church J: *Childhood and Adolescence.* New York, Random House, 1968

Strang R: *An Introduction to Child Study.* New York, Macmillan, 1959

Templin MC: *Certain Language Skills in Children: Their Development and Interrelationships.* Minneapolis, University of Minnesota Press, 1957

Tennis KH and Lampl EE: Stranger and separation anxiety in infancy. *J Nerv Ment Dis* 139:247-254, 1964

Watson EH and Lowrey GH: *Growth and Development of Children.* Chicago, Year Book Publishers, 1967

Wolman BB, Egan J and Ross AO (eds): *Handbook of Treatment of Mental Disorders in Childhood and Adolescence.* New Jersey, Prentice-Hall, 1978

Yates AJ: *Theory and Practice in Behavior Therapy.* New York, John Wiley, 1975

INDEX